Epidemiology
in Veterinary Practice

Epidemiology in Veterinary Practice

CALVIN W. SCHWABE, D.V.M., M.P.H., Sc.D.

HANS P. RIEMANN, D.V.M., Ph.D.

CHARLES E. FRANTI, Ph.D.

Department of Epidemiology and Preventive Medicine
School of Veterinary Medicine
University of California
Davis, California

Lea & Febiger · 1977 · *Philadelphia*

Library of Congress Cataloging in Publication Data

Schwabe, Calvin W
  Epidemiology in veterinary practice.

  Includes index.
  1. Communicable diseases in animals. 2. Veterinary medicine—Practice.
I. Riemann, Hans P., joint author. II. Franti, Charles E., joint author.
III. Title. [DNLM: 1. Disease vectors. 2. Epidemiology. 3. Veterinary
medicine. SF745 S398e]
SF781.S38 1977   636.089'44   76-15960
ISBN 0-8121-0573-7

PRINTED IN THE UNITED STATES OF AMERICA

The veterinarian, from the start, has been accustomed to the concept of the protection of populations against crowd disease.

REGINALD ATWATER

To the memory of
K.F. Meyer, D.V.M.
1884-1974
Giant among epidemiologists,
Rare among men.

PREFACE

EPIDEMIOLOGY complements other medical disciplines by providing the means to describe disease patterns and events in large or small populations; it is also the means to obtain a succession of closer and closer approximations to an understanding of how and why such events occur. An epidemiological approach is suitable to a wide range of problems encountered in the private or public practice of veterinary medicine. This book introduces methods and concepts appropriate to veterinary practice situations.

Upon first consideration, epidemiology might appear to be much more directly relevant to the prevention, control, or investigation of diseases than to their diagnosis or treatment. We would dispel that notion quickly and maintain that an epidemiological approach will suggest itself to the veterinary practitioner whenever he attempts to diagnose or treat animals on a "herd" basis, even, for example, in the context of a hospitalized *population* of sick dogs or cats. Further uses will be evident to any veterinarian whose practice is part of some *system* for provision of curative or other types of veterinary services.

In using epidemiology in veterinary practice, an inability to distinguish clearly between practice and research is soon apparent. This problem is not surprising for, even in its practice aspects, epidemiology *is* a kind of field-based research. We believe it useful, therefore, to point to the different emphasis customarily given acquisition of field-research skills in training individuals to practice "plant medicine" versus animal medicine. *Most* plant pathologists are trained in experimental design and interpretation, and are oriented to problems of production. They know how to carry out prospective field trials in which the effects of different variables upon disease occurrence—and upon production—may be examined systematically. Further, the plant pathologist's study variables generally include not only different manifestations of disease-resistance and the like, but also *management* variables such as irrigation levels, fertilization levels, planting times, and rotation patterns. Field trials in plant medicine demonstrate new approaches and ideas to farmers; at the same time they provide the "pathologist" with a fuller understanding of a particular disease process and the means for making various predictions and recommendations concerning it. However, such a systematic field-research approach to problems is not often enough applied to animal diseases in relation to production. This different emphasis is only partly explainable by the complexity of animal diseases. Mostly, it simply reflects the lack of appropriate training for many veterinarians. This situation is unfortunate and serves to emphasize that epidemiology is the principal educational ingredient required for realization of a more integrated, production-oriented, "herd"-based system of practice in veterinary medicine.

We hope that this book of field methods and herd concepts helps to remedy this situation. It is the product of our collected experiences in teaching epidemiology and medical statistics to students of veterinary medicine, human medicine, and public health; but it especially results from our team teaching of this approach to disease in the program for the Master of Preventive Veterinary Medicine (M.P.V.M.) degree in the University of California. Our respective inputs into and responsibilities for the book's contents broadly reflect our individual backgrounds in three historic schools of epidemiology—the ecological, the medical detection, and the mathematical. From somewhat different perspectives, training, and experiences, we have attempted to evolve a practical approach to problems of disease in animal populations.

We assume that users of this book have taken a beginning course in statistics or are pursuing one concurrently with their study of epidemiology. We regard a basic understanding of statistics as essential to all veterinarians, if for no other reason than as a basis for comprehending the literature. To apply the statistical methods we have illustrated requires no mathematics background beyond algebra. However, epidemiology is a field which encourages cross-disciplinary efforts generally; and, in our experience, most practicing epidemiologists will choose to work collaboratively with biostatisticians as well as with a variety of other nonmedical specialists.

This book was designed to support epidemiology courses conducted at two different levels. The first 12 chapters, which introduce the principal concepts and some of the most-used methods, are suitable for a first course. Slightly more advanced methods are considered in Chapters 13 through 16, while Chapter 17 explores in some detail the principal subject areas for heightened epidemiological inputs into veterinary practice.

A number of problems are interspersed throughout the book. We feel that use of these and others which the teacher may supply are useful to test a veterinarian's ability to apply epidemiology to practice situations. For solving most of them, it is suggested that the problem be uncovered line by line, exposing a new question only after the preceding question has been answered fully. In our experience, the value of such problems is enhanced considerably if, after an opportunity to work them out individually, a class discusses them together.

Our references to specific diseases and disease management programs are only to illustrate concepts, methods, and problems. They are not intended to be sources of "best information" about these individual diseases, critical appraisals of existing programs, or the like. In other words, this book is intended solely as a guide to ways to develop and use information about diseases rather than as a source for specific data about diseases.

Part of the enjoyment and excitement of studying and teaching epidemiology, we find, is the extent to which it involves interactive learning encounters between students and teacher. Certainly, much of our own understanding has come from exchanges of ideas with our students and colleagues. To them all we are abundantly grateful and, with some difficulty, single out for thanks several special contributors to this book. First of all, contributions of material and helpful comments by our colleagues, Dr. Roger Ruppanner and Dr. Wayne Martin (the latter formerly of this department and now at the University of Guelph), have been especially numerous and are much appreciated. They and our other colleagues, Dr. Al Wiggins and Dr. Jess Kraus, reviewed portions of the manuscript in some detail; and Dr. Dick Howitt of the Department of Agricultural Economics on our campus read Chapter 15. Dr. Michael Burridge of this department helped with Chapter 13. Several classes of M.P.V.M. students in the University of California have served as guinea pigs for much of our material. To them we are particularly grateful. Others to whom we owe a very special debt include Mrs. Margie Roth and Mrs. Linda Fink for their patient typing of our difficult-to-read drafts and Mrs. Alyne Lavoie-Ruppanner for her illustrations. We hope this book will prove useful to veterinary students, practitioners, and teachers; and we welcome comments or suggestions from one and all.

CALVIN W. SCHWABE
HANS P. RIEMANN
Davis, California   CHARLES E. FRANTI

CONTENTS

Part 1

ORIENTATION

"Herd health
means disease control
means field research
means epidemiology"

Chapter 1

THE MEANING AND SCOPE OF EPIDEMIOLOGY

EPIDEMIOLOGY is the study of diseases in *populations*.* It is still a fledgling field, even though its empirical expression as a philosophical approach to disease has persevered through a long history of waxing and waning. Fortunately, veterinary practice is one area of medicine in which a reasonably high level of interest in the population aspect has been sustained over a considerable period of time.

USES OF EPIDEMIOLOGY

Epidemiology has two principal uses. It serves as the investigative or *diagnostic* discipline for population or herd medicine, and it supports various forms of *directed action* against diseases. These uses are not mutually exclusive.

Epidemiology as a diagnostic discipline

Three parent diagnostic disciplines—clinical diagnosis, pathology, and epidemiology— are available to the student of disease.[2] They complement one another; and their distinctly different tools may be applied sequentially to the solution of diagnostic problems, although use of all three may not be necessary in each instance. Their availability provides the veterinarian with a varied and powerful armamentarium for describing diseases and investigating their causes. Some of the characteristics of these disciplines are summarized in Table 1–1.

The epidemiological approach to diagnosis is a *holistic* one, which contrasts with the more *reductionistic* approaches of clinical diagnosis and pathology; that is, epidemiology is concerned with the whole forest as well as with the trees and the leaves. Its basic unit of concern—its patient—is the herd, the flock, or the drove rather than the single sick animal. This *population* unit includes the well animals as well as the sick and dead ones.

The objectives of these three diagnostic disciplines differ appreciably. Since disease in an individual animal is marked by observable signs and the two possible outcomes of recovery or death, the object of clinical diagnosis is to gain knowledge necessary for the treatment and recovery of this sick individual. The usual object of pathological diagnosis, on the other hand, is acquisition of knowledge to treat future cases. In contrast to both, the epidemiologist's diagnosis is concerned less with individual patients *per se* than with the *frequency* of these events of disease and death in a population, along with their *patterns* and *probabilities* of occurrence. An immediate object of epidemiologic diagnosis is to identify determinants of particular disease or death frequencies. These determinants are then used to define a web of causation, with the ultimate objective being acquisition of knowledge necessary to reduce these frequencies.

Even though its main objective is the prevention or control of a disease *en masse* rather than the cure of a sick individual, the practice of epidemiology nevertheless shares with the practice of clinical medicine a distinctly humanitarian content. However, it manifests this approach as a general exercise of social responsibility on the part of the health professions rather than through a series of individual benevolent acts. In practice, the beneficial results of this social role of epidemiology tend to be permanent. As George Bernard Shaw and others have long argued, the worth of health practitioners generally might better be judged by the death rates of the populations they serve rather than by the numbers of sick individuals they treat.

The *settings* in which the epidemiologist diagnoses diseases also differ from those of the clinician and the pathologist (see Table 1–1). Much of the epidemiologist's work is carried out initially in the field, under the actual circumstances and in the same environment in which the disease occurs and is being acquired. These observational data then may be subjected to further handling in the statistics laboratory or computer center.

---

*Chapter notes are collected at the end of the book. They elaborate upon statements in the text or document their source.[1]

Table 1–1.   Complementary Sequence of Diagnostic Disciplines in Veterinary Medicine

	Clinical Medicine ⟶ Pathology ⟶ Epidemiology		
Unit of concern	Sick *individual*	Dead *individual*	*Population* (well, sick, dead)
Usual setting	Hospital or clinic (i.e., often removed from circumstances and environment where disease occurred)	Laboratory	"Field" (farm or feedlot, etc.) (i.e., the setting in which the disease occurred)
Primary objective	R_x individual	R_x future individuals (i.e., obtain information)	Control disease or prevent its future occurrence
Diagnostic procedure	Naming disease on basis of signs and symptoms; largely an organoleptic procedure	Naming the disease on basis of host responses	Determination of frequency and patterns of occurrence of disease
Questions asked	What is it?	What is it?	What is it (i.e., the nature and frequency of the population event)?
	How do I treat it?	What is its mechanism (i.e., pathogenesis)?	Which individuals have it (i.e., frequency by host characteristics)?
		What "caused" it (i.e., identify specific etiologic agent)?	Where is it occurring? When does it occur (i.e., its pattern of occurrence)?
			What "caused" it (i.e., determinants of the event directly or indirectly associated with frequency and pattern of occurrence)?
			Why did it occur (i.e., required combination of circumstances)?
			How it is controlled or prevented?

Despite such basic differences, useful bridges between the three diagnostic approaches have been or are being created. The clinical pathologist bridges the original gap between the clinical diagnostician and the pathologist by applying some of the tools and perspectives of the latter to the living patients of the former. Similarly, the clinical epidemiologist makes an effort to see sick animals in the herd and on the farm rather than exclusively in the clinic or hospital, and draws epidemiological inferences from his observations. In human medicine, a hospital epidemiologist is another type of person fulfilling this bridging role within an already hospitalized population.

In the same way, the pathologist who examines animals in the setting in which they have died or who attempts to generalize his individual experiences from case to case by drawing inferences from populations of case histories or autopsy files builds other bridges in the epidemiologist's direction. Geographic pathology is one name sometimes given to an expression of this effort.

A "medicine in the field" approach is the way most veterinarians have practiced throughout the history of

their profession. In fact, unique features of veterinary practice have always been the extent to which it is field oriented and almost wholly dependent upon the practitioner's abilities as an observer.[3] Modern epidemiology merely attempts to bring a more rational, orderly format and a somewhat more sophisticated methodology to such largely empirical and *ad hoc* efforts of veterinarians of the past. The necessity for order and new methods grows as the complexity of population problems faced by veterinarians increases. Further comment upon these problems appears in Chapter 17.

Diagnostic uses of epidemiology have two interrelated avenues for their initial expression: *intensive follow-up* and *surveillance*.[4] As the name implies, *intensive follow-up* is a detailed, multifaceted study of all seemingly relevant aspects of a disease event in a population unit. One of its commonest forms is the *outbreak investigation*, an area in which fairly standardized protocols of procedure have evolved for some types. *Surveillance* is the opposite of intensive follow-up. As technically defined, surveillance is an *active* disease accounting process, i.e., a broad, overall, organized approach to the collection, collation, analysis, expression, and dissemination of *data* about disease in large or small populations. Some like to call it "information for action."

Surveillance data for large-scale efforts include such passively acquired items as reports of cases of disease or causes of death from institutional veterinary clinics, diagnostic laboratories, and food protection services; morbidity reports from individual veterinary practitioners; outbreak reports from livestock disease control personnel; and reports of invaders detected or intercepted by international quarantine authorities. Other data include items derived from more *active* efforts, such as detailed information resulting from instances of intensive follow-up of cases or outbreaks, results of special one-time or repeated prevalence surveys, and evaluation reports and other active feedback from continuous disease control or prevalence monitoring programs. These important subjects of intensive follow-up and surveillance are considered in greater detail in Chapters 3 and 14.

One practical diagnostic question is how we come to know things about particular diseases in veterinary medicine. In the past, books about diseases often consisted largely of an author's store of *clinical impressions*. In effect, through his personal experience of a number of individual cases of a particular disease, the author had built up a store of information in his brain, from which he retrieved the general descriptions given in his text. Every clinician goes through such a mental retrieval process each time he carries out the differential diagnosis of a case. However, no matter how experienced a clinician may be, this "home system" type of data storage and retrieval is always a far more acceptable procedure for making individual case diagnoses than for indicating definitively anything about the general characteristics of a given disease.

Now, fortunately, medical books based entirely on clinical impressions are rare, and books about diseases tend to rely more for their descriptions upon quantitative or semi-quantitative statements of particular disease characteristics. These statements are usually based upon a series of written clinical case records, autopsy records, or other forms. Typically, these latter types of data tell us that, for example, given a series of clinical or autopsy records on, say, arthritis of the horse, X% of these cases involved the fetlock joint, Y% the stifle joint, and so on. That record of data is fine so far, and most would believe that this type of information about a disease is superior to that based solely on a mental impression and the frailties of the human brain.

On the other hand, the preceding statement, for example, does *not* mean, as some authors would state it, that *in horses*, X% of cases of arthritis occur in the fetlock joint and Y% in the stifle joint; that is, that

the frequency of risk of involvement of these joints in the universe of horses is X% and Y%, respectively. Why? Well, for one reason, because there is no way to determine whether the author's series (sample) of arthritis cases is typical or representative of the universe of arthritis cases in horses. If it is, good; but usually there is no way to tell, so his data merely suggest an hypothesis to investigate. Suppose then he makes the same sort of statement of proportions for the breeds of arthritic horses in *his* record series and then states that "arthritis of horses occurs much more commonly in thoroughbreds than in Arabians." Now he really is on thin ice. Not only do the qualifications already stated about representativeness of data also apply here; but, even if the cases in his series *are* completely representative, how can anyone know whether all thoroughbred horses outnumber all Arabian horses in the universe of horses from which our sample came, to the same extent as, or to a greater extent than, in our arthritic horses? Were that the case, his statement of breed association would be completely wrong.

The preceding kinds of frequency of risk statements are made commonly in the literature from studies of clinical or autopsy records. They are called proportional morbidity (or proportional mortality) rates, and often they do not mean what their authors say they mean.

To obtain better answers to such questions, it is important to examine the clinical data *together* with similar data from the universe, or a valid sample of it. Therefore, one of the more important ways that epidemiology can aid us is in providing suitable means to describe and characterize diseases. Methods for achieving this include (1) recording and quantifying appropriately collected disease data, (2) comparing them to suitable universe or community data, and (3) stating results in a way that indicates their validity and accurately reflects an analytical process and its limitations.

Even more important, these same epidemiological techniques can be applied in veterinary practice. They can be used to diagnose the causes of a number of cases of a disease occurring simultaneously, or nearly so, in the herds or other populations of animals for which a veterinarian may be responsible.

Epidemiology in directed action

In an epidemiological sense, directed actions are *doing things* about herd diseases in systematic and logical ways. These actions include (1) studies on the nature and extent of the *disease problems present* in a given population; (2) studies on the overall behavior of *particular* diseases in different populations, with investigation of their determinants and patterns of occurrence; (3) *planning* and *evaluation* of efforts to *prevent* or *control diseases*; and (4) research on *new methods* or approaches for the investigation and control of crowd diseases.

HISTORIC APPROACHES TO EPIDEMIOLOGY

Existing books about epidemiology commonly define and treat the field in terms of one particular historical tradition or approach to its overall development. Thus, there is the approach that considers epidemiology largely in terms of its *medical detection* dimension. This avenue grew mostly from the experiences of clinicians and pathologists in the last century as they first considered population aspects of commonly occurring diseases of man and other animals.

Other authors consider epidemiology from the standpoint of *medical ecology*. The traditional exponents of that approach were those veterinarians and physicians who first discovered that (1) the life cycles of parasites of vertebrates often were biologically complex, (2) zoonoses and many other infections shared among vertebrate species were relatively non-specific, and (3) some infections were transmitted from vertebrate to vertebrate by invertebrate vectors. Ecologists, entomologists, parasitologists, zoologists, and others have all contributed both to the efforts to unravel the intricacies of such biologically complicated diseases and to the development of the ecological school of epidemiology.

Still other epidemiological works consider the field almost solely in terms of *mathematical methods*, which have been applied mostly in identifying the determinants of "diseases of unknown etiology." This relatively large group of diseases has proven unresponsive and unyielding to the traditional diagnostic thrusts of the clinician and the pathologist. Until now, this mathematical approach to epidemiology has been used primarily by statisticians and public health workers.

Finally, lesser yet important inputs to modern epidemiology have come from persons whose training or bent has been more geographical or economic than medical, from geneticists, and from individuals in such human practice specialties as occupational medicine.

The important thing to realize is that epidemiology does not owe its accomplishments to, nor derive its present strengths from, any single historic approach. While these different aspects of epidemiology may have been fairly distinct in the past, representing as they did different interests of epidemiologists and differences in their training and background, they have shared important basic elements. In the practice of epidemiology today, distinctions between these medical detection, ecological, and mathematical schools tend to blur; and contributions derivative of each often go into the solution of a particular problem. As a result, modern epidemiologists tend to

view their field more comprehensively than in the past and also tend to identify parts of their total strategy in functional or strategic terms. Epidemiology's future lies in this continued melding of relevant inputs and in the continued development of newer and more probing methodologies.

STRATEGIES OF EPIDEMIOLOGY

The *overall* strategy of epidemiology is the "scientific method" applied to problems of diseases in populations. This approach usually involves collecting and evaluating preexisting data and hypotheses; making personal observations; using this information inductively to suggest relationships or associations, that is, to form new hypotheses; and finally, analyzing observational data and/or data obtained from specific experiments, in order to accept or reject these hypotheses, in either case a deductive approach.[5] The essential aspect of the last step is to test the predictive value of the hypothesis. The stages in this overall process are often referred to as *descriptive*, *experimental*, and *analytical* epidemiology.

It has been said with good reason that while "art is I, science is we." In other words, to advance the scientific knowledge of any particular disease, the cycle just described is often repeated again and again, frequently by different persons. Thus, application of the scientific method almost always involves a systematic stepwise series of processes, a series of successive approximations. Thus, almost any alert individual in a field such as medicine is *frequently* in a position to advance knowledge in modest yet substantial ways. An epidemiological perspective enhances these possibilities.

Finally, there is one other implied input that must be used well, i.e., the published *literature*. It is a vital aspect, but it is beyond the scope of this book to consider use of the many available *bibliographic tools* that enable the epidemiologist to systematically locate the results of colleagues' efforts, past and present. Introductions to these varied tools—current literature scans, article indices, abstract compilations, subject reviews, bibliographies, and computerized search inputs to the literature of population medicine—are to be found in several available guides.[6]

Descriptive epidemiology

Descriptive epidemiology means making *observations in the field* in order to describe a particular disease event or disease phenomenon as fully as necessary. These efforts usually are intended not only to identify the problem but also to characterize it fully: its extent and spatial distribution; its temporal relationships; the host species involved; the populations affected or at risk and *their* relevant characteristics; the frequency of illness or occurrence of new cases; the possible agent, environmental, or host determinants of the phenomenon or event; and a mode of transmission, in the case of infections. The questions asked include: *what* is the event or phenomenon, *which* are the animals involved, *when* did it take place, *where* did it take place, and finally, *how* and *why* did it occur?

The observational process involved in such descriptive studies should be neither a mere "fishing expedition" for clues nor indiscriminant "data dredging" operations just for the sake of obtaining data. Instead, they should be planned, systematic, multifaceted, intensive follow-up and/or surveillance efforts (depending upon the nature and dimensions of the problem of concern). Descriptive studies yield qualitative data of the several types mentioned, as well as certain kinds of quantitative information. These latter usually are expressed in the forms of tables, graphs, maps, and rates, or as statements of central tendency and dispersion.

By their nature, descriptive studies are expected to lead to hypotheses about the particular event or phenomenon, e.g., its possible determinants.

FORMULATION OF EPIDEMIOLOGICAL HYPOTHESES. A hypothesis is an explanation or a proposition that can be tested by facts that are known or can be obtained. In general, an epidemiological hypothesis should specify (1) the population or other group to which the hypothesis applies; (2) the determinant or other maneuver being considered; (3) the expected effect or response (e.g., the disease); (4) the time-response relationship (e.g., the time that will lapse between exposure to a cause and observation of the effect); and (5) the dose-response relationship, to the extent that such information is obtainable.

The following methods are useful in formulating epidemiological hypotheses.[7]

Method of difference. If the frequency of a disease differs appreciably under two sets of circumstances and some factor can be identified in one circumstance but is absent in another, this factor (or its absence) may have caused the disease. An example is the high prevalence of congenital malformations in offspring of sheep grazing in areas where *Veratrum californicum* grows and the low prevalence in similar areas where *Veratrum californicum* is absent.

Method of agreement. If a factor is common to a number of different circumstances that have been found to be associated with the presence of a disease, this factor may be a determinant of the disease. During a routine analysis of surveillance data on salmonellosis, nearly all isolations of *Salmonella new brunswick* from human patients were found to come from infants who, at different times and in different geographical locations, had consumed reconstituted dry cows' milk. The agent was later isolated from that product.

Method of concomitant variation. This method involves the search for some factor whose frequency or strength varies with the frequency of the disease. This method is used in retrospective and prospective studies, but is of less value than the first two methods in outbreak investigations. An example would be an observation of increased frequency of a disease with increasing rainfall.

Method of analogy. The distribution of one disease may be sufficiently similar to that of some other disease to suggest a common cause. A peculiar age and geographic distribution of pernicious anemia in Scandinavians was similar to the distribution of infection with the fish tapeworm, *Diphyllobothrium latum*, in the same population. This factor first suggested that the two diseases might have a common cause, which in this case turned out to be the consumption of raw freshwater fish. In this example, a more immediate or direct cause-effect relationship resulted from the fact that this tapeworm deprives its human host of vitamin B_{12}. It is important to note that the latter fact may be most useful for *treating* the individual patient, while knowledge of the first less-direct cause is essential for *prevention* or *control* of the disease.

In addition to hypotheses, descriptive studies sometimes identify natural experiments, which then may be analyzed. This particular aspect of descriptive epidemiology can be made clear by referring to one of the classic studies with which veterinarians and all epidemiologists should be at least somewhat conversant.[8]

JOHN SNOW ON CHOLERA. Although human cholera is not a zoonosis and therefore not of direct interest to most veterinarians, one of its early students was the great French veterinarian, Edmond Nocard, who served as a member of the Asian Cholera Commission in the last century.

In the mid-1800's, an English physician named John Snow set about to explain the then-unknown cause of human cholera. Of particular interest is that he succeeded in doing this some 30 years before Robert Koch discovered a specific bacterium, *Vibrio cholerae*, and its etiological relationships to cholera. That situation may sound paradoxical, but it is important to recognize that, when the clinician or pathologist talks about a disease's cause, he is usually referring to an *immediate* cause, often a specific living or nonliving *agent*—such as the tapeworm in the previous example—which, if combatted in the sick individual through some therapeutic regimen, may result in a clinical cure. However, what the epidemiologist means by cause also *includes* more remote causes, such as eating raw freshwater fish. In other words, *any determinant* of disease (specific agents included) that, if eliminated or altered, results in a decrease in the incidence of a disease in a population, that is, in the risk of individuals in the population acquiring the disease, is a cause. These conceptions of cause are two quite different things (see Table 1–1).

Based on his observations on the clinical manifestations of cholera (a profuse watery diarrhea) and on its common occurrence among family members and its virtual absence among attending physicians and nurses, Snow hypothesized that cholera was an enteric disease contracted by mouth and thus was not directly contagious. Diarrhea was prominent in cholera, and he postulated that it was probably associated with transmission of the disease.

Snow then proceeded to show that cholera occurred when people drank water mixed with the feces of infected individuals. At the same time he demonstrated that, if the sources of this contaminated water could be found and cut off, the frequency of occurrence of the disease would decline drastically. The best-known instance of the latter was his now-famous recommendation to remove the handle from London's Broad Street Pump!

How did John Snow go about establishing the validity of his hypotheses? Was he able to feed people sewage or contaminated water, as a veterinarian would probably have considered doing in a similar situation of animal disease? No. Instead, he decided to examine the death certificates for London at the time of the 1832 cholera epidemic and to convert these data into death rates. Then, from plotting these deaths and rates on maps of London, he noted that excessive mortality was associated with those districts supplied with water by the Southwark Water Works, a private company that, he discovered, drew its water from the Thames River *downstream* from the city's sewage outflow. The cholera death rate of that district was higher than the death rate of most other districts of the city. That observation encouraged Snow's belief in the validity of his sewage-water hypothesis. He, therefore, made similar observations on cholera deaths during the epidemic of 1849. From these observations he concluded that other water companies, such as Vauxhall (then merged with Southwark) and the Lambeth Company, were probably involved since these companies also drew their water from below the city's sewage outflow. What Snow did in these two epidemic years was to carry out what would now be considered rather crude retrospective epidemiological studies.

Then, when he was able to take a third look at similar statistics from yet another London cholera epidemic in 1853, Snow noticed a small difference in the situation, and *proceeded to take the fullest advantage of* his findings. He found that between 1849 and 1853, the Lambeth Company had moved its water intake upstream on the Thames to some distance above the sewage outflow of London and the intakes of the other companies. Moreover, he noted

that in one subdistrict of about 15,000 people served by the Lambeth Company exclusively, not one cholera death had occurred. In some other districts, however, he observed that the water was supplied by *both* the Lambeth Company and the Southwark and Vauxhall Company, and these districts had a level of cholera death rates intermediate between the level for those served exclusively by either company. Upon further inquiry and much field work, Snow found that, in the districts served jointly, the pipelines of both companies often ran down the same streets. About 300,000 people drew their water from the supplier whose water they preferred or from whichever happened to be connected to their taps. The situation was rather like choosing a dairy's home-delivery routeman from among those available in cities in the United States today.

To his great credit, Snow realized that he had stumbled upon a natural experiment on a large scale. Two populations from the same environment, similar to one another with respect to sex and age distribution, socioeconomic conditions, and other factors, clearly differed, insofar as he could tell, *only* with respect to the source of their water. Thus, by comparing their cholera death rates, he was able to carry out what epidemiologists now call a cohort study using preexisting data.[9] The results of that study gave strong support to his earlier observations of an apparent association between contaminated water and cholera; and he strengthened his hypothesis still further when he showed that, by altering this hypothesized link, such as by removing the handle from the Broad Street Pump, he could greatly alter the frequency of occurrence of the disease among the population at risk.

Thus, the usual objectives of descriptive studies in epidemiology are, as in John Snow's case, to define patterns of a disease's behavior and occurrence, then formulate hypotheses about possible determinants of these observed patterns, and, if possible, discover the prior occurrence of natural experiments through which one can test the hypothesized associations.

Experimental epidemiology

In contrast, the strategy of experimental epidemiology involves designing specific population experiments to test epidemiological hypotheses. These experiments are often prospective and proceed from the postulated cause to the observable effect.[10] Commonly performed types of prospective epidemiological experiments include vaccine trials and drug trials as well as various other so-called clinical trials.

An early classic example to illustrate this strategy was the series of field experiments carried out by the American veterinarian, Frederick Kilborne, between 1889 and 1892. He wanted to test an hypothesis, advanced first by American cattlemen, that Texas fever of cattle was caused by ticks. All epidemiologists should be familiar with this study since Kilborne demonstrated for the first time that disease-producing microorganisms can be transmitted between vertebrates by invertebrate vectors.[11]

FREDERICK KILBORNE ON TEXAS FEVER. By 1885, Daniel Elmer Salmon, the founder of veterinary services in the U.S. government, had shown that the patterns of occurrence of Texas fever in American cattle could not be explained by any known mechanism for disease transmission and that this disease did not originate in cattle located north of a line that he had determined. Kilborne believed that the cattle tick's natural range coincided with Salmon's Texas fever line, and he urged the testing of the cattlemen's tick hypothesis. Salmon approved this study by Kilborne and at the same time directed Cooper Curtice, another Bureau of Animal Industry (B.A.I.) veterinarian, to work out the life history of the cattle

tick, and also directed Theobald Smith, a young physician in the B.A.I., to study the pathology and possible microbial etiology of the disease.

In the summer of 1889, Kilborne divided the B.A.I.'s experimental farm into well-separated fenced fields, as shown in Figure 1–1. Susceptible northern cattle were distributed in groups in these fields (Table 1–2), with two different possibilities for their exposure to ticks as well as to North Carolina (southern) cattle from which all ticks had been removed. The result was that *only* the susceptible cattle exposed to the ticks developed the disease.

These types of experiments, which strongly supported the tick hypothesis, were repeated in the summers of 1890, 1891, and 1892. In the meantime, Smith's work showed that the responsible agent, or *immediate* cause of Texas fever, was a blood protozoan now called *Babesia bigemina*. Kilborne and Cooper Curtice then postulated that Smith's agent

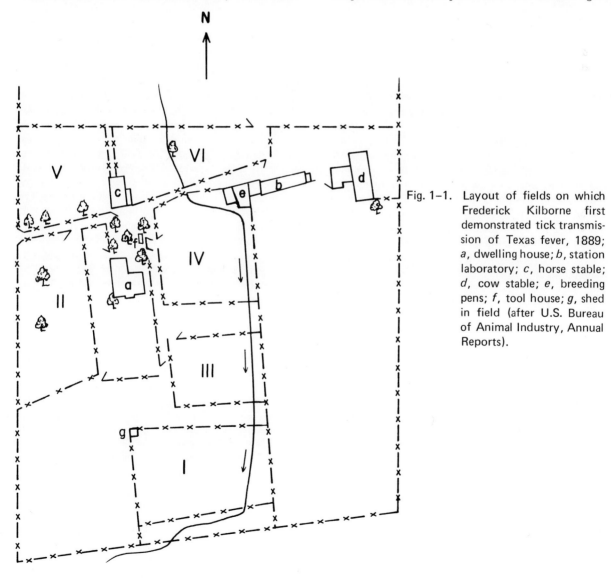

Fig. 1–1. Layout of fields on which Frederick Kilborne first demonstrated tick transmission of Texas fever, 1889; *a*, dwelling house; *b*, station laboratory; *c*, horse stable; *d*, cow stable; *e*, breeding pens; *f*, tool house; *g*, shed in field (after U.S. Bureau of Animal Industry, Annual Reports).

Table 1–2. Texas Fever Tick Experiments by F. L. Kilborne, 1889 (after U. S. Bureau of Animal Industry, Annual Reports)

	No. resistant North Carolina cattle infested with ticks (no. ill or dead)	No. initially tick-free susceptible northern cattle (no. ill or dead)	No. resistant North Carolina cattle freed of all ticks (no. ill or dead)	No. free adult ticks distributed on field
1st Series				
Field I	4 (0)	14 (12)		
Field II		4 (0)	3 (0)	
2nd Series				
Field III	3 (0)	3 (1)[+]		
Field II*	3 (0)	3 (2)[+]		
Field IV		4 (0)[+]	3 (0)	
Field V		4 (3)[+]		Several thousands

*Subsequent to other experiment in Field II

[+]Experiment carried out in autumn

was being transmitted from ticks to cattle; Curtice further suggested that it was being maintained from one generation of ticks to another. Therefore, northern susceptible cattle were also exposed to larval ticks hatched in the laboratory. The results of one of these latter experiments are shown in Table 1–3.

The cumulative result of all of Kilborne's experiments was the positive establishment that a tick was a determinant of Texas fever in that the disease could not occur in its absence. Moreover, the progeny of such ticks were also shown to be a cause of the disease. Disclosure of the relationship of a tick to a parasite and its vertebrate host was a major breakthrough in the progress of medical science. Generally, this experimental epidemiological approach may be resorted to much more often in veterinary medicine than in human medicine.

Analytic epidemiology

While simple descriptive mathematical techniques, such as rates and measurements of central tendency and dispersion, have long been used to describe observational and experimental data in epidemiology,

the strategy of analytical epidemiology goes beyond this purely descriptive process to draw statistical inferences about diseases in populations from available samples of the populations.

The results of nature's experiments on cholera, as observed by John Snow, and the man-made epidemiological experiments designed by Frederick Kilborne and Cooper Curtice to determine the cause of bovine piroplasmosis were both clear-cut. A relative abundance of data convinced even the most skeptical. However, no statistical analyses were undertaken by these early epidemiologists to strengthen or support the validity of their particular conclusions. There will often be similar situations in which a careful inspection of data will be all that is required. Certainly, this step should never be overlooked because of eagerness to undertake some more sophisticated form of analysis that may not only take time and effort, but also obscure some valid but purely common-sense conclusion.

On the other hand, retrospective observational studies or prospective experimental studies commonly yield either less clear-cut results than Snow's or Kilborne's, or data which, on inspection only, may

Table 1–3. Experiment by F. L. Kilborne with Larval Ticks and Texas Fever, 1891 (after U. S. Bureau of Animal Industry, Annual Reports)

	No. susceptible northern cattle to which larval ticks were applied (no. ill or dead)	No. initially tick-free susceptible northern cattle (no. ill or dead)	No. resistant North Carolina cattle to which larval ticks were applied (no. ill or dead)	No. resistant North Carolina cattle infected with ticks (no. ill or dead)
Field I	3 (3)		1 (0)	
Field VI		8 (7)*		4 (0)

*The one clinically unaffected animal was a calf.

mask a less-than-obvious conclusion. Yet they may contain the answers. In these situations, analytical epidemiology, the most recently developed major strategy of epidemiology, uses mathematical tools to help determine, for example, the statistical significance of hypothesized associations between possible determinants of disease and observed rates of disease frequency. Mathematical tools help us decide whether such associations are likely to have occurred by chance.

Specific mathematical methods toward these ends include the sampling techniques themselves as well as techniques for (1) determining the strength of epidemiological associations, e.g., the method of relative risk, (2) determining the importance of associations, e.g., the method of attributable risk, or (3) determining the *statistical significance* of associations, e.g., the chi-square test. Analytical epidemiology also offers more complicated mathematical methods, such as life table studies and mathematical modeling, as well as techniques for the identification of multiple determinants (e.g., factor analysis, discriminant analysis, multiple regression). The particular example of cholera and sewage is considered further in this regard on page 16, and the general subject of analytical methods is discussed beginning in Chapter 5.

Chapter 2

DISEASES IN POPULATIONS

TRADITIONALLY, medicine has been taught with primary emphasis on the individual sick animal and only secondary emphasis on the affected herd or population, despite the fact that medical *practice* in its broad sense involves studying diseases and controlling them, in addition to treating individual cases. In human medicine, neglect of the population as a basic unit of concern was so complete in many countries that, to afford a partial remedy, schools of public health had to be created as separate institutions. Recently, there have been shifts in emphasis in medical education still further down the "holistic-reductionistic" spectrum to the levels of the organ system or even the cell as primary units for attention. It is beyond the purpose of this book to discuss scientific or social implications of these facts beyond indicating that most of the well-defined social problem areas that the veterinary profession has addressed—whether food production, public health and consumer protection, or ecological imbalances and environmental threats—are problem areas in which the population unit of concern demands emphasis. These areas are discussed in detail in Chapter 17.

POPULATION UNITS

First, what is the population with which we are concerned? The question cannot be answered without first stating the circumstances of the practice of veterinary medicine, since the unit of concern could just as well be six birds in a private aviary or 20 fish in a city aquarium tank. It could be a 100-cow dairy herd in New York or a 2000-cow dairy herd in California. It might be a 50,000-steer feedlot in Colorado, the 2 million broilers of a single Delmarva producer, all 3.9-million swine in Minnesota in 1975, or the more than 25 million dogs in the United States in 1975. Finally, it could even be a population of unknown size, e.g., skunks or ticks in a veterinarian's practice area. The particular range of species or magnitude of their numbers is not fundamentally important because the epidemiological concepts applicable to each and the methods of approach to problems of disease would *generally* be similar even if, in some special instances, specifically different. For most purposes in epidemiology, it is an advantage to know the size of the particular population being considered, although at times it is sufficient to observe known samples of that universe or even to work with lesser knowledge of a population.

POPULATION AT RISK

An initial part of many descriptive studies in epidemiology is the counting of population events such as disease or death. The object is usually to express these data, if possible, as frequencies (i.e., as relative frequencies, proportions, or probability statements). However, to perform this function involves relating the enumerated events to the population in which the events took place. The denominator value for such *rates* is called the *population at risk*. What does "at risk" mean?

When virulent Asian Newcastle disease virus, apparently introduced into this country by imported wild birds intended for the pet-bird trade, escaped into the immense chicken population of southern California in 1971, all chickens in the designated quarantine area were regarded as susceptible or at risk because this exotic virus apparently did not discriminate among chickens by age, sex, or breed, and none of the chickens had been immunized against it. Therefore, the whole population was potentially at risk of acquiring the infection.

If, however, the general population of concern is a large cattle herd in Texas and the problem is abortion, the population at risk would not be this entire herd population because the male animals are not at risk of abortion, the disease event. Even more specifically, the population at risk would be only the *pregnant* females in this herd. More will be said about populations in Chapter 7.

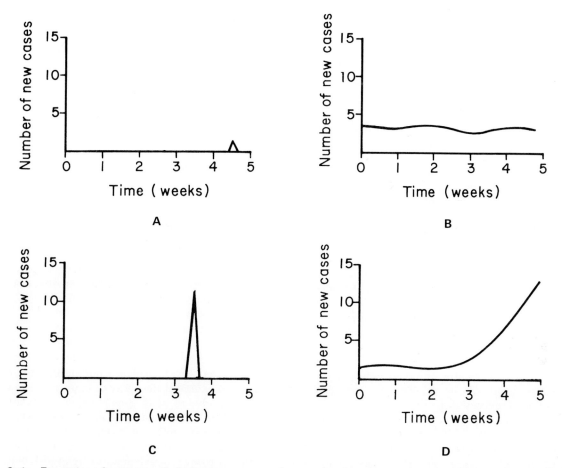

Fig. 2–1. Examples of patterns of disease occurrence. *A* sporadic; *B* endemic; *C* point epidemic; *D* propagating epidemic.

PATTERNS OF DISEASE OCCURRENCE

There are three commonly recognized patterns of disease occurrence in populations—sporadic, endemic, and epidemic (Fig. 2–1).

Sporadic disease

If a disease occurs rarely and without regularity in a population unit, it is said to occur *sporadically*. In the case of infectious diseases, a sporadic pattern of occurrence suggests the question, "Where *is* the disease when it is apparently not around?" Possible explanations might be that (1) infection exists in the population *inapparently* and only in occasional animals do signs of disease evidence themselves; (2) the infection is generally absent and the disease is noted only when an infected animal is introduced into the population from outside; or (3) the infection is being maintained in another species of animal in the same general environment and only occasionally do conditions for interspecies transmission and observable disease arise. In the first instance, one

might wonder further, "What is different about these occasional symptomatic animals?" or, in the latter instance, "What about these particular animals or their environment made interspecies transmission possible?"

Endemic disease

If, on the other hand, a disease occurs with predictable regularity in a population unit with only relatively minor fluctuations in its frequency pattern over time, it is said to occur *endemically* in the population, or to be endemic or native to the area. With the world as the universe, endemic disease represents a clustering of disease events in space but not in time. A disease may be endemic at any level of occurrence. For particular diseases, it is possible to define specific frequencies of occurrence as *holoendemic* (most animals affected), *hyperendemic* (a high proportion of animals affected), *mesoendemic* (a moderate proportion of animals affected), or *hypoendemic* (a relatively small proportion of animals affected).

Epidemic disease

Finally, a disease is said to occur *epidemically* if its frequency in a given population during a given time interval *is clearly in excess of its expected frequency*. The epidemic occurrence of disease has nothing to do *per se* with absolute numbers of cases; it is a purely relative term for unexpectedly high frequencies of disease occurrence. Thus, whether an observed frequency of any particular disease constitutes an epidemic would vary from one place and one population to another. For instance, one district in Kenya might *normally* experience new cases of foot-and-mouth disease in 5 to 10% of its cattle each year. Were 5% of the cattle affected in one month, however, that occurrence would be considered an epidemic, whereas 1% affected in one month probably would not. One confirmed case of foot-and-mouth disease in Florida, on the other hand, would represent an epidemic occurrence, too, because the expected frequency of occurrence there is zero. Epidemicity represents a clustering of disease in both space and time. "Outbreak" is a somewhat less precise term, roughly synonymous with epidemic.

A *pandemic* is a very large-scale epidemic, usually involving several countries or even continents. A truly global pandemic can be thought of as the clustering of disease events in time but not in space.

EPIDEMIC CURVES

All of these population patterns of disease are statements of disease event frequencies against time. The graphic expression of such data, particularly from an epidemic or outbreak, in the form of a frequency histogram or frequency polygon for a defined time interval is called an *epidemic curve*. Plotting an epidemic curve is one of the most useful ways to visualize the dynamics of a particular disease event in a population. Examples of different types of epidemic curves are given in Figures 2–1 and 6–1 to 6–3.

FREQUENCY OF OCCURRENCE OF DISEASE

Occurrences of disease events in a population are usually expressed as frequency *rates*, which represent the proportion of affected animals in the population, or state the statistical probabilities of disease occurrence. One way to indicate disease frequency is as an *attack rate*. This is a general term for the proportion of a specific population affected during a particular *outbreak* or some other defined but usually short period of time. The denominator is the population at the onset of the outbreak. More precise expressions of disease frequency are morbidity rates which indicate the *prevalence* or the *incidence* of an illness.

Prevalence

The most commonly used *prevalence rate* is called the *instantaneous*, or *point*, prevalence rate (I.P.R.).

It is expressed as follows:

$$\text{I.P.R.} = \frac{\begin{array}{c}\text{No. cases of a disease existing}\\ \text{in a population at a point in time}\end{array}}{\begin{array}{c}\text{No. animals in that population}\\ \text{at that same point in time}\end{array}}$$

Prevalence, therefore, is a cross-sectional measure of the amount of an illness present in a population at any given moment. As often applied in practice, however, a moment may be some fairly short interval of time.

Incidence

By contrast, a morbidity frequency may also be expressed as an *incidence rate* (I.R.):

$$\text{I. R.} = \frac{\begin{array}{c}\text{No. } new \text{ cases of disease which occur in a}\\ \text{population during a stated period of time}\end{array}}{\begin{array}{c}Average \text{ number of animals in}\\ \text{that population during the} \quad \times \quad \begin{array}{c}\text{Length of time}\\ \text{period}\end{array}\\ \text{same time period}\end{array}}$$

Incidence is a measure of the *likelihood* or *risk* in a population of an individual acquiring an illness during a stated *period* of time. The denominators of both of these morbidity rates should be the population at risk. More will be said in Chapter 5 about what these two distinctly different morbidity rates mean, how they are related to each other, and what the respective values and limitations are of each one.

DETERMINANTS OR CAUSES OF DISEASE OCCURRENCE

To reiterate an important statement from Chapter 1, when an epidemiologist refers to a disease determinant, he means *any* variable—a specific agent, a host factor, or an environmental factor—which directly or indirectly increases frequency of occurrence of a disease. If this variable can be eliminated or altered, the frequency of the disease will decline and its importance as a population problem will decrease. To illustrate this statement, one can consider that tubercle bacilli are present in several cows in a dairy herd. Tuberculosis cannot occur in their absence; and at least a few of these animals will probably show active disease. Thus, *Mycobacterium tuberculosis bovis* must be regarded as *a* casual variable, or a determinant of the frequency of active tubercular disease in this herd. However, it is not the only determinant.

Another determinant would be the housing of these cattle, particularly as it might affect population density or their closeness to one another. If this herd is confined to a barn one-third the size of the adequate barn it is now using, the probability of transmission of the tubercle bacilli would rise, the numbers of organisms acquired by some animals would be greater, and the animals might be under greater stress. As a result, one could expect both an increased frequency of infection and an increased frequency of disease.

Then, if one appreciably reduces the nutritional quality of this herd's currently adequate diet, the resistance of individual animals might decline and there might be another increase in the frequency of active tubercular cases. Clearly, then, things like suboptimal nutrition and crowded housing, in addition to the tubercle bacillus, can *all* be determinants of bovine tuberculosis as a herd or population problem. Moreover, while the tubercle bacillus is a specific living *agent*, nutritional state is a *host* variable and housing density is an *environmental* function. Diagrammatically, tuberculosis as a herd disease can be visualized as an interaction among all three of these classes of determinants (Fig. 2–2), the result of which is a given frequency of disease.

Multiple determinants of smog disease

Another illustration of the interrelationships of multiple determinants in diseases involves cattle exhibited at the Smithfield Fat Stock Show in London in December, 1873. Veterinarians observed that many fat cattle being exhibited suffered cardiopulmonary failure and had to be sent for emergency slaughter. The attendant veterinarians attributed these cardiopulmonary illnesses to the effect of an unusually dense and acrid chemical-laden fog. This event is important because it marked the first demonstration of the dangers to health of what is now called *smog*. In describing this episode in a contemporary veterinary journal, one veterinarian noted that "if anyone, a few weeks ago, had suggested the possibility of a London fog doing serious damage to cattle ... submitted to its influence, he would have been looked upon as supplying in himself a melancholy instance of intellectual fogginess. All the inconvenience and discomfort of a metropolitan fog, with its palpable flavour and pungency, dwellers near the city realize full well; but in all our experience there could be found no grounds for serious apprehension. Nevertheless, it is beyond question, that a number of animals did suffer seriously from the inhalation of the fog-clouded

atmosphere which prevailed during the second week of December."[1]

While a detailed news report also appeared in the London *Times* of December 12, 1873, physicians overlooked the possible human health significance of this event and no one questioned whether this smog might also have affected Londoners who were forced to breathe it. Only when the same thing rather remarkably recurred 79 years later in the Smithfield Fat Stock Show of December, 1952, was the curiosity of public health officials piqued. Their now-famous retrospective study of excessive London deaths for that week in December showed that over 4000 people also died in that particular smog disaster. Most of them were either very young or very old or were already cardiopulmonary invalids.

Much more is known about the circumstances of such epidemics today. What, then, is the cause of smog deaths in cattle and people? Is it a specific chemical *agent* such as $SO_2^=$ emitted into the air in high concentrations (Fig. 2–3*A*)? Is it perhaps a specific climatic *environmental* change resulting in an inversion layer of cool air that traps the warm air below and produces the dangerous levels of pollutants that build up near the ground? Is it the fact that associated deaths occur only in individual cattle or people with already overburdened hearts or in other cardiac or pulmonary invalids, that is, only in individuals with some inherent *host* liability or defect? Would it be most nearly correct to regard all three of these factors as interrelated determinants of the frequency of death in smog episodes (Fig. 2–3*B*)?

Modern epidemiology rests on the premise that diseases in populations do have multiple determinants and that these determinants usually include one or more specific animate or inanimate agents, as well as factors associated with the host animals themselves and their environment. Therefore, it follows that, in the prevention or control of a disease, attention should be directed to the relative importance of and the ease of approach to *all* identifiable determinants.

EPIDEMIOLOGICAL ASSOCIATIONS

An important area of epidemiological practice and research is the identification of associations between frequencies of disease events and their possible

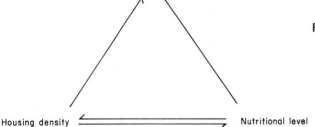

Presence of
Mycobacterium tuberculosis bovis

Housing density
of animals

Nutritional level
of animals

Fig. 2–2. Diagram of possible multiple determinants of a given frequency of new tuberculosis cases in a dairy herd.

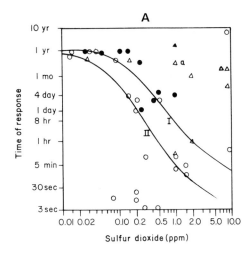
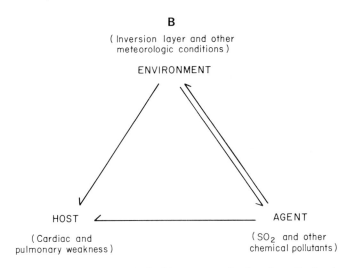

Fig. 2–3. *A,* Effects of sulfur oxides on health; the symbols refer to specific incidents, e.g., the London, England smog of 1952 is represented by *a*; (O)=morbidity in man; (●)=mortality in man; (△)=morbidity in animals; (▲)=mortality in animals. The area above curve I indicates range of concentrations and exposure times in which deaths have been reported in excess of normal expectation; the area above curve II indicates range of concentrations and exposure times in which significant health effects have been reported (redrawn from Munn, R. E. 1970. *Biometeorological Methods.* Academic Press, New York; after U.S.D.H.E.W. 1967. Air quality for sulfur oxides. Public Health Service, Washington).

B, Diagram of interaction of host, agent and environmental determinants of smog disease in animals and man (redrawn from Schwabe, C. W. 1969. *Veterinary Medicine and Human Health,* 2nd ed. The Williams & Wilkins Co., Baltimore).

agent, host, and environmental determinants. In the more or less remote past, clinicians and pathologists tended to have little regard for such epidemiological evidence about disease determinants. They considered it circumstantial evidence; and by that they meant weak, nonscientific evidence, insusceptible to proof and invalid as a basis for scientific conclusions. Necessity was again the mother of invention, however; and the very fact that many diseases of unknown etiology failed to yield to more traditional diagnostic inputs prompted epidemiologists to seek the help of mathematicians for ways to determine the *probability* associated with observed relationships between possibly causal variables and diseases. As a result, there are now a number of analytical tools with which to help identify and strongly support certain types of epidemiological evidence about causes or determinants of sometimes complex and obscure diseases.

This situation is fortunate in that the possible determinants of a disease in many instances may not be as apparent as those cited for tuberculosis or smog disease. One might ask, for example, what are the important determinants of present levels of occurrence of mammary tumors in dogs, or neonatal deaths in calves, or emphysema in horses, or even of mastitis in dairy cows? Trying to discover some of the determinants of such complex diseases involves an

initial search for apparent *associations* between some factor(s) and the disease. This association then becomes the basis for a causal hypothesis. Such an hypothesis can often be tested from observational data (nature's experiments) or from experimental data.

Table 2–1 shows Snow's cholera death data from 14,632 persons in three subdistricts of London. In 1853, this group was served only by the Lambeth Water Company. Here, apparently, is an absolute association: no one who drank Lambeth water died, *but* there is no group with which to compare this population. Would any of these people have died if they had drunk Southwark and Vauxhall water? Who knows. Thus, *one basic rule for demonstrating epidemiological associations is that there must be both a case population and a comparable control population.*

Suppose Snow had chosen to compare cholera deaths among inhabitants of these three subdistricts with deaths in another 12 London subdistricts that were supplied only Southwark and Vauxhall water. This is essentially what Snow did with the data from the 1832 and 1849 epidemics, but how could he or anyone else be certain that the water source was the only relevant difference between the two populations from different parts of London? Suppose there were socioeconomic differences, or something else that related to the likelihood of dying of cholera. Thus,

Table 2–1.   Cholera Mortality in London in Area Supplied with Water by Lambeth Company (data from John Snow)*

	Died of cholera	Did not die of cholera	
Drank Lambeth water	0	14,632	14,632
Did not drink Lambeth water	0	0	0
Total	0	14,632	14,632

*See Chapter 1, Note 8.

another rule in such situations is that *the populations to be compared should, insofar as possible, differ only with respect to the variable being examined.*

Luckily, Snow did not have to make the preceding comparison in the 1853 epidemic because he discovered then that the people in 16 other subdistricts were being supplied with water by *both* companies. These data gave Snow two parts of the *same* population that apparently differed *only* in their water source. Data for this natural experiment could be expressed as in Table 2–2.

This situation is susceptible to statistical analysis for significance of the hypothesized association. For example, calculating the chi-square statistic and testing whether the two proportions (525/181,868 and 94/118,245) differ significantly produces $\chi^2 = 152$.[2] This chi-square value is statistically significant at the 0.0001 level; that is, it is unlikely that such differences in these proportions would have arisen by chance in this population more often than once in 10,000 times! Note that such an analysis requires data on those who did not die as well as on those who died. Methods to analyze epidemiological data are considered in more detail in Chapters 5, 11, 12, and 13.

Statistical and biological significance

An important point to emphasize is that a *statistically* significant association need not necessarily be a *biologically* significant one. Epidemiologists must resist an automatic temptation to regard all statis-

tically significant associations between factors and disease as *causal* associations because, for various reasons, they may not be.[3]

There are other types of epidemiological evidence that may strengthen our *belief* in the causal nature of an hypothesized association, though not necessarily prove it. In addition to ones stated in connection with the derivation of hypotheses, these types include: (1) a biologically meaningful association; (2) a *temporal sequence*; that is, the cause precedes the effect (which is not, however, the same as saying that one *leads* to the other); (3) a *dose-response* relationship; that is, the disease event varies in incidence as the factor does, or the first is a *function* of the second; (4) a related proposition; namely, if the factor is eliminated, the frequency of the event declines; and (5) repetitions of the study yield the same or similar results. Retrospective and prospective studies as well as *associations* and *causal associations* reappear in Chapters 11 and 12.

INFECTIONS AND INFECTIOUS DISEASE

Certainly, the epidemiologist is not concerned exclusively with infectious diseases although government veterinary services have been slower than public health services in visualizing population-oriented approaches to important diseases of other types. Infections still remain as important problems in both fields, however; and from the epidemiological standpoint, there are a number of factors to understand about them.

Table 2–2.   Mortality from Cholera in One Area of London Supplied with Water by Both Southwark and Vauxhall and Lambeth Companies, 7 Weeks Ending August 26, 1854 (data from John Snow)*

	Cholera deaths	Population not dying	
Southwark and Vauxhall	525	181,343	181,868†
Lambeth	94	118,151	118,245†
Total	619	299,494	300,113

*See Chapter 1, Note 8.
†Populations supplied by each company estimated from proportions of households served by each, as determined by Snow.

First, there is the difference between *infection* and *infectious disease*. Infection is a state of symbiosis. It simply means that the body of one living organism, the host, is invaded by another living organism, the symbiont. If the relationship benefits the symbiont and does not harm the host, the relationship is said to be commensal[4] and the infection inapparent or subclinical. If, however, this relationship between symbiont species and host species harms the host so that it manifests signs and symptoms, the symbiotic relationship is one of *parasitism* and the result is infectious disease. These relationships are shown as part of a biological continuum or spectrum in Figure 2–4.

Last, *infestation* is a more loosely applied term that is limited to superficial invasions of a host's skin or haircoat by ectoparasites. It also applies to instances when inanimate objects harbor these and other "vermin," e.g., when an animal's blanket or bedding straw is infested with mites or a barn is infested with rats.

Infection: Conflict or harmony?

Most students of infectious diseases have likened this process within individual animals, as well as that between populations of parasites and populations of hosts, to a struggle or conflict between two opposing forces. Such commonly used terms and expressions as

invading agents and *mobilization* of body *defenses*, the designation of veterinarians and physicians as disease *fighters*, and their efforts as directed toward the *conquest* of disease also suggest the military nature of this conflict. In fact, the American veterinarian, Maurice C. Hall, wrote a book on disease control[5] in 1936, and expressly described the processes of disease and the possibilities for disease control in terms of military strategy and tactics.

After remarking that laboratory workers generally lack "the basic knowledge of topography, climatology, farm practice and other things essential in translating laboratory findings into control measures" and suggesting similar deficiencies among hospital-oriented clinicians, Hall advocated training a distinct group of disease fighters who "could employ to advantage the principles developed by men of military genius in *making an estimate of a situation and [applying] the strategical and tactical principles of warfare* to the resolution of the problem [of disease]" (italics ours). What Hall was calling for, if not by name, was a force of *epidemiologists* who (1) could carry out and interpret diagnostic intelligence programs of surveillance and intensive follow-up and (2) could use these tools and this knowledge to select and support appropriate strategies of directed action. The value of these analogies of disease and disease control to conflict and survival is beyond dispute.

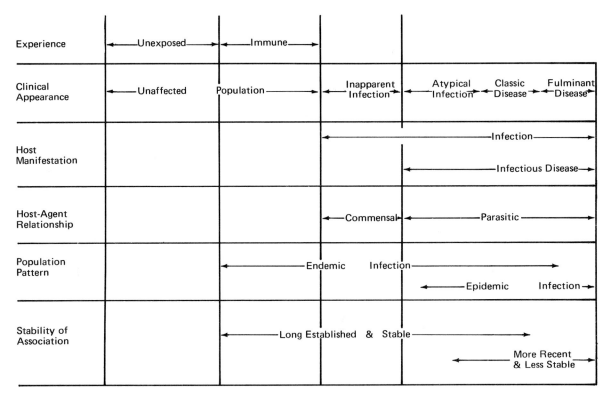

Fig. 2–4. Biological continuum of herd infections (redrawn from Schwabe, C.W. 1969. *Veterinary Medicine and Human Health*, 2nd ed. The Williams & Wilkins Co., Baltimore).

Despite this predisposition of clinicians, pathologists, and epidemiologists to adopt a warlike attitude, René Dubos,[6] among others, has pointed out that the evolutionary process in infections actually suggests that peaceful coexistence or "commensalism . . . [rather than conflict] should be regarded as the normal expression of interrelationships between the microbial world and other living things." He stressed the frequency with which infection occurs in the absence of disease and the further belief "that among men and animals the ability to prevent microbial agents from expressing their pathogenicity is much more common than the ability to ward off infection." Without belittling the ability of particularly virulent agents to produce disease almost straightaway, Dubos noted that whether an inapparent infection becomes a disease is a function not so much of an organism's virulence (an *agent* factor) but of the immunologic state and constitution of the *host* and the conditioning or stress-provoking circumstances of its *environment*. This point of view is basically epidemiologic.

Epidemiologists generally believe that, at the population level, commensal relationships between particular infectious agents and their hosts evolve from frankly parasitic and often epidemic beginnings, but that selection for the less virulent population of agents and the more tolerant population of hosts results first in the evolution of endemic patterns of disease and, ultimately, endemic patterns of inapparent infection—or commensalism (see Fig. 2–4).[7] Dubos went on to suggest the little-explored possibility that ways (other than some forms of immunization) to accelerate these evolutionary processes to advantage might be discovered. This possibility is considered when discussing the genetics of disease resistance and the basis of herd immunity in Chapter 9.

Latent infections and carriers

In the common circumstance of infection without disease, such infections have been referred to as inapparent or subclinicial, and the host-parasite relationship as commensal. Two special conditions of inapparent infection in individual hosts should be recognized. The first of these is the *latent* infection.

The word latency carries the connotation of dormant or *potential*. Therefore, a latent infection is an inapparent infection of an individual animal that has the potential to develop signs and symptoms. The responsible triggering mechanism for manifest infectious activity is usually some altered host response, for example, an endocrine response to stress that, in turn, commonly reflects some environmental force to which the individual has been subjected. A common example is infection of the human or simian mouth with a herpes virus, an infection that manifests itself as cold sores or fever blisters or more severe disease only when the host-parasite balance is tipped by some

external factor. Certain usually silent parainfluenza virus infections in calves bear a similar relationship to occasionally manifest disease.

The second special case of inapparent infection is the *carrier* animal. As used epidemiologically, a carrier is the inapparently infected individual which is also a transmitter (or potential transmitter) of the infectious agent. The so-called *healthy* or true carrier is an individual in which the infection remains inapparent during its entire course and never manifests itself. In contrast, the *incubatory* carrier is an individual that is capable of transmitting an infectious agent while it is still in the incubatory stage of an infection that will manifest itself clinically. Last, a *convalescent* carrier is an individual that continues to shed infectious organisms after the signs and symptoms of disease have disappeared and a clinical recovery has taken place. The existence of these silent carrier animals immeasurably complicates many surveillance and control efforts against infections.

A final subject of epidemiologic importance in considering infections in populations is that of the linkages or connections between the infected individuals and the susceptible individuals in a population, that is, the mechanisms for transmission of infectious agents.

Transmission of infections

A *transmissible* or *communicable* infection is one that can be passed from infected animals to other susceptible animals. Transmission of infection can be accomplished by *contact* between animals, or through contamination of inanimate *vehicles* (such as water or food) by infectious secretions and excretions, or through the intermediary of an invertebrate animal *vector*.[8] The epidemiological patterns and the approaches to control of these three groups of communicable infections are quite different.

Another common, but less-used term, *contagious*, also means transmissible but connotes transmission only as the result of an intimate association or contact with infected animals or their excretions or secretions. More information about these respective modes of transmission appears in Chapters 3 and 4.

Other epidemiologically useful terms are applied to transmission of infections. *Horizontal* transmission means transmission of an infectious agent between contemporaries, or animals of more or less the same generation. *Vertical* transmission, on the other hand, means transmission from infected animals of one generation to animals of the succeeding generation, sometimes transovarially, *in utero* or with colostrum.

APPLICATION OF SOME BASIC POPULATION CONCEPTS

The following situation is the first of several problems which test the ability to apply some of the epidemiological concepts and methods discussed.

Problem 1. Consultation in a dairy herd

Suppose you are an extension veterinarian called for consultation by a local practitioner. A disease characterized by high fever, pulmonary and pleural effusion, anuria, and rapid death occurred on R. and L. Dairy Farm beginning June 2, 1967. This farm consists almost entirely of cleared improved pasture and abuts on a state forest. The animals are all purebred Jerseys or Brown Swiss. Cows being milked are housed in Barn A. Dry cows also are kept in one section of Barn A but a few days before calving are transferred to Barn B, located on another part of the farm. One day after calving, the fresh cows are moved back to Barn A and the calves kept in pens in Barn B for about one month. Older calves are kept in Barn C at some distance from both of these buildings. Animals from Barns A and C are pastured separately. Other data on the herd and this disease episode are given in Table 2–3.

You learn that two other herds in the county were also affected. This county includes a portion of a forested state park. To your knowledge, no other cases of a similar disease have occurred recently in the state or elsewhere. However, you and local veterinarians note the similarity between this disease on these three farms and several other occurrences of disease in this same county in the summer of 1959. At that time several R. and L. calves (N4378, N4380, and N4382) were sick but they recovered. No agent was isolated from the 1959 outbreaks and the condition was undiagnosed. Insofar as is known, this disease has *never* been seen anywhere apart from these two occurrences in cattle in your county. The springs and summers of both 1959 and 1967 were unusually dry.

UNCOVER AND ANSWER ONE QUESTION AT A TIME

(1) Plot an epidemic curve for the occurrence of this disease on R. and L. Farm, beginning June 2.

(2) Would you describe the pattern of occurrence of this disease as sporadic, endemic, or epidemic? Could you characterize it further?

(3) Describe the population at risk.

(4) What was the attack rate in Barn A for the week of June 8 through June 14? For the week of June 15 through 21? Although, for outbreak investigations, attack rates are usually calculated rather than incidence rates, what were the incidence rates for these same periods? Write formulas and show your calculations.[9]

(5) What was the prevalence of illness in Barn A at the end of June 18? Write the formula and show your calculations.[10]

(6) Do you think this disease was infectious? Why?

(7) If so, what was the possible incubation period?

(8) Why did no cases appear in Barn A between June 23 and August 24?

(9) If this disease is an infection, what is its probable mode of transmission? Why?

(10) How did it originate in this county? In this herd?

(11) Attempt to explain the three recoveries and the unaffected animals in Barn A.

(12) Suggest explanations for the cases on August 15, August 24, and August 26.

(13) If this disease is an infection, is it being transmitted vertically?

(14) The examination of what host associations, if any, might be relevant in attempting to explain the epidemiology of this disease? How do you think you might examine your hypothesized host associations retrospectively using June's data? Be specific but do not make any actual calculations.

(15) The responsible virus was isolated during a similar outbreak on another farm on September 24, 1967. How do you think you might design an experimental prospective study to test further or prove a host factor association that you may have hypothesized in this outbreak?

(16) A serological test for this infection was developed in 1968. Would you be interested in making epidemiological use of it and/or of the virus isolation procedure? How? Explain fully.

Table 2–3.   Chronology of Unknown Disease on R. and L. Dairy Farm (Problem 1)

Cow no.	Breed	Age (yrs.)	Date animal added to herd	Date of onset of symptoms	Date animal died
Barn A (milking cows and dry cows)					
A15674	Jersey	3	May 30, 1967	June 2, 1967	June 6, 1967
R325	Jersey	4	Oct. 2, 1965	June 14, 1967	June 18, 1967
D1754	Jersey	8	Dec. 4, 1963	June 14, 1967	June 19, 1967
R758	Jersey	5	Jan. 18, 1964	June 14, 1967	June 18, 1967
C175	Jersey	4	Apr. 4, 1967	June 15, 1967	June 18, 1967
Z1926	Jersey	5	May 30, 1967	June 16, 1967	June 19, 1967
B328	Jersey	7	Apr. 22, 1960	June 16, 1967	June 19, 1967
12C35	Brown Swiss	3	Nov. 22, 1966	June 22, 1967	Recovered
R478	Jersey	3	Jan. 3, 1967	June 22, 1967	June 25, 1967
?	Jersey	Ca. 9	Unknown	June 22, 1967	Recovered
M1572	Jersey	8	Aug. 22, 1960	June 23, 1967	June 26, 1967
B1320*	Brown Swiss	9	Sept. 15, 1960	June 23, 1967	Recovered
A3257	Jersey	4	Nov. 4, 1966	June 23, 1967	June 26, 1967
D591	Jersey	3	Apr. 4, 1967	June 23, 1967	June 27, 1967
10C59	Brown Swiss	3	Jan. 18, 1965	Not affected	—
B7624	Brown Swiss	3	Jan. 18, 1965	Not affected	—
N4378	Jersey	8	Aug. 12, 1959	Not affected	—
8D142	Brown Swiss	7	Aug. 22, 1960	Not affected	—
?	Brown Swiss	Ca. 5	Unknown	Not affected	—
N4382†	Jersey	8	Aug. 12, 1959	Not affected	—
7F82	Brown Swiss	5	Dec. 4, 1963	Not affected	—
42C891	Brown Swiss	9	Mar. 15, 1962	Not affected	—
C358	Jersey	5	Aug. 6, 1967	Aug. 24, 1967	Aug. 28, 1967
C359	Jersey	4	Aug. 6, 1967	Aug. 26, 1967	Aug. 29, 1967
Barn B (calving and calf raising barn; springer cows, dams and young calves)					
Z1581††	Jersey	6	July 30, 1967	Aug. 15, 1967	Aug. 19, 1967
Calf of Z1581	Jersey	<1	Aug. 2, 1967 (born)	Aug. 15, 1967	Recovered
Calf of B1320	Brown Swiss	<1	Aug. 3, 1967 (born)	Not affected	—
Calf of N4382	Jersey	<1	July 6, 1967 (born)	Aug. 16, 1967	Recovered

Barn C (older calves)

No cases

---

*B1320 was moved to Barn B on August 1, calved normally on August 3, 1967, and was transferred back to Barn A on August 4th.

†N4382 was moved to Barn B on July 1, calved normally on July 6, 1967, and was transferred back to Barn A on July 7th.

††Z1581 was bought on July 30th and placed in Barn B. She calved on August 2. This cow was kept in Barn B because she had developed severe diarrhea on August 1 and was being kept off the milking line during treatment.

Part 2

BASIC CONCEPTS AND METHODS

"Here's good advice for practice:
go into partnership with nature;
she does more than half the work
and asks none of the fee."
MARTIN H. FISCHER

Chapter 3

MEDICAL DETECTION APPROACH

MEDICAL detective work is an inherently exciting activity.[1] It involves going out into the *field* to seek clues about disease events and then following through to orderly conclusions. Medical detection was the original "school" of epidemiology, but its significant development occurred primarily in the last century when clinicians and pathologists were first called upon to set up government veterinary services and local health departments. As they began to follow up cases of diseases in animals and man in the field, they evolved methods to investigate contacts and outbreaks and to carry out systematic case-finding surveys.

That this school of epidemiology is a *field*-based activity is evident from the colloquial expressions associated with it. Thus, the mass case-finding technique, which developed early in veterinary services and has figured prominently in most successful disease control and eradication programs since, was familiarly dubbed "down the road" testing. Furthermore, just as detectives of all types bear such sobriquets as "gumshoe" and "flatfoot," this medical detection approach came to be known as "shoe-leather" epidemiology.

Shoe-leather epidemiology has been applied mostly to the investigation of outbreaks of infections transmitted either by contact or by vehicles and to the control of these rather straightforward types of diseases. This basic kind of field epidemiology still provides the grist for the day-to-day lives of many veterinarians and physicians involved in public health or livestock disease control work.

This school of epidemiology has also figured prominently, if empirically, in the private practice of food-animal veterinary medicine. As a consequence, it is not hard to find experienced veterinary practitioners who feel that epidemiology is really nothing new or is in no way different from what most of them already know how to do and, in fact, do. They are correct, although relatively few private or public veterinary practitioners make use of anything like the full range of epidemiological tools available to them.

TRANSMISSION OF INFECTIONS BY CONTACT AND BY VEHICLES

Practitioners of the medical detection school of epidemiology have been concerned largely with infectious diseases transmitted by *contact* between animals or through the medium of contaminated *vehicles*. Contact transmission includes:

(1) Direct contact, that is, physical contact between animals, as in venereally or other touch-transmitted infections.

(2) Indirect contact, that is, contact with the fresh feces, urine, saliva, or fetal membranes of infected animals, including contact with objects such as bits, drinking bowls, or instruments very *recently* contaminated by often still-visible secretions or excretions of an infected animal.

(3) Droplets, for example, those sprayed from the mouth or nose of a coughing, sneezing, or bellowing animal directly onto the mucous membranes of the nose or mouth or the conjunctivae of another animal. These droplets are large infectious particles that are propelled only short distances.

(4) Droplet nuclei, that is, via an aerosol of the dry residua of droplets from an infected host. These small particles can travel considerable distances through the air (Table 3–1).

Vehicle transmission, on the other hand, is the passage of infectious agents between animals through the medium of inanimate substances such as feed and food; water; generated aerosols (e.g., those produced in the hosing-down of barns, slaughterhouses, and rendering plants); dust; soil; fomites such as blankets, bits, harnesses, or instruments; or through serums, whole stored blood, plasma, or other biologicals. The time interval for fomite transport is longer than for indirect contact; that is, the fomite vehicle is not usually visibly contaminated with *fresh* saliva, pus, or other infectious material.

Alternatively, some epidemiologists prefer to group these different forms of transmission as: (1) *direct*, only by direct or indirect contact or droplets; (2)

Table 3–1. Comparison of Dust, Droplets, and Droplet Nuclei in Disease Transmission (from Wells, W.F. 1955, Airborne Contagion and Air Hygiene. The Commonwealth Fund and Harvard University Press, Cambridge).

	Dust	Droplets	Droplet nuclei
Mode of transmission	Vehicle	Contact	Contact
Sources of material	Solid matter, fabrics, etc.	Fluids from nose and throat	Solid residues of evaporated droplets
Production	Attrition	Atomization of fluids	Evaporation of droplets
Mode of suspension	Air wafted	Projected into air by sneezing, etc.	Caught in air by evaporation
Particle diameter	10–100 μ	$>100\,\mu$	2–10 μ
Settling velocity	1 ft./min. to 1 ft./sec.	>1 ft./sec.	<1 ft./min.
Time of suspension	Limited by settling velocity	<3 sec.	Limited indoors by ventilation
Flight range	Hovers in clouds	Immediate in space	Dispersed throughout confined atmospheres
Concentration	Locally high	Immediately intense	Dispersed throughout confined atmospheres
Types of organisms	Most saprophytic	Parasitic and pathogenic	Parasitic and pathogenic
No./cu. ft.	Normally <100	Indeterminate	Normally below 1
Inhalation	Trapped in nose and throat	Indeterminate	Penetrate to lung
Mode of infection	Endemic infection of nose and throat	Contact infection	Epidemic contagion
Pattern of infection	Static	Indeterminate	Dynamic
Vulnerability	Resistant	Indeterminate	Vulnerable to chemical and physical agents
Removal	Filtration and electrostatic precipitation	Best by face mask	Electrostatic precipitation
Control	Air cleanliness, oiling, etc.	"Spacing out"	Sanitary ventilation (air change and equivalent air disinfection)

airborne, by droplet nuclei, generated aerosols, and dust; and (3) *vehicle-borne*, as described in the preceding paragraph, but excluding dust and aerosols.

In either case, vehicle transmission represents several epidemiologically different possibilities:

(1) Mechanical transmission (as in indirect contact)—the infectious organism does not multiply in or on the vehicle, but merely survives the transmission interval, as do leptospires in water.

(2) Propagative transmission—the organism undergoes multiplication in the vehicle, as do staphylococci in milk.

(3) Developmental transmission—the organism undergoes a necessary period of development in or on the vehicle, as do many nematode eggs and larvae in soil.

(4) Cyclopropagative transmission—both multiplication *and* development of the organisms occur in or on the vehicle. Examples are in the transmission of *Strongyloides* spp. and certain mycotic organisms.

Concepts about vehicle-borne and contact infections

Vehicle-borne infections often occur explosively in a population through the simultaneous exposure of numbers of animals to a *common source* of infection (i.e., the vehicle). The epidemic curve for such a "point" or common source epidemic is characteristic (see Figs. 2–1C and 6–1).

For an infection transmitted by direct contact, droplets, and droplet nuclei, a measure of its communicability within a restricted population or herd is its *secondary attack rate* (S.A.R.). This rate, useful in outbreak studies, is expressed as follows:

$$\text{S.A.R.} = \frac{\text{No. cases in an outbreak minus the primary (index) case(s)}}{\text{Total no. susceptible animals minus the primary case(s)}}$$

DIAGNOSTIC METHODS OF SHOE-LEATHER EPIDEMIOLOGY

Two useful diagnostic methods developed by practitioners of shoe-leather epidemiology are intensive follow-up and epidemiological surveillance (mentioned briefly in Chapter 1).

Intensive follow-up

Certainly the most common application of the medical detection approach in veterinary medicine is in the diagnosis of a herd illness, or *outbreak*, on the farm. Here, the veterinarian may be concerned with describing the outbreak and its causes, including traceback of the primary case; that is, he tries to establish the origin of the first sick animal in the herd or possible linkages between several sick animals in different herds, e.g., a common sales yard. Perhaps he can trace back an affected lot of animals from the slaughterhouse to the farm, or the movement of affected animals from one farm to another. All these events may relate to protection of the remainder of the herd, or other herds or populations. Each is a common situation for an intensive *follow-up*.

Similarly, intensive follow-up is necessary when pursuing reports of possible introductions into a country of an exotic infection such as with foot-and-mouth disease virus, or of a new vector of disease, such as some African tick. The U.S. Department of Agriculture veterinary services have specially trained teams for this type of intensive follow-up.

Other situations for intensive follow-up are the problem herds which are sometimes disclosed in the final stages of a disease eradication effort. In the bovine tuberculosis eradication program in the United States, for instance, one large problem herd in California was continually being infected with the tubercle bacillus from a mixed feral swine and European wild boar population on the same ranch. In other problem herds, nontuberculous cattle have been shown to react to the tuberculin test as a result of their sensitization to locally occurring species of soil mycobacteria.

Intensive follow-up is also required in approaching the control of epidemiologically complex multicausal disease problems on a farm unit basis. These types of disease problems are certain to gain increasing importance in the future and to demand high control priorities. They include bovine mastitis, "shipping fever" and similar stress-related disease complexes, neonatal loss problems, reproductive inefficiencies, multiple parasitisms, diseases with genetic components, many metabolic diseases, and those many disease syndromes in which opportunistic pathogens or malnutrition may play ill-defined parts.

Usually required both in the problem herd situation and with the latter type of multicausal disease problems are systematic observations leading to the formulation of hypotheses about possible causes, the conduct of appropriate retrospective studies, and/or the design of a series of prospective field studies for positively identifying specific determinants and their effects upon the frequency of the disease, the frequency of an immunodiagnostic test result, or the frequency of other events.

Besides personal observations, outbreak investigations (and other epidemiological studies) often depend heavily on interviews and questionnaires. Since unusable answers are a common feature of questionnaire surveys, specific attention to this form of data collection is desirable.

INTERVIEWS AND QUESTIONNAIRES.[2] Design of a questionnaire or interview form requires care, first in determining the nature of the information sought and then in deciding on the specific questions that will elicit that information. Whether a questionnaire is to be sent by mail or used as a checklist during a personal or telephone interview, questions should be simple, straightforward, and precise. Questions should be interpretable in only one way. For example, when a farmer is simply asked for the total number of cattle on his farm, he might answer 40 when there were actually 70, because 20 of the animals did not belong to him and the remaining 10 were on a piece of land he had leased to a neighbor. In personal interviews, such ambiguities can be corrected; but in mail questionnaires, they may become major sources of errors. For such reasons, it is essential to pretest a questionnaire by having several persons in the target population answer it, and then rephrase any questions that may be unclear.

If a questionnaire becomes lengthy, it may be better to construct two questionnaires. The more detailed one should contain questions addressed only to a sample of the total persons interviewed. The shorter one, containing the most essential questions, would be addressed to all persons interviewed.

The following are guidelines for devising questionnaires for use in mail, telephone, or personal interviews. General contents should include:

(1) Title of the project.

(2) Name and address of the interviewee and date of interview.

(3) Brief explanation of the project (may be on a separate sheet).

(4) Assurance to the interviewee of the degree of confidentiality.

(5) Indication of beneficial results to the interviewee, e.g., what information might be expected

from the study and what feedback the interviewee will receive.

(6) Explanation of the format of the questionnaire, the interpretation of questions, and the format of the answers.

(7) Space for personal comments by the interviewee.

In designing the questionnaire *per se*, the following should be considered:

(1) Means of communication (mail, telephone, or personal interview).

(2) Type of investigation, e.g., hypothesis testing or formulation.

(3) Objective of study, e.g., opinion or precise facts.

(4) Subsequent analysis required. For example, if a statistical analysis is considered, data should be of the numerical type, or categorical data should be expressed as numbers (see Chapter 5). If the data are to be analyzed by computer, the questionnaire should have spaces for coding answers.

(5) Time available (to the interviewer for carrying out the project, and to the interviewee for answering the questions). For example, at certain times it may be easier to obtain the interviewee's cooperation than at others.

(6) Cost of the interview (usually personal interview > telephone interview > mail interview).

As to the questions themselves, they should be simple, clear, precise, and comprehensive. Open-ended questions should be avoided if possible. Commonly used questions are:

(1) Enumerative questions, which can be answered with a number or by a check (√) in a category:

Number of horses	8			
or				
Number of horses	0 1-5 6-10 11-15 >15			
	√			

(2) Yes-no type questions, which should provide space for "I don't know" and "not applicable" answers. This practice will help to avoid the possibility of nonresponses. It is important to insist on the necessity of answering all questions.

(3) Narrative (subjective) questions.

Some questions may be included to cross check particularly important information. These apparently different questions relate to the same thing so that the interviewer can check on information given by the interviewee. For example, in census interviews, these questions might be "How old are you?" and later "What is your birth date?"

Additional considerations in interviewing and submitting questionnaires include the desirability of choosing interviewees at random, the consideration of comparison groups wherever appropriate, and the possibility of sending questionnaires to interviewees before a personal visit to give them a chance to think about the subject.

Other forms of data collection during an intensive epidemiological follow-up study should be similarly systematic and detailed, and should reflect equal forethought and design. As mentioned, the commonest form of intensive follow-up, and one of the most routine program activities in public veterinary practice and in some of the newer forms of population-based private veterinary practices, is the *outbreak investigation*.

OUTBREAK INVESTIGATION. Outbreak investigations are often carried out in response to dramatic disease events such as an acute infectious disease or an intoxication. Food poisoning is a typical subject of outbreak investigation, and public health epidemiologists have developed standard procedures for this purpose.[3] The purpose of outbreak investigations is to find out what is going on, generally in order to be able to take corrective action. The methods applied in outbreak investigations are basically the same as those used in other forms of intensive follow-up.

(1) Clinical and pathologic work-up or verification of diagnosis. Clinical and necropsy findings are reviewed to arrive at a clinical diagnosis or possible diagnoses and to offer guidance in specimen collection for laboratory testing (see Table 1–1).

(2) Descriptive epidemiologic work-up. The objectives of the study are clearly formulated. All possible variables of interest are identified. For example, information available with respect to affected and unaffected individuals (and herds) is surveyed; and data about place (environment) and time of disease onset are recorded, appropriately reduced, and displayed. Tentative hypotheses to explain causes, source of agent, distribution of cases, or other unknowns may be formulated at this stage.

Additional information needed is determined on the basis of this preliminary evidence; and other possible sources of data are identified, as required. Conduct of the common-source outbreak type of investigation illustrated next (see Disease Outbreak on a Mink Ranch) is based mainly on personal observation, on interviews with persons who have been in a position to make observations pertinent to the outbreak, and on existing records. Other types of data collected may include weather conditions, treatments, or population characteristics. Samples are taken for laboratory examination, if deemed necessary. Hypothesis refinement continues.

(3) Analysis and interpretation of data. The data from these field investigations (and, if already available, the laboratory examinations) are collected and assembled in tables, maps, and graphs. The initial hypotheses are then subjected to a visual analysis and, if necessary, to statistical tests. If an hypothesis is rejected, another hypothesis must be developed. For this purpose, it might be necessary to gather additional information. This process of hypothesis formu-

lation and testing is cyclic. Broad hypotheses may be developed first, and some of them accepted or rejected concomitantly with the formation of new ones as the investigation and examination proceed. This method can be described as one of successive approximations.

(4) Reporting of results and implementation of control measures. The completing steps in an outbreak investigation usually are to implement appropriate control measures or other objectives of the study and to compile the type of report required.

The following example illustrates a typical outbreak investigation.

Disease outbreak on a mink ranch.[4] The mink ranch of an Agricultural Experiment Station housed approximately 5000 mink. On Sunday, July 13, about 300 mink were found dead and many more were sick. By Monday, about 500 more animals had died. Unfortunately, the consulting veterinarian was not called in until Wednesday morning. His previous records showed that the *usual* level of combined morbidity and mortality among mink on this ranch during this phase of their producing season was 0.9% per week.

These mink were all housed in one large building, divided into sections by movable walls. March was the breeding season. Kits were born in May and were weaned at about eight weeks of age. July, therefore, was a critical month because there were several categories of mink to be cared for: (1) lactating females with suckling kits; (2) females with kits on starting ration, (3) growing kits, (4) dry females, and (5) males (Table 3–2).

The diet of these mink consisted mainly of meat, fish, cereals, and fat, supplemented with powdered milk, bone meal, vitamins, and minerals. They were fed once a day except on weekends, when they were fed on Saturday afternoon only. Protein feeds (raw meat or fish) usually made up 40 to 60% of the mink's diet. At the time of the disease outbreak, a feed trial was being conducted to determine the least expensive source of protein feed. As part of this feed trial, a separate ration was prepared for each of the five categories of mink. Three categories were divided into three experimental groups each (see Table 3–2). The protein part of the ration for each of these groups came from a different source, the rest of the ration being the same for that category. Table 3–3 shows the composition of the various rations being fed in July.

The protein fraction of these rations (except the supplements) was usually frozen fish or meat. Liver was obtained in plastic bags and frozen. After thawing for a day at room temperature, these items were weighed, ground, and mixed with the other ingredients of the ration. The protein supplement, dried blood, bone meal, and vitamin-mineral mix were supplied in various forms (pellets, granules, powder) in 50-pound sacks. Oats, wheat, corn, bread, and skim milk were supplied in sacks of 50 pounds. The fat was received in barrels of various sizes and stored in a refrigerator. The rations for each category of mink were prepared separately. First, the ingredients that occurred in equal amounts for all three groups in one category were mixed. One-third of this mix was then mixed with the appropriate amount of frozen feed.

By Wednesday, July 16, 1096 of a total of 4907 mink had died, and 862 others were sick (Table 3–4). The signs displayed were: group 1, starvation (kits); group 2, dehydration (females) and starvation (kits); group 3, bite injuries (kits); group 4, starvation (kits); groups, 5, 6, 7, 8, and 9, squinting of the eyes, paralysis of front and/or hind limbs, dyspnea, and coma-prostration. Necropsy did not reveal any lesions.

In this outbreak, only *groups* of animals could be considered with respect to time of onset. It was observed that mink in groups 6 and 7 had been the first ones to become ill (Sunday). Peak mortality occurred on Monday morning among mink in groups 6, 7, and 9 and later in groups 5 and 8. After Wednesday, very few mink died.

From these observations and information, it was possible to determine: (1) the most commonly occurring signs, (2) an approximate incubation period, and (3) feed items fed to each group of mink. The most common signs tabulated were paralysis and dyspnea, followed by pallor of mucous membranes, squinting of eyes, starvation and trauma in kits, and dehydration (in one lactating female). These findings suggested botulism. As the illness occurred very suddenly, the outbreak was believed to have a common source, the nature of the disease suggesting some feedstuff. To obtain information on which feed item was associated with this outbreak, the veter-

Table 3–2.   Distribution of Mink by Age and Sex in 11 Experimental Groups, July 12.

Group no.	Females and suckling kits			Females and starting kits			Growing kits			Dry females	Males
	1	2	3	4	5	6	7	8	9	10	11
No. adults	100	100	100	100	100	100				300	220
No. kits	430	415	438	428	414	415	418	420	409		

Table 3–3.   Composition of July Ration (in Percentage of Feed Items in Ration) for the 11 Groups of Mink.

Feed item	1	2	3	4	5	6	7	8	9	10	11
Fish										62	62
Fish and protein supplement	47			52			55				
Fish and red meat		47			52			55			
Red meat			47			52			55		
Liver	10	10	10	5	5	5	5	5	5	5	
Cereals	16	16	16	14	14	14	10	10	10	12	17
Blood and bone meal	4	4	4	6	6	6	5	5	5		
Horse fat				10	10	10					
Fish fat	22	22	22				10	10	10	20	20
Vegetable fat				12	12	12	14	14	14		
Vitamins and minerals	1	1	1	1	1	1	1	1	1	1	1
Total	100	100	100	100	100	100	100	100	100	100	100

inarian resorted to the following fairly standard methods for common source outbreak investigations.

(1) Compilation of an attack rate table

The attack rate (A.R.) is more or less the same as an incidence rate, the time being the short period during which mink affected by the outbreak got sick, and the denominator being the population at risk at the onset of the outbreak. The data so expressed for mink that did eat and those that did *not* eat each feedstuff are shown in Table 3–5. Thus, the 3445 mink that ate fish were at risk with respect to this feed item. Of these, 1214 got sick; therefore, the attack rate was 35.2%.

Table 3–5 shows that the attack rate was highest for mink that ate vegetable fat, and suggests the possibility that that item was the cause. The rate was also high for red meat and horse fat. The lowest attack rate was found in mink that did not eat liver. This finding, in turn, would suggest this item as the possible culprit. This difference indicates the importance of constructing an attack rate table for both the animals that were exposed to each possible determinant (i.e., feed item) *and* those that were not.

The risks associated with eating vegetable fat, liver, or other feeds can be derived from fourfold tables (Table 3–6). The χ^2 test can be used to calculate the likelihood that the difference in attack rates between mink that ate and did not eat vegetable fat, or liver, could have happened by chance. For example, in analysis of the data in Table 3–6 by the χ^2 test,

$$\chi^2 = \frac{[(41)(887)-(1917)(2062)]^2(4907)}{(1958)(2949)(2804)(2103)}$$

= 2,211 > 12.12; that is, a difference of this magnitude (68.4% vs. 1.9%) could have occurred by chance less than once in 2000 times.

(2) Further observations on the lowest attack rates, the background levels of illness, and the actual numbers of animals involved

This step is important because careful inspection of the data may obviate a time-consuming analysis of

Table 3–4.   Health Status of Mink in the 11 Experimental Groups on Morning of July 16.

Group No.	1	2	3	4	5	6	7	8	9	10	11
No. well	526	509	535	520	48	40	43	93	143	274	218
No. sick	3	4	3	8	360	165	30	220	46	22	1
No. dead	1	2	0	0	106	310	345	107	220	4	1
Total	530	515	538	528	514	515	418	420	409	300	220

Table 3–5.   Attack Rates (A.R.) for Feed Items in Outbreak of Disease in Mink.

Feed item	Mink eating feed				Mink not eating feed			
	Total	Sick & dead	Well	A.R.(%)	Total	Sick & dead	Well	A.R.(%)
Fish	3445	1214	2231	35.2	1462	744	718	50.9
Protein supplement	1476	387	1089	26.2	3431	1571	1860	45.8
Red meat	2911	1543	1368	53.0	1996	415	1581	20.8
Liver	4687	1956	2731	41.7	220	2	218	0.9
Cereals	4907	1958	2949	39.9	0			
Blood and bone meal	4387	1930	2457	44.0	520	28	492	5.4
Horse fat	1557	949	608	61.0	3350	1009	2341	30.1
Fish fat	3350	1009	2341	30.1	1557	949	608	60.9
Vegetable fat	2804	1917	887	68.4	2103	41	2062	1.9
Vitamins and minerals	4907	1958	2949	39.9	0			

the data, a process that could even produce misleading conclusions.

The lowest attack rates among those mink that did not eat particular feed items are indicators of a possible source of poisoning. In this example, the liver, the vegetable fat, and the dry blood-bone meal would be likely candidates, the most likely one being the liver. Only two mink not eating liver got sick or died. For those not eating vegetable fat, however, 41 animals were sick or died. As pointed out, the expected level of sickness and death on this ranch was about 0.9% per week. Observe that the attack rate for mink *not* eating liver is the same as this expected level. The attack rate for those mink not eating vegetable fat is twice the expected level. This fact suggests liver as the feed item to incriminate. It can be interpreted as follows: If liver is removed from the mix, the attack rate should be back to expected levels. This corrective action is exactly what was recommended at this point in the investigation. Morbidity and mortality then subsided to expected levels.

For feed items liver, cereals, blood and bone meal, vegetable fat, and vitamins and minerals, the actual numbers sick or dead account for all or almost all of the animals that became sick or died in the outbreak.

(3) Greatest difference

At times the difference between the attack rates among those that ate and those that did not eat different items is considered. The items with the largest differences are usually the ones to be incriminated as the cause of the outbreak. The largest differences were found for vegetable fat, liver, and dried blood-bone meal. If the factor considered *is* a causal one, this difference is called the *attributable risk*. In this example, however, vegetable fat *appears* to be a likely determinant *because its feeding is related to the feeding of liver*. As a result, feeding vegetable fat was statistically associated with disease occurrence; however, the association was not causal. This problem is considered further in Chapter 11.

(4) Further inspection of data in light of possible circumstances

This classic method of investigation of common source outbreaks would almost invariably yield the answer quickly (1) if only one feed item were contaminated, and uniformly contaminated besides, and (2) if all susceptible animals ingesting that item became sick and those not eating that feed item remained well. By applying these standards to data in Tables 3–2 and 3–3, one can see that the distribution

Table 3–6.   Fourfold Table for Calculating Risk of Sickness among Mink Eating Vegetable Fat (Data from Table 3–5).

	Sick & dead	Well	Total
Ate vegetable fat	1917	887	2804
Did not eat vegetable fat	41	2062	2103
Total	1958	2949	4907

of vegetable fat among groups of mink better fits the distribution of sick mink than does the distribution of liver, since five out of six groups that ate fat experienced high mortality. This high mortality rate was not the case with any of the groups not eating fat. In the case of liver, many groups that ate this item experienced low morbidity and mortality.

However, pathogenic agents, whether micro-organisms, toxins, or other disease-producing sub-stances, are not always distributed uniformly in feed or food. Furthermore, not all animals may be susceptible to the same extent because of vaccination or natural variation in resistance, and not all of them necessarily receive the same dose of the pathogenic agent, either because they do not eat the same amount of a given feed item or because different batches of the same item were used in the preparation of the ration. This latter was the case in this outbreak, a fact confirmed finally by the laboratory studies.

Additional follow-up investigations, such as second-stage relative risk (outlined in Chapter 11) and laboratory methods, make it possible to obtain further evidence as to which possible determinants to incriminate; but even this basic type of epidemiologic outbreak investigation often permits corrective action to be taken with minimal time delay. As exemplified by the outbreak investigation, the medical detection route in epidemiology is mainly an observational and descriptive process leading in most instances to some form of analysis and to logical inferences, often statements of probability.

Surveillance

The shoe-leather school of epidemiology also gave birth to another quite different approach to medical detection, namely *surveillance*, at least in its data collection aspect. Surveillance is organized epidemiologic intelligence on a broad scale. In government agencies concerned with animal health or human health, this development initially had two disparate beginnings, one directly related and active and the other indirectly related and primarily passive.

When public health departments first came into existence in the last century, government or eccle-siastic registers of human births and, often, deaths already existed in some countries. It was soon realized that these vital statistics, based on the official *reporting* of events in peoples' lives, had medical value; and epidemiological studies based on them began in public health (as for example, in John Snow's study on cholera in London, recounted earlier). Thus, before the turn of this century, public health authorities, both medical and veterinary, were sensitized to the disease intelligence possibilities inherent in the official reporting of demographic information. This circumstance resulted in the designation of certain so-called scheduled or quaran-

tinable diseases, new cases of which were made legally reportable to public health departments. Thus began the reporting of morbidity incidence and the essentially passive acquisition by health departments of such incidence-type data about disease occurrence. Veterinarians who were commonly represented in local health departments during that early period utilized such data to justify and initiate programs directed against meat- and milk-borne diseases of man. Incidence-reporting mechanisms, which have both inherent strengths and weaknesses, are still the backbone of most public health disease surveillance programs.

This situation does not exist in livestock disease control agencies, however. In contrast, when the agriculturally based veterinary services were created in government, also in the 19th century, they lacked vital statistics for animals; and the circumstances of husbandry were, and largely still are, such that, except for specific well-confined and controlled populations of animals, they are impossible or difficult to obtain. In addition, most food-producing animals experience a truncated life cycle—ending, often at an early age, in the slaughterhouse.

Morbidity incidence reporting, therefore, seemed even less likely in veterinary medicine *per se* than birth or death reporting. Consequently, at the onset, veterinarians had to consider other approaches to the acquisition of population morbidity data for animals. For example, when Daniel Elmer Salmon established government veterinary services in the United States (the Bureau of Animal Industry (B.A.I.)), he did so to provide, in the words of the enabling legislation he drafted, the "means for the suppression and extirpation of . . . contagious diseases of domestic animals" from this country. Salmon thus formulated a bold concept of regional disease eradication and then proceeded to apply it immediately, and successfully, to the eradication of contagious bovine pleuro-pneumonia (bovine mycoplasma pneumonia) from the United States.

That first large-scale disease control program in this country was based on a shoe-leather effort that has been called "down the road" testing ever since. B.A.I. and state veterinarians actually set out to visit every farm in the affected areas of several states, to examine every cow, and to slaughter every affected animal. They succeeded; as a result, the two weapons of *prevalence survey* and regional disease eradication became established in the veterinary armamentarium. A similar approach in several European countries was directed against rinderpest in cattle.

Soon afterwards, Bernard Bang in Denmark demon-strated the diagnostic testing value of tuberculin in cattle. This discovery was followed immediately in Europe and the United States by the inauguration of large-scale, systematic, mass skin testing of cattle, that is, surveys of tuberculosis prevalence. Similar efforts were directed to other diseases. For example, dourine of horses was eradicated from the United States in 1916 when B.A.I. scientists succeeded in developing high-speed laboratory techniques for running very large numbers of complement fixation tests in a single day. Thus was born the technique of *seroepidemiology* and another demonstration of the value of this approach of mass testing or prevalence surveillance of disease.[5]

This *active* survey process was more directly the scientific precursor of the modern idea of overall epidemiological surveillance—as formulated in the U.S. Center for Disease Control by Alexander Langmuir during and after World War II—than was the more traditional public health approach of incidence reporting.

Thus, by different processes of evolution, incidence reporting became the basis of public health intelligence and prevalence surveillance the basis of veterinary intelligence for a long time. In both cases, the alternative approaches were considered either more difficult or less practicable.

One important facet of diagnostic surveillance may be illustrated by an on-going cattle disease prevalence monitoring program in the United States.

U.S. MARKET CATTLE IDENTIFICATION PROGRAM. Various means of livestock identification have been practiced for many years for the purpose of proving animal ownership. When organized programs for combatting livestock diseases such as brucellosis and tuberculosis were established, there was a strong need for a system that would make it possible to trace infected animals back to their herds of origin. This ability for backtracing animals varies among countries. In some countries, for example Denmark, where swine and other livestock are shipped directly to slaughter, mainly in cooperative slaughterhouses, the owner marks each animal so that backtracing is simple and rapid. The owner also is paid according to the health status of the animal he sends to slaughter; and this inducement improves cooperation in disease control programs.

In other countries, such as the United States, which have a more complicated market chain (Fig. 3–1), backtracing is much more difficult; and no reliable method existed until the development of the Market Cattle Testing Program, later renamed the Market Cattle Identification Program. Impetus for the Market Cattle Identification (M.C.I.) Program was the need for traceback of brucellosis reactors, but it has also been used for backtracing animals when tuberculosis-like lesions are found during meat inspection. The M.C.I. program began as a pilot program in the state of Washington in 1955; similar programs were introduced in Oregon and Montana in 1957, with the purpose of substituting a brucellosis sampling approach to beef cattle populations for "down the road" on-the-ranch brucellosis testing of all animals. The latter procedure was to be retained for dairy herds and for all cases in which infection was traced back to beef herds by the M.C.I. program or in which there proved to be insufficient surveillance of the

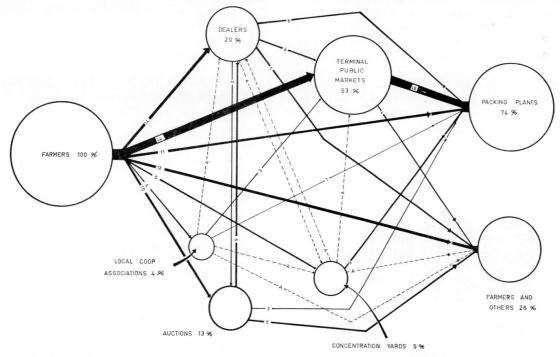

Fig. 3–1. Patterns of movement of cattle from farmer to market in the United States (redrawn after U.S. Department of Agriculture).

herd through M.C.I. slaughter-testing of culled animals.

The M.C.I. program relies on the participation of livestock sales establishments. Their personnel, directed by the brand inspectors, apply a federal-state backtag made of specially prepared paper (Fig. 3–2). This tag is fixed to the animal's back with a strong glue and will remain in place for more than a month if correctly applied. Each livestock sales establishment has an assigned backtag prefix that does not change. This backtag number and readable permanent markings (e.g., firebrands) are recorded on a brand inspection master sheet. All previously applied tags are removed, and their numbers are also recorded on this master sheet.

The types of animals eligible for backtagging differ from state to state. In California, usually only beef breeding animals two years of age and older are backtagged. This sample is not a random sample of the cattle population, but for the purpose of brucellosis surveillance it is desirable to obtain a biased sample. The animals covered by the M.C.I. program are probably good sentinel animals since they are culls, are older than the average, and have been in the herds for a considerable period of time. In the slaughterhouses, meat inspectors collect blood samples from backtagged animals. These samples are submitted to a central (state-federal) laboratory with the backtag attached to the tube, or else the tube number is recorded on an accompanying form. The laboratory report is forwarded to a central office, which then locates the herd of origin and the name of the owner, his addrèss, county, herd number, and other pertinent information. Computer systems are sometimes used not only to store and retrieve these data but also to print postcards giving each owner information about the outcome of the blood-testing.

Tracing of animals in the M.C.I. program can generally be completed within a week. However, errors do occur in the livestock sales establishments, in the slaughterhouses, or elsewhere; and backtracing is not always successful. There can be significant differences among livestock sales establishments and among slaughterhouses in the same area with respect to the percentage of infected herds that can be identified.

In spite of the difficulties encountered, there is no doubt that the M.C.I. program is a valuable tool for surveillance for bovine brucellosis and tuberculosis in the United States. This program also has potential use for epidemiological surveillance of other cattle diseases and has been used in recent years in a series of studies of anaplasmosis in California (referred to in Chapter 14). It could also be used for the study of other infectious and noninfectious conditions that can be monitored by analysis of blood, serum, or samples of organs; for example, the study of vitamin and mineral deficiencies, blood types, serum enzymes, and pollutants. In fact, systems like the M.C.I. could become the backbone for an overall animal disease surveillance program for the United States.[6]

METHODS FOR DIRECTED ACTION AGAINST DISEASE

Most successes in the *prevention, control,* or regional *eradication* of diseases have been achieved by practitioners of the medical detection approach to epidemiology. Thus, it is appropriate to compare these three general avenues of directed action and consider some of the specific methods that shoe-leather epidemiologists have developed.

Prevention of disease, in an epidemiological sense, means all measures to exclude disease from an unaffected population of animals. It usually includes (1) measures for the exclusion of an infectious organism from geographic areas in which it is now absent and (2) measures to protect a given population from diseases that already occur in its geographic area. The usual method for the former is *quarantine,* and for the latter *mass immunization, mass prophylactic treatment,* and *environmental control.* Education is a further and broadly applicable approach to disease prevention.

Disease *control,* on the other hand, is a term to describe all measures used to reduce the frequency of

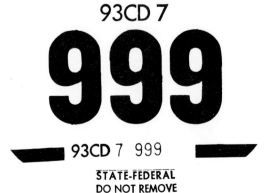

Fig. 3–2. Backtag used in the U.S. Market Cattle Identification Program (1/2 actual size).

illnesses already present in a population, by reducing or eliminating causes of illness, ultimately to levels of little or no consequence. Prevention and control programs usually represent continuing efforts.

Eradication of disease is a bolder concept of directed action in which the object is the extinction of a species of infectious microorganism. For several years, it was believed that this goal had been accomplished globally only in the special case of vesicular exanthema of swine (although that virus was preserved in the Plum Island Laboratory of the U.S. Department of Agriculture); now it is not certain whether even that has been the case.[7]

On the other hand, *regional* eradication of disease, a concept first developed by Daniel Elmer Salmon, has been accomplished a number of times in veterinary medicine by combinations of case-finding surveys, selective slaughter, herd depopulation, quarantine, mass immunization, mass treatment, environmental control, biological control, vector control, and education. Biological control, reservoir control, and vector control will be considered in the discussion of medical ecology in Chapter 4.

In addition to the idea of mass case-finding surveys and the much older approach of deliberately killing a sick minority of animals to protect a well majority,[8] veterinarians in the government services visualized, developed, and first successfully applied most of these specific methods for combatting diseases in populations. Subsequently, many of these methods for directed action were used to advantage by public health authorities as well. Among these several methods to combat herd disease, the oldest by far are selective slaughter and quarantine.

SELECTIVE SLAUGHTER. The deliberate killing of a minority of infected animals to protect the well majority has been a disease control measure employed in veterinary medicine for a long time. Its beginning probably coincides with the first vague recognition of contagion, the observation that animals appear to contract diseases from one another. Certainly, by Roman times veterinarians recognized contagion, and some individuals had speculated about the existence of microbes. Marcus Terentius Varro,[9] writing about animal husbandry in the 1st century B.C., said about swamps, "... there are bred certain minute creatures which cannot be seen by the eyes, which float in the air and enter the body through the mouth and nose and there cause serious diseases." Varro, like Virgil, then discussed the practice of slaughtering sick animals or animals exposed to such contagions in order to abort plagues before they could spread throughout the entire herd.

The selective slaughter of diseased animals or reactors to immunodiagnostic screening tests has featured prominently in many successful, modern, large-scale campaigns against animal diseases. In past instances, the costs involved in this seemingly drastic procedure have always been far outweighed by the monetary benefits realized. The limiting factors have been how great a percentage of animals would be involved initially, how temporarily disruptive such an approach would be to the economy, and whether replacement animals were available. Such considerations sometimes have suggested that a high frequency of disease first be reduced substantially by mass immunization or some other measure and then that the disease be stamped out by selective slaughter.

DEPOPULATION. When a diagnostic test cannot be applied to an affected population in order to carry out selective slaughter, when the population is inaccessible for other measures, when an infection is spreading in a population too rapidly to cope with it otherwise, or when no other approach works, complete depopulation of an affected restricted population may be the only available procedure to protect the species at large.

Thus, when foot-and-mouth disease became established in the deer population of the Stanislaus National Forest in California in 1924, there was no alternative but deer depopulation. Of 22,214 deer killed in that successful campaign, 2279 were found to have foot-and-mouth disease. On the other hand, needless depopulation of many wild animal species took place in parts of Africa early in this century in efforts to combat trypanosomiasis. With the advent of the precipitin test method for examining the blood meals of biting arthropod vectors and identifying the species of vertebrates on which they feed, it has been shown that some of the mammal species depopulated then did not normally serve as hosts of particular tsetse flies and therefore were not reservoir hosts of trypanosomes.

QUARANTINE. Quarantine is the physical separation of sick animals from healthy ones, or the placing of a restraint on the movements of exposed or infected animals or items that they may have contaminated. That quarantine was also commonly employed by Roman veterinarians is clear from the 1st century writings of Columella[10] and other authors. In referring to the introduction of a plague among cattle, Columella wrote that, "those which are infected [must be] segregated from the healthy, that no infected animal may come into contact with the rest and destroy them with the contagion." He further advised that "sheep whose breathing is asthmatic ... be transferred to other districts, a precaution which, in my opinion," he wrote, "ought to be taken in all diseases and plagues."

The term quarantine itself is of much later origin. It is derived from *quarantinas*, stations set up in the late Middle Ages in some Mediterranean seaports, where voyagers from plague-infested areas abroad were segregated for 40 days. The figure 40 was a purely arbitrary one, reflecting the biblical 40 days and 40 nights.

Quarantine is applied at the international level to prevent transmission of infections or vectors from one country to another. The veterinary services of the U.S. Department of Agriculture, for example, operate quarantine stations for this purpose at Clinton, New Jersey; Miami, Florida; and Honolulu, Hawaii. In the first 45 years of Britain's rabies quarantine, 23 animals developed symptoms of rabies while in quarantine; in the United States, *Brucella melitensis* infection, surra and exotic tick vectors of piroplasmosis and Nairobi sheep disease have been among the infections and infestations intercepted at quarantine stations. The Office International des Epizooties was established in Paris in 1924 to standardize veterinary quarantine procedures and regulations throughout the world. Quarantine also is applied interstate and locally in the United States. In one recent year alone, more than 367 violations of interstate quarantine regulations were detected in this country. Strict local quarantine is an established facet of most veterinary efforts directed against exotic infections and other instances of focal disease situations of an emergency nature.

MASS TREATMENT. With successful applications of mass disease detection techniques in veterinary medicine in the late 19th century, mass treatment was suggested as a way to combat diseases occurring at very high levels of prevalence because total depopulation of affected herds or the deliberate slaughter of individual affected animals or reactors was not feasible economically. The mass treatment approach to disease control depends upon the availability of safe and cheap therapeutic agents. Its first application on a large scale was against tick infestation of cattle in the U.S. South. This effort, in which all cattle in the affected population were dipped in an arsenic solution, was first successfully applied by Cooper Curtice in North Carolina in 1906. The same approach was then directed against scabies in sheep and other ectoparasitic infestations of livestock.

Subsequently, development of safe drugs for mass chemoprophylaxis has resulted in the routine medication of feeds, water, and salt. Thus, diseases such as psittacosis in caged birds have been combatted with antibiotic-treated feeds, coccidiosis in chickens by sulfonamides in drinking water, and gastrointestinal helminths in cattle by broad spectrum anthelmintics incorporated in salt licks.

MASS IMMUNIZATION. Mass immunization has been one of the most effective forms of directed action against diseases undertaken in veterinary medicine. Its successes have been numerous, but discussion of the principles involved and products available lies outside the subject area of this book. If anything, past veterinary research and disease control programs have focused too exclusively upon this attractive avenue of attack on diseases to the neglect of other potentially valuable approaches to infections and to the development of population approaches to important noninfectious diseases of animals.

Often the full potential of mass immunization in disease control is not realized because of widespread lay and professional misuse of veterinary vaccines in some countries (e.g., improper storage and administration of vaccines and lack of aseptic techniques) and sometimes because of inadequate potency and safety controls over vaccine manufacture and distribution. In addition, the public is generally overconfident about vaccines as a panacea to disease problems. A further point of growing concern is that use of certain live vaccines beyond a point of initial necessary disease reduction may in itself preclude the total elimination of a given infectious agent from a population or may seriously complicate surveillance and control monitoring programs based upon serologic testing.

Among the more interesting areas for future development of mass immunization as a disease control tool are methods for mass administration of vaccines that dispense with problems of needle hygiene (such as use of jet injection guns) or that eliminate the need to handle animals individually (e.g., stable vaccines incorporated in water or feed, and vaccines administered by the mucosal route as aerosols).

ENVIRONMENTAL CONTROL. Some of the first organized environmental control measures against disease were the provision of safe public water supplies and facilities for the removal and treatment of human sewage and other urban wastes. These efforts commenced in the 19th and early 20th centuries, and were largely contributions of engineers who were brought into the newly developing public health departments for those purposes.

Earlier, some European cities had begun to require that animal slaughter be confined to central abattoirs and, in the 1800s, meat inspection legislation was introduced generally. Veterinarians were recruited into newly created public health departments at that time; and men such as Robert von Ostertag laid the ground rules for the field of food protection in general. Before the turn of the century, veterinary and medical attention was also directed to the production and marketing of safe milk. The method for heat-treating wine, developed by the French chemist and microbiologist, Louis Pasteur, was applied to milk; and some of the first public health laboratories were established by physicians, veterinarians, and others, largely for the microbiological examination of milk, water, and meat. This active period in the development of major environmental controls against water-borne and food-borne infections of man is often called the "Great Sanitary Awakening."

Early environmental control advances in veterinary medicine *per se* included an approved sanitary regimen for production of certified milk, the standards of which were later modified for production of milk intended to be pasteurized. A similar advance was the proposal of the so-called McClean County System of Swine Sanitation by a B.A.I. scientist, B.H. Ransom, in the 1920s. This program involved environmental disinfection, sow disinfection, moveable farrowing houses, use of uncontaminated forage fields, and provision of clean water, nutritional supplementation, shade, and creeps for baby pigs. These combined measures were directed chiefly against *Ascaris lumbricoides* infections, including verminous pneumonia; but they also effectively reduced the incidence of and losses from other swine helminths, as well as from necrobacillus. Under this widely adopted system, American producers began to market more generally uniform and healthy pigs at six months from two sows than they had previously been able to market from three sows.

A similar program of using portable pens for rearing calves free of heavy parasite burdens was introduced widely in the southern U.S. in the 1940s. Pens for individual calves were arranged on the lower part of a grassy slope and moved further up the slope frequently enough to disrupt the transmission cycles of prevalent helminths and coccidia. In another broad environmental effort, heat disinfection of animal feeds was successfully applied to garbage fed to swine during national eradication campaigns against vesicular exanthema and hog cholera in the United States.

Like these programs, most veterinary environmental efforts have been directed toward disinfection; pasture rotation (including moveable pens); manure disposal; and housing improvements, such as adequate shelter, ventilation, and lighting. A principal advantage of disease control measures directed to the physical environment is that they often need not involve handling or doing anything at all to the susceptible or affected population. This advantage is perhaps greater in public health than in veterinary medicine.

EDUCATION. With rare exceptions, education has been the least successfully applied approach to disease control in veterinary medicine. Much more attention has been paid to its importance in public health; and an instructive public health literature on social sciences in relation to public programs exists for the veterinarian's use. This subject is not developed here, but the reader is referred elsewhere for instances of veterinary failures in education of the public.[11]

This overall medical detection approach to directed action against diseases may be illustrated by the hog cholera eradication program in the United States.

Hog cholera eradication program in the United States

Hog cholera is a viral disease affecting pigs. The disease was observed first in the Ohio River Valley of the United States before 1850. It subsequently spread to other parts of the United States and to other nations. Until the initiation of the hog cholera eradication program in 1963, it was the major swine disease in this country, with an annual cost of over $60 million. Approximately 80% of this cost was for control by vaccination. The much higher cost of the completely uncontrolled disease in the absence of vaccination is impossible to estimate.

Canada, Denmark, and Australia have successfully eradicated hog cholera; and the U.S. eradication program was based on similar technical principles. Congress authorized this cooperative federal-state program in 1961. As designed, it consisted of four phases:

I. Preparatory-legislative
II. Initial reduction of the prevalence of disease by vaccination, quarantine, and other regula-

Table 3–7.   Annual Number of New Cases of Hog Cholera in United States, 1967–75 (Data Available from U.S. Department of Agriculture as Numbers of Cases, not as Incidence Rates).

Year	No. new cases
1967	689
1968	849
1969	1055
1970	1231
1971	468
1972	76
1973	163
1974	2
1975	2

tion of animal movements

   III. Elimination of infection by depopulation of affected herds (after termination of vaccinations)

   IV. Protection against reinfection.

Theoretically, hog cholera would seem a fairly easy disease to eradicate since swine are the only *known* reservoir of the virus, and the virus usually does not survive long in nature (although *unusual* instances have been reported of its survival, e.g., 85 days in ham and sausage casings and up to seven weeks in manure water!). The virus is also readily destroyed by heating and disinfectants.

The progress of this eradication program is roughly illustrated in Table 3–7 in terms of the numbers of new infected animals by year throughout the United States. During the first few years of this campaign, a rapid decline in incidence occurred; but by 1966 the program seemed to have lost some of its momentum and an increase in incidence followed. In retrospect, it can be seen that 1966 might have been the optimal year for a nationwide shift from phase II to phase III of the program. Vaccination was terminated in 1969, and this action automatically moved the program into phase III. The immediate result was an increase in incidence of infected herds, which then dropped rapidly again. Part of the reason for a fairly dramatic increase in disease occurrence in 1969 was that the vaccines not only had had a protective effect, but also some vaccines had actually caused outbreaks in herds because of a content of infective virions. By the end of 1970, part of the remaining reservoir of infection had been removed through depopulation of infected herds, an effort that began in 1969.

The initial 1972 target year for complete eradication could not be met, and after 1972 the program showed symptoms of "last phase difficulties." There were probably several reasons. Some previously unknown facts about the disease's epidemiology had become evident. Another last phase discovery was that flaws existed in the diagnostic procedure. It was learned, for example, that pregnant sows can transmit hog cholera virus to pigs without themselves showing symptoms ("pregnant sow syndrome"); and these pigs then may not appear ill until they are exposed to stress. It was also learned that hog cholera may occur in a mild chronic form. "Junk" pigs, in particular,

may develop chronic, hard to detect, atypical disease (see Fig. 2–4). In addition, the relative importance of sources of infection began to change, with herd addition and garbage feeding both becoming more important. In some areas, spread of virus by biting flies assumed local importance.

Numerous "problem herd" situations were available for intensive follow-up studies; and outbreaks continued to occur in a few states. During this stage of outbreaks and problem herds, information was rarely available for calculating true incidence rates, nor were data collected for studies of possible effects of different host and environmental variables on either maintenance of inapparently infected populations or spread of the virus.

This overall sequence of events for the hog cholera program is depicted in Figure 3–3. In the last phases, when clinical detection alone proved insufficient, the need was for a sensitive and specific test that was simple enough to apply in mass screening. However, such a test has not been available for detecting atypical and inapparent hog cholera infections. Despite such difficulties, the U.S. eradication program against hog cholera continued to progress slowly and, by 1975, all 50 states were in phase IV of the program.

The following problems reflect some of the additional concepts and approaches presented in this chapter.

Problem 2. An unexpected level of mortality in a chicken breeding flock

Suppose in a pedigreed breeding flock of laying hens being trapnested, the hatching eggs are handled in such a way that each can be related to the hen that produced it. The expected hatchability rate on a daily basis is 90 to 96%. An epidemic of a specific teratogenic defect is observed in eggs in which chicks develop to term but are unable to hatch from their eggs. The nature of this defect is such that it is believed to arise very early in the development of the embryo. As the result of your intensive follow-up investigation of this marked deviation from expected hatchability rates, you have hypothesized a number of management procedures applied to these laying hens *or* their eggs, which could be determinants of this disease episode. Your retrospective study of this

Fig. 3–3. Situation in the late phase of eradication of a disease in which subclinical and difficult-to-detect infections occur.

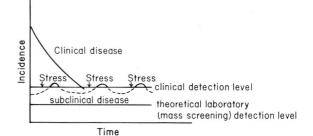

Table 3–8.   Attack Rates for Epidemic in Hatching Eggs in Chicken Breeding Flock.

Procedures applied to:	Eggs exposed to management procedures			Eggs not exposed to management procedures		
	Total	Not hatched	A.R. (%)	Total	Not hatched	A.R. (%)
Hens producing eggs						
Newcastle vaccine lot 225	922	443	48	1330	407	31
Newcastle vaccine lot 89	458	250	55	1794	600	33
Newcastle vaccine lot 362	872	157	18	1380	693	50
Insemination with pooled semen sample 4	321	280	87	1931	570	30
Insemination with pooled semen sample 6	675	192	28	1577	658	42
Insemination with pooled semen sample 8	83	71	86	2169	779	36
Insemination with pooled semen sample 10	1173	307	26	1079	543	50
Eggs themselves						
Tylosin dip, A&D brand	421	215	51	1831	635	35
Tylosin dip, Ri brand	680	513	75	1572	337	21
Heat treatment at 115° F.	1972	828	42	280	22	8
Injection with antibiotic R	1221	122	10	1031	728	71

situation results in compilation of the attack rate data shown in Table 3–8. Note that the antibiotic solutions used to dip eggs usually contain a disinfecting agent.

Determine which of these factors, if any, were responsible for this epidemic. Are there good alternative possibilities? If these data were all that were available to you, what corrective action would you recommend?

If any data are lacking for analytical procedures that you might wish to apply, indicate precisely what data you would want and *how you would intend to use them*. Add any clarifying description that will explain your line of investigation or conclusions.

Problem 3. Investigation of a disease outbreak in a cattle feedlot

A beef-feedlot complex in southern California consists of approximately 42,000 cattle in 56 pens. You are a consulting epidemiologist called in on December 12. It has been reported to you by telephone that the average daily mortality number in this whole complex has been 15 for the past month, with a monthly range of eight to 21 deaths. Then on December 11, 1822 cattle died and on December 12, 1483 others. Your task is to identify the source and/or cause of this epidemic and to control it *as quickly as possible*.

The intent of this exercise is not merely to test your ability to obtain a "correct" answer or answers,

but to check your ability to approach an epidemiological problem logically and systematically and to use what you have learned. In seeking information, be practical as to the effort and time that would be required to obtain this information *under field circumstances*.

(1) With the information you possess upon arrival at the feedlot, first record fully your initial reasoning and any hypotheses.

Now, you may obtain the other information that you will need. This information is hidden in the chapter notes at the end of this book. The key to each piece of information is found in the index. Obtain only *one* type of information at a time, and in a *logical* order. At *each* such step, again record your further reasoning, hypotheses, and conclusions. For example, say you wish to know *first* what color these cattle are. Think of *how* this information could be indexed, for example, "color of cattle" or "cattle color." Look up one alternative possibility in the index of this book. Under "color of cattle" (problem 3), the index may refer you to page 221. On page 221, a note will say: "All of the cattle were red with white faces." If there is no index listing "color of cattle," try the alternatives, e.g., "cattle color." If you exhaust reasonable indexing alternatives, assume the information requested is not important or unavailable and proceed to another information category.

(2) At this point, record the information category *you* sought first, and record your further reasoning,

hypotheses, conclusions, or actions; for example, the first information requested might be the color of cattle. Your conclusion may be: These animals are grade Herefords, but this information seems to add nothing to my knowledge of this situation.

Carry this process through in *stepwise* fashion; that is, obtain information (3), (4), (5), etc., or *as far as you need to go to take reasonable practical* actions that will terminate this outbreak as quickly as possible.

Regarding the continuing value of this basic shoe-leather approach to field problems of disease, the English medical statistician, Bradford Hill, pointed out almost poetically that its past use shows well how "the highest returns can be reaped by imagination in combination with a logical and critical mind, a spice of ingenuity coupled with an eye for the simple and the humdrum, and a width of vision in pursuit of facts that is allied with an attention to detail that is almost nauseating."

Chapter 4

THE ECOLOGICAL APPROACH

Medical ecology as an epidemiological school is probably as old as medical detection. However, it was more the creation of researchers and academicians than of government practitioners of veterinary medicine or public health, and its evolution was somewhat less orderly.[1] Ecological perspective and ecological methods first came into epidemiology when it was realized that the transmission of disease agents was sometimes more complicated than by contact or by food and water vehicles; and also that the same infections could exist in nature in more than one species of animal.

Thus, in 1790, the Danish veterinarian, Peter Abildgaard, showed that some trematode parasites *required* a succession of different host species to complete their life cycles. Similar observations with other helminths caused the veterinarians, physicians, and zoologists who were creating the science of parasitology to realize that the epidemiological aspects of some infectious diseases were inherently complex. Thus, they proceeded to develop useful vocabularies and methodologies to describe the phenomena they observed.

Others, such as the German physician, Rudolf Virchow, who coined the term *zoonosis*, noted the frequency with which newly described infectious microorganisms were transmissible in nature from lower vertebrates to man. At the same time, many veterinarians began to appreciate that this phenomenon of sharing the same pathogen among different vertebrate host species was a common one.

Finally, from 1888 to 1892, Frederick Kilborne carried out the series of experiments (mentioned in Chapter 1) that proved that some microorganisms were transmitted from an infected vertebrate animal to a susceptible vertebrate animal by an arthropod species. He also proved that, in ticks at least, an infectious agent associated with disease in vertebrate animals could be maintained in nature from one generation of invertebrate "vectors" to the next. Following closely upon these revelations about Texas fever were similar discoveries of vector transmission of malaria, yellow fever, and other diseases of man and lower animals. The concept of vectors introduced a whole new dimension to the subjects of epidemiology and disease control.

The result of all of these disclosures was to impress upon more biologically minded disease investigators the ecologically complicated nature of many infectious disease processes. Eventually, these independent lines of approach of the parasitologists, the students of zoonotic and other animal diseases, and the students of vector-borne infections began to coalesce in individual careers with some of the insights of ecologists *per se*. Thus, an ecological approach to the study of infections and their often complex patterns of transmission and maintenance in nature was created collectively by veterinarians like Karl F. Meyer in the United States and Robert Daubney in East Africa; zoologists such as Eugene Pavlovsky in the Soviet Union; physicians, including Howard Ricketts in the United States and David Bruce in Malta and Africa; and a few ecologists *per se*, such as Charles Elton in England. As an aid to conceptualizing this approach, ecology's relationships to other scientific disciplines are indicated in Figure 4–1 and Table 4–1.

SOME BASIC CONCEPTS IN MEDICAL ECOLOGY

As a result of these developments, medical ecology gained useful concepts with which the practicing epidemiologist in veterinary medicine must be conversant.

Ecosystems, biotic communities, and biotopes

Pathogenic microorganisms and other parasites, together with the vertebrate and invertebrate species they infect, are components of identifiable ecosystems. An *ecosystem* may be defined as a biotic community living in its biotope.

Biotope refers to the smallest geographic area that provides uniform conditions for life. Examples of biotopes would include a swamp, a hummock arising from the swamp, a burrow in one of these hummocks, an open pasture, and a hedgerow between two pastures. A biotope can be looked upon conveniently as the physical address of either a particular

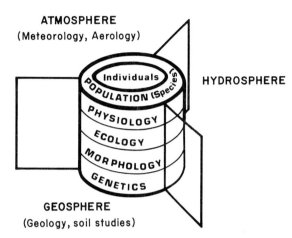

ENVIRONMENT
(Biosphere)

ATMOSPHERE
(Meteorology, Aerology)

HYDROSPHERE

GEOSPHERE
(Geology, soil studies)

Fig. 4–1. Position of ecology and its relationship to other sciences (redrawn from Naumov, N.P. 1972. *The Ecology of Animals.* University of Illinois Press, Urbana).

species of organism or a biotic community of organisms.

A *biotic community*, or biocenosis, is the assemblage of animals, microorganisms, and plants inhabiting any given biotope. Thus, cattle, sheep, deer, rabbits, snails, leafhoppers, katydids, nematodes, various plants, bacteria, yeasts, molds, and viruses might all be part of a biotic community present in the same pasture biotope.

Certain ecosystems of which specific infectious agents form a part are the "type" ecosystems of those agents; that is, they are a particular agent's natural *nidus* or nest, in other words, the maintenance ecosystem for that particular parasite in nature. It follows that infections themselves may be thought of as being part of characteristic maintenance ecosystems. Specific efforts to locate and describe these natural, as opposed to syanthropic or man influenced, nidi or foci for different infections have sometimes been referred to as the practice of *landscape* epidemiology.[2]

Climax, niche, and biome

When a succession of different species of animals, plants, and microorganisms in a geographic area of some size have evolved in their relationships to one another to a state of environmental "homeostasis," the resulting balanced ecosystem is spoken of as an ecological *climax*.

Climate is considered to be the overriding force that determines the end result of most such ecological successions. Thus, a climax results from efforts of a succession of animal, plant, and microbial species to adapt and adjust to a particular climate and habitat, with the eventual survival of the several species most fit to occupy such a physical and biological area. In this overall process, food-chain and food-pyramid relationships between predator and prey, between

competitors, and between symbionts and hosts eventually reach a balance. Such climax relationships between organisms may differ seasonally with the weather, as shown diagrammatically for the tundra biome in Figure 4–2.

Evolution to a climax can be visualized by imagining an area of recent lava flow. First, certain types of microorganisms and simple plants would appear (reappear); these groups, in turn, would attract and support a few forms of animal life. As pockets of soil were created, some of these plants would be competed with or succeeded by other plants. New animals would also enter. If the competitor, predator, or parasite pressure on any species became too great, these species could lose their positions of dominance or might disappear entirely. As particular prey and host species lost out, so usually would the parasite and predator species that were sustained by them, and so on.

Considering the specific roles of parasites and hosts in such a succession, one could reason teleologically that it would seldom be to a parasitic species' advantage to kill its host species, because each individual host's death would decrease the parasite's probability of survival. With respect to host-parasite relationships in any ecological succession, it would be expected, therefore, that more resistant or tolerant animals of any host species would tend to be selected genetically, and the same selective pressure would favor the least virulent parasite strains. What would be expected then in an ecological succession is an evolution from an epidemic disease relationship to an endemic disease relationship and, eventually perhaps, to a state of inapparent or symptomless infections or commensalism (see Fig. 2–4).

A *pro-climax* is an alternative end stage of an ecological succession reached when man intervenes to prevent an eventual climax from being attained. For example, man's annual burning of the savannah

Table 4-1.　Ecology in Relation to Other Biological Sciences (from Wright, S. 1959. Genetics and the Hierarchy of Biological Sciences. Science, 130:959)

Biological level	Climax phase		History		
	Description	Dynamics	Description	Dynamics	
Ecologic system					
World biota	Biogeography	Biostability	Paleontology	Biotic evolution	Multiplication
Local biota	Ecology (community)		Ecologic succession		
Interbreeding population					
Species	Taxonomy	Species stability	Phylogeny	Macro-evolution and transformation	Species cleavage
Deme	Demography	Population genetics		Micro-evolution and population genetics	
Multicellular organism					
Individual	External characters	Behavior and genetics of behavior	Life history		Physiology of reproduction and formal genetics
Organ	Anatomy	Gross physiology	Descriptive embryology	Morphogenesis	
Tissue	Histology			Developmental genetics and histogenesis	
Cell					
Cytoplasm and nucleus	Cytology	General physiology and physiological genetics	Cytogenetics		Mitosis
Autonomous macromolecule					
Gene	Gene chemistry	Gene physiology	Theory of gene		Gene duplication
DNA			Gene mutation / Descriptive process		
Nonautonomous molecule	Biochemistry				

FEED			PREY	PREDATORS			
Marine mammals fish and invertebrates	Tundra vegetation			Polar fox	Wolf	Ermine	White owl
	●		Northern reindeer	●	●		
	●		Lemmings	●		●	●
	●		Ptarmigan	●	●	●	●
	●		White hare	●	●		●
		PREDATORS					
●			Polar bear				
●			Polar fox				
●			Wolf				
●			Gulls				

Winter

Fig. 4–2. Food relationships in winter and summer in Arctic tundra climax ecosystem (redrawn from Naumov, N.P. 1972. *The Ecology of Animals*. University of Illinois Press, Urbana; after Sdobnikov, 1958).

grasslands in parts of East Africa maintains the dominance of certain grasses and prevents a succession of the brush species (as well as their associated tsetse flies and game animals) from realizing their natural ecological potentials. Overgrazing by livestock, or other agricultural or technological practices, also can maintain specific pro-climax states and, sometimes, result in synanthropic or other secondary infectious cycles. Such is the case, for example, with yellow fever virus, man, and *Aedes aegypti* mosquitoes in cities.

What also happens in an evolving climax is that each animal, plant, or microorganism comes to occupy a well-defined ecological *niche* or "slot" with respect to its competitors, its enemies, and its food. Therefore, just as an organism's biotope is its physical address, its niche can be thought of as its occupation, its *functional* position in the community. Its niche is

what the organism does. Another way to conceptualize niche is to consider that a particular niche has boundaries that are determined by the species' overall relationships to the various competitor, synergist, parasite, host, predator, and prey species with which the organism lives (Fig. 4–3).

More than one species of animal or parasite may be capable of occupying essentially the same niche (Table 4–2); and given proper circumstances, one may replace the other, just as historically one powerful nation has tended to occupy a "power vacuum" or place left by the decline, withdrawal, or defeat of another nation. For example, a population of *Streptococcus agalactiae* may occupy a well-defined niche in the udders of certain individuals in a herd of dairy cattle. If a program of specific mass chemotherapy is used to eliminate these parasites from their niche and the niche itself remains (perhaps

FEED			PREY	PREDATORS						
Marine mammals fish and invertebrates	Tundra vegetation	Water and soil invertebrates, and fishes		Polar fox	Tundra wolf	Ermine	White owl	Falcon	Hawk	Gull
	•		Northern reindeer	•	•					
	•		Lemmings	•	•	•	•	•	•	•
	•		Ptarmigan	•	•	•	•	•	•	•
	•		Sparrows	•		•	•		•	•
	•		Geese, Brants	•	•			•		•
	•		White hare	•	•		•			
	•	•	Snipe	•		•	•	•	•	•
•		•	Loons, Eiders, Ducks	•	•			•		•
			PREDATORS							
•			Polar bear							
•			Polar fox							
•			Guillemots							
•			Gulls							

Summer

Fig. 4–2. Food relationships in winter and summer in Arctic tundra climax ecosystem (redrawn from Naumov, N.P. 1972. *The Ecology of Animals.* University of Illinois Press, Urbana; after Sdobnikov, 1959). (Continued)

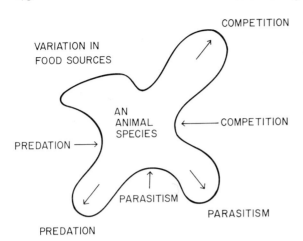

Fig. 4–3. Conceptualization of niche "boundaries" of a species as determined by mutual predation, competition, and parasitism.

because of continued traumatizing of the udder tissues by a faulty milking machine), what might sometimes be observed is that the streptococci's vacant niche is filled by another bacterial species that is not susceptible to the antibiotic being used.

Finally, to be distinguished from climax and niche, is *biome*, which is a large, climatically determined area characterized by a distinctive stable flora. The relatively few recognized biomes include tundra, savannah-like grassland or steppe, tropical rain forest, and desert.

Interfaces and mosaics

An ecological *interface* is a border between two ecosystems, for example, the border between a hummock and a surrounding swamp, the border between a forest and a plain, or the border between a cultivated river valley and brush-covered foothills. Interspecies spread of infection is facilitated at such interfaces.

To illustrate this concept, in parts of India where low foothills rim cultivated plains, rabies outbreaks occur in domestic animals and man in the plains villages each year following the monsoon. The sequence of events is that the monsoon rains serve to flood and seal off jackal dens on the hilly slopes. As a result, starving, sometimes rabid jackals penetrate the ecological interface into the edges of the adjacent plains in search of food and thus are brought into contact with and bite villagers and their dogs and cattle. Rabies transmission is rare in these plains areas of India at other seasons of the year.

Such conditions for interspecies transmission of infections are even greater when one ecosystem is interspersed throughout another, for example, in instances in which man creates clearings for himself and his domestic animals in a forest in order to practice a "slash and burn" kind of agriculture. These patterns of interspersed ecosystems are called *mosaics*.[3] Transmission of Kyasanur Forest disease, for instance, has occurred in India in recent years at the edges of such forest clearings. This particularly interesting situation is described later in the chapter.

Indicator species

Just as the experienced fisherman or hunter can say with authority that "this is a good stream for trout" or "this is quail country," so the medical ecologist learns to say with equal confidence that "this is fascioliasis country" or "we'll find plague here." Both possess the power of observation and stored knowledge of any skilled and experienced naturalist. Such a person might have difficulty explaining just how he knows a specific fact about a certain landscape, because more often than not his ability was derived empirically from a long and varied experience.

In medical ecology, an effort is made to describe in a systematic fashion the natural ecosystems of different infections. In this process, *indicator species* often identify themselves, and these species are then able to serve as clear markers for a particular ecosystem. Thus, specific disease ecosystems can often be spotted, at least tentatively, by noting the occurrence of a characteristic plant or animal indicator.

RESERVOIRS AND THE RELATIVE SPECIFICITY OF INFECTIONS

There are about 918,000 *species* of animals for the world's 200,000 veterinarians to consider. Every day, most of these animal species pick up a variety of potential pathogens either from their physical environments directly or through their social relationships with other animals. Many of these pathogens establish themselves typically and produce recognized diseases. Fulminant disease sometimes results too; and, as the host quickly dies, the parasite in effect pulls the temple down upon itself.

Other pathogens establish atypical or partially abortive infections in certain hosts. As examples, nonspecific clinical infections with schistosomes, hookworms, or ascarids are of particularly common occurrence. Finally, some of these invaders may reside silently or inapparently in certain host species (see Fig. 2–4).

All of these types of interactions are so common that there is absolutely no reason to regard the

Table 4–2.   Some Niche Equivalents in Mammals in Different Grassland Communities (from Allee *et al.* 1949. *Principles of Animal Ecology.* W.B. Saunders Co., Philadelphia)

Strata categories	Asia	Africa	N. America	S. America	Australia
1. Saltatorial, herbivorous mammals: habitat niche on floor and feeding niche in herbaceous stratum	Asiatic gerboa	Springhaas	Jack rabbit		Red kangaroo
2. Fossorial, herbivorous mammals:					
a. Habitat niche in subterranean and floor strata; feeding niche in herbaceous stratum	Suslick, hamster	African ground squirrel	Ground squirrel	Viscacha, pampas cavy	European rabbit (introduced)
b. Habitat and feeding niches in subterranean stratum	Mole-rat	Golden mole	Prairie mole, pocket gopher	Tucotuco	Marsupial mole
3. Cursorial, herbivorous gregarious mammals: habitat niche on floor; feeding niche in herbaceous stratum	Saiga antelope, goitered antelope, gazelle, maral stag, wild ass	Zebra, eland, springbok, gazelle, black wilde-beest, blue wildebeest, (30 genera of antelopes)	Pronghorn antelope, bison	Pampas deer, guanaco, marsh deer	Pig-footed bandicoot
4. Cursorial predators: habitat and feeding niches on floor stratum	Manul cat, corsac fox, cheetah	Lion, serval, caracal, cheetah, hunting dog	Coyote, wolf, puma	Pampas cat, wolf	Tasmania wolf

laboratory guinea pig, a gentle mammal native to the Andes of South America, as a species *uniquely* susceptible to an unusually wide spectrum of infectious agents since, given suitable conditions, interspecies transmission of infectious agents appears the rule in nature rather than the exception. For example, at least four-fifths of all known infections of man are shared in nature with at least one other species of vertebrate animal.

The suspicion that most infections are not strictly host specific is, or should be, axiomatic among epidemiologists. However, that statement does not mean that all possibly susceptible species fulfill the same epidemiological roles. For example, one species might serve a *reservoir* role and another might represent a biological "dead-end" host in which an essential phase of development of the parasite does not occur or, for some other reason, transmission cannot take place.[4] In other instances, a particular vector species may be inefficient and affect transmission only in the presence of a large and heavily infected population of vertebrate reservoirs, but may not be otherwise capable of perpetuating that infectious cycle.

Animal species that can perpetuate a particular infection in nature are called maintaining or *reservoir* hosts. It is these host species upon which the infectious agent depends ultimately for its own survival, and at least some of these species form part of its natural nidus or type ecosystem.

However, things other than animals also serve as reservoirs of infection. For example, reservoirs of *Histoplasma capsulatum* and *Cryptococcus neoformans* appear to be bird feces or soil enriched with bird feces. A reservoir, therefore, is considered to be *any* animate or inanimate substance in which an infectious agent multiplies or develops and upon which it depends as a species for survival in nature. Any one infectious agent can have more than one reservoir. For example, man and cattle are both reservoir species of *Taenia saginata*, because different stages of the parasite depend on each. On the other hand, foxes and bats may both serve a more or less identical reservoir role for rabies virus in the same locality or in different localities.

In studying diseases of man and of economically important mammals and birds, epidemiologists have neglected to consider fully the innumerable epidemiological possibilities for reservoir hosts. Kilborne's fortuitous discovery that ticks—extremely distant relatives of cows—share a particular protozoal parasite with cattle in nature should have indicated the virtually limitless biological possibilities available. This idea of a possibly broad range of reservoir hosts is suggested even more strongly by the fact that different, easy-to-detect helminthic parasites of cows and other mammals also spend portions of their life cycles in other animal species as different as snails, earthworms, snakes, fish, and crustaceans. One might well ask whether mammalian viruses might not do likewise.

So far, epidemiologists have rarely considered even the poikilothermic land vertebrates in veterinary and medical epidemiology; though whenever they have looked at them, as in studies of salmonellosis,[5] leptospirosis, and a few of the viral encephalitides, the results have often been significant or at least interesting. The much further-out possibilities suggested by the occurrence of mycoplasmas as pathogens of plants and by the reported resemblance of vesicular stomatitis virus to certain plant viruses (and the fact that in this instance the heterothermic sandflies that may transmit vesicular stomatitis virus between vertebrates also feed on plants) suggest prospects that are more than intriguing to the medical ecologist. The single well-studied facet of the relative specificity of infections involves the classic zoonoses.

Zoonoses

The zoonoses are infections shared in nature by lower vertebrate animals and man or, according to the World Health Organization definition, infections naturally transmissible between lower vertebrate animals and man.[6] As already indicated, a great majority of human infections are zoonoses.[7]

The zoonoses are a large and rather disparate group of infections. From the epidemiological standpoint, they are therefore classified by the following criteria, which reflect differences in their infectious cycles and prospects for control.

(1) *Direct zoonoses* are those transmitted by contact or vehicle and that biologically *require* only a single vertebrate reservoir species to maintain the infectious cycle. Important examples of direct zoonoses are rabies, brucellosis, and trichinosis.

(2) *Cyclozoonoses* are those zoonoses that biologically *require* at least two species of vertebrate animals to complete their infectious cycles. Examples of cyclozoonoses are the taeniases and hydatid disease.

(3) *Metazoonoses* are those zoonoses that are transmitted to vertebrate hosts by invertebrates and depend upon invertebrate vectors or intermediate hosts for completion of their infectious cycles. Metazoonoses include the arbovirus infections, fascioliasis, plague, and the piroplasmoses.

(4) *Saprozoonoses* are those zoonoses that require organic or other inanimate matter as a reservoir. Examples of saprozoonoses are cutaneous larva migrans and coccidioidomycosis.

Some few zoonoses, clonorchiasis for example, are not easily classified.

Zoonoses may also be separated into two large groups, anthropozoonoses and zooanthroponoses, depending upon whether lower animals or man serve as reservoirs of infection for the other. Unfortunately, these two terms have been used for their alternative meanings; thus the literature can be confusing.

TRANSMISSION OF INFECTIONS BY VECTORS

The subject of transmission of infections by the contact and vehicle routes has been introduced in Chapter 3. The remaining alternative is *vector* transmission, a subject of particular interest to ecologically oriented epidemiologists.

As already mentioned, the term vector is used epidemiologically to refer to an *invertebrate* animal that carries or transports an infectious agent between vertebrates.[8] This vector role may be a direct one, in which the invertebrate animal actually picks up the infectious agent from an infected vertebrate and subsequently passes it directly to a susceptible vertebrate, as in cases of vector transmission by biting flies. However, a vector may also function more *indirectly* by picking up the agent from the excreta of an infected vertebrate or by passing it on to the water or food of a susceptible vertebrate, or some combination of these alternatives. In some instances, the vector itself is eaten by the susceptible vertebrate. There are many different possibilities and examples of such indirect transmission, e.g., housefly transmission of salmonellae, earthworm transmission of metastrongylid lungworms, and snail transmission of fascioliasis.

Vector transmission, like vehicle transmission, takes place by one of several possible mechanisms:

(1) Mechanical transmission—the vector acts as a "flying needle," as in the case of tabanid flies or mosquitoes and certain hematogenous infections such as anthrax or myxomatosis; or acts as a "flying swab," as when noctuid moths, which feed on the lachrymal secretions of cattle, transmit infectious keratitis. The transmission interval is usually short and depends upon the survival time of the agent upon the body or mouth parts of the vector (see also paratenic host, defined later).

In other situations, the vector also serves an essential *biological* function in the life of the parasite. As with vehicles, these relationships may take several different forms:

(2) Propagative transmission—the infectious agent multiplies in the vector, as does the plague bacillus, *Yersinia pestis*, in the flea.

(3) Developmental transmission—the infectious agent undergoes an essential phase of its development in the vector, as with the dog heartworm, *Dirofilaria immitis*, in mosquitoes.

(4) Cyclopropagative transmission—both multiplication and development of the parasite occur, as in the case of *Babesia* spp. in ticks.

Transovarial vector transmission is a special situation in which the parasite is passed vertically from the infected vector to its own offspring through the ovary, as happens with Nairobi sheep disease virus

and *Babesia bigemina* in ticks. This phenomenon introduces important epidemiological complications with respect to the control of such an infection.

Transstadial vector transmission occurs when the infectious agent is picked up by one stage of the vector, say, the larva of a mite, as in scrub typhus, and then persists in the vector as it metamorphoses through successive stages.

Epidemiologically, a further important distinction between vectors is whether they are flying vectors and therefore can actively seek out their vertebrate hosts. For those that can, as is the case with mosquitoes, the flight range of the vector and its biting patterns may determine the extent and rapidity of spread of an infection and the rapidity of its build-up in an outbreak.

Nonflying vectors, such as ticks and mites, although dependent upon passive contact with the host, sometimes position themselves favorably for such contacts and respond actively to vibrations and other stimuli. With such vectors, factors such as transovarial transmission or the length of the period between blood meals may assume considerable epidemiological importance.

Similarly, swimming or other water-inhabiting vectors, such as some snails, may release the infectious organisms into water, thus enabling them to be actively or passively disseminated, as in the schistosomiases or fascioliasis. In such instances, transmission to a susceptible vertebrate may occur remotely from the vector.

Parasitologists have contributed some additional but slightly different terms to this general area of medical ecology. Thus, many vectors also are *intermediate hosts* (or, less often, *definitive hosts*) of the infectious agent. The definitive host is the animal in which an agent, such as a protozoan or helminth, undergoes its sexual phase of reproduction. This sexual phase is occasionally in the invertebrate vector, as in the case of piroplasms and malarial parasites in arthropods. More often, however, the invertebrate is the intermediate host in which nonsexual phases of development occur. The further term, *paratenic* host, refers to purely mechanical transport without further development of an agent, as when a small fish harboring plerocercoid larvae of *Diphyllobothrium* sp. is eaten by a larger fish and the plerocercoids reencapsulate in the latter.

Some useful concepts about vector-borne infections

Chapter 2 makes reference to inapparent infections. A related term applied to vectors is *masked* infection. A masked infection is the infection of an individual vector in which the infectious agent cannot be demonstrated with present tools.

Another commonly used term that is relative to vector transmission and has epidemiological meaning is "extrinsic incubation period." This term refers to the period of time between infection of an individual biological vector and the vector's ability to transmit the infectious agent to another susceptible vertebrate host.

ALTERNATIVE MODES OF TRANSMISSION OF INFECTIONS

As when considering other aspects of the epidemiology of diseases, it is important to maintain an open mind about *all* possibilities or alternatives for disease transmission in any situation. Early in his field studies of Texas fever, Daniel E. Salmon recorded that the pattern of spread of that disease could not be explained by any known mode of disease transmission. When he supported Kilborne and Curtice in their testing of the bizarre theory of a tick connection with that disease, he recognized at the same time that John Gamgee and other well-known veterinary authorities had already dismissed the idea as too preposterously *unprecedented* for any scientist even to consider.

Rigid acceptance of definitions, classifications, and other presumptions about diseases and their agents may thwart creative epidemiological investigations of diseases and approaches to the disruption of their transmission. For example, with regard to infections caused by rickettsiae (organisms once defined as being transmitted only by arthropods), the work on Q fever first showed the possibilities for, and in that disease the importance of, alternative nonvector routes for rickettsial transmission. In another instance, Donald Cordy recognized that the agent in the helminth-transmitted "salmon poisoning" infection of dogs (discussed later) possessed virtually all the properties of a rickettsia; yet it could not be so designated officially until there was a change in the internationally accepted definition of rickettsiae as being limited to arthropod-transmitted organisms. One wonders, in this connection, how many rabies experts even considered the *possibility* that rabies virus might have alternative nonbite routes for transmission before Constantine and his associates clearly demonstrated its air-borne transmission in caves.

"NEW" DISEASES OR ESCAPES FROM NICHE BOUNDARIES

While some infectious diseases were recognized in antiquity, the first known occurrences of a number of others have been comparatively recent. For instance, hog cholera apparently was unknown until it was seen in pigs in the Ohio River Valley in 1833. A swine industry in that area was just developing.[9] The source of this virus still is not known, but several potential reservoir species have been examined unsuccessfully.

Similarly, African swine fever was seen in domestic swine only after they were introduced into East Africa in the early 1900s. In this instance, it is now known that the virus had existed there commensally in indigenous African wild pigs. Again, bluetongue disease of sheep was first observed when Merino sheep were introduced into South Africa. They, too, immediately developed a "new" disease. In this case, bluetongue infection was subsequently found to occur subclinically in African wild blesbok and, more recently, the virus has been isolated from apparently unaffected African rodents.

A few examples of "new" diseases and their possible explanations follow.

KYASANUR FOREST DISEASE. This disease, now known to be caused by a virus of the Russian Spring-Summer Encephalitis group, was first observed among the human and monkey inhabitants of new agricultural clearings in an evergreen rain forest in Mysore, India, in 1955. It is now known that the natural focus or type ecosystem of this virus includes an assemblage of forest shrews and rodents and their associated ticks. The principal tick vector and the only one known to bite man is *Haemaphysalis spinigera*. Its preferred hosts, however, are cattle. Man became infected with the Kyasanur Forest virus following his cultivation of "slash and burn" clearings within this ecosystem, thereby forming ecological *mosaics*. Seasonally, he entered the surrounding forest to collect forest products. Additionally, his cattle browsing in the forest edges (i.e., at ecological *interfaces* of the forest and clearing) caused dense populations of *H. spinigera* to build up in these interface locations. Cows probably also introduced the infected tick into the clearings themselves. A "new" disease of man resulted.

PIROPLASMOSIS. As another example, different tick vectors of *Babesia* spp. bite man with differing frequencies, and man cohabits or frequents some of the ticks' extensive ecosystems. If these ticks do bite man, they probably can inject the parasite. What happens? Do infections result? Does disease occur?

As with most such possibilities, virtually nothing was known. Then in 1957, a Yugoslav cattle farmer became seriously ill with what was diagnosed as *Babesia bovis* infection. As often happens with new observations, two other instances of human piroplasmosis were brought to light in short order. All three of these initial infections were in previously splenectomized individuals. Then, in 1969, the first clinical case of piroplasmosis was diagnosed in an apparently healthy American woman with an *in situ* spleen. She lived on Nantucket Island off the coast of Massachusetts. In 1973, a second case of human piroplasmosis, also in a nonsplenectomized person, occurred, *also* on Nantucket Island. Between July 17 and August 28, 1975, five additional human cases were reported from Nantucket. An epidemic occurrence of a new disease! But is latent babesial infection in man really as rare as these few diagnosed clinical cases suggest? Must the clinically affected individual possess some rare characteristic? Why should this sizeable epidemic have occurred on that one small island?

These two examples are instances in which a parasite has been able to escape its customary niche boundaries when a new but susceptible vertebrate host was introduced into or at the edges of the ecosystem of the parasite. But there are still other possibilities.

MARBURG AGENT. In 1967, the previously unknown "Marburg agent" caused illness in 25 people; seven of them died. These persons were European laboratory workers who had been handling tissues of vervet monkeys imported from Uganda. Of greater interest, however, was the fact that six secondary human cases resulted from contact with these primary cases, and one of these man-to-man transmissions was shown to have been by the venereal route.

In this instance, an infected host species was removed from its natural ecosystem and introduced into the "laboratory ecosystem" of a susceptible host—man. Here, intimate exposure of man to infected tissues (such as could also have occurred had people eaten these monkeys) resulted in infections then capable of direct man-to-man transmission. Other human infections caused by a Marburg-like virus, but of unknown origin, were reported from South Africa in 1975.

EOSINOPHILIC MENINGOENCEPHALITIS. In another instance, Shoho in Japan during World War II made serial sections of the entire spinal cords of affected horses to show that a strange new epidemic equine encephalomyelitis was caused not by a virus as suspected but by an arthropod-borne filarid worm of the genus *Setaria*, which normally lives *commensally* in the serous cavities of cows. Why this strange interspecies transmission began and assumed relatively large proportions, no one knows. Some parasitologists wondered at the time just how common such a strange occurrence might be.

Their wait was not long; in 1961, another previously unknown disease, this time an eosinophilic meningoencephalitis of man, occurred epidemically in the Society Islands, and it has been diagnosed since in many other parts of the Pacific and Southeast Asia. Its etiologic agent also was suspected of being a virus, but is now known to be another nematode parasite whose natural ecosystem includes rats and land snails. The life cycle of this parasite, *Angiostrongylus cantonensis*, had been worked out in rats in Brisbane only in 1955. It involved an *obligatory* cerebral migration by the parasite in its normal rat host. Rats are infected by eating land snails that contain the larvae of the parasite.

Some investigators now believe that these epidemics of human infection resulted from the intentional and unintentional spread of the giant African snail, *Achatina fulica*, throughout the Pacific. Opportunities for human infection were created in part by differing food prejudices about eating this snail cooked or raw and by the secondary introduction of the larval infection into paratenic hosts, such as freshwater crustaceans, which were commonly eaten uncooked by some of the affected peoples. As with the Marburg agent, this example is probably an instance of a parasite's escape from its usual niche boundaries as the result of the introduction of an infected host species, a snail, into a new ecosystem, where the existence of particular dietary habits favored infection of a new species—man.

PLAGUE IN THE UNITED STATES. Among the possibilities for initiating new patterns of interspecies transmission are less direct ecological changes. One mechanism is illustrated by the plague, which exists silently and endemically in wild rodent populations of the western United States. Plague, of course, is *not* a new disease, although in man it pops up anew whenever circumstances allow.[10]

In 1965, the largest human plague epidemic known in the United States since 1924 affected children on the Navajo Reservation at Gallup, New Mexico. It coincided with an epidemic occurrence of plague and mass die-off in prairie dogs. It appears that either a prairie dog or other rodent population build-up resulting in decreased social distances may have exposed prairie dogs to small rodents (and their fleas) that are the natural reservoir hosts of plague. This situation happened with sufficient frequency to establish and spread epidemic plague among the dense prairie dog population. This sequence was facilitated by the fact that the reservoir rodents often cohabit burrows dug by prairie dogs.

Indian children, in turn, found that sick prairie dogs could be caught readily as pets or for food. Thus, several human and many prairie dog infections occurred in one summer in an environment in which human and prairie dog exposure is typically rare and highly sporadic. This occurrence was an example of interspecies transmission—of escape of a parasite from its niche boundaries—that probably resulted from changed population dynamics of a nonreservoir host. This change, in turn, brought unusual opportunities for contact between man and the plague bacillus.

MYXOMATOSIS AND BOUTONNEUSE FEVER. A similar situation, but in reverse, seems to have occurred in France. There, epidemiologists noted that, coincident with the intentional introduction of myxoma virus into the wild rabbit population of southern France in 1953, there was a marked decline in the human incidence of Mediterranean tick typhus or boutonneuse fever. The intriguing explanation suggested at the time was that certain field rodents serve as inapparently infected reservoir hosts of the boutonneuse fever rickettsia, with the organism transmitted from rodent to rodent by their ticks. These rodents and their ticks commonly inhabit old rabbit burrows. Ordinarily, man or other susceptible species such as dogs would not come into contact with rodent ticks in their rabbit burrow ecosystem. However, rabbits that take refuge from predators in these old burrows commonly pick up infected ticks and thus serve to transport the ticks and their rickettsiae to hunters and hunting dogs. These relationships are shown diagrammatically in Figure 4–4. The hypothesis advanced for the relationship between myxomatosis and the disappearance of boutonneuse fever was that the myxoma virus, by decimating this population of rabbits, secondary hosts of the vector tick, removed the vital ecological link in transmission of the boutonneuse fever rickettsia from reservoir rodents to man or dogs.

TRYPANOSOMIASIS IN EAST AFRICA. Another mechanism for escape of an infectious agent from its niche boundaries is illustrated by trypanosomiasis in East Africa. In this instance, two ecosystems were separated by another disease, rinderpest, and subsequently reestablished their interface. In the 1890s, a great rinderpest epidemic swept down through East Africa from Egypt and the Sudan.[11] It left such devastation in its wake that it is easy to understand why, when rinderpest also ravaged Europe in the late Middle Ages and after, the Roman Church issued papal bulls in a frantic effort to halt its spread. In East, Central, and South Africa, vast populations of antelopes and other game were destroyed by this plague; and the large cattle populations of the nomadic tribes practically ceased to exist. One observer described the extent of this carnage by noting that "the vultures had forgotten how to fly."

A strange consequence of this rinderpest disaster, now recognized in retrospect, was that trypanosomiasis ceased to exist in large African areas in which formerly it had been endemic. What happened over a large area is that the tsetse flies perished with their wild mammalian hosts; as a consequence, so did the trypanosomes themselves. The result was that a "wild game-tsetse fly, savannah-woodland ecosystem" and a "man-cattle, savannah-cultivation ecosystem," which had previously shared extensive *interfaces* in East Africa, were pushed far apart. The early students of human and animal trypanosomiasis in East Africa observed the disease mostly *after* this ecological event. They felt that host-specific trypanosomiasis infections normally existed completely independently in East Africa in man, in domestic animals, and in wild game. There are now reasons to disbelieve this explanation. Ford[12] has described how these two separated ecosystems gradually expanded toward one another in succeeding years until finally, about 1925, they began to reestablish interfaces over a broad front, and possibilities for an active transmission of trypanosomes from game species to cattle and man were recreated. Thus, the trypanosome again had the opportunity to escape from its customary niche boundaries, particularly when agricultural clearings (mosaics) were cut in the bush. By 1946, when equilibrium was reestablished between these two ecosystems, the result was a stabilization of the previously growing cattle population.

ANISAKIASIS. A pathogen also may escape its niche through purely technological changes initiated by man. For example, a previously obscure ascaroid nematode of marine mammals and fishes was brought into contact with man in the 1950s by technological changes in the European herring industry and in Japanese fisheries. In 1955, the first human case of a serious intestinal granulomatous disease of man caused by larvae of *Anisakis* spp. was diagnosed in the Netherlands. After many subsequent occurrences in Holland and elsewhere, it was shown that this new human disease resulted from "improved" icing procedures on the fishing boats (including the use of

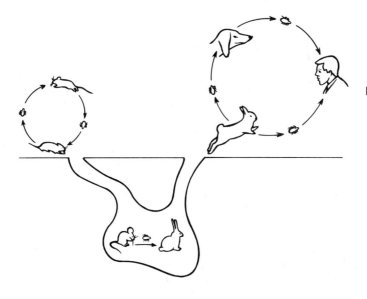

Fig. 4–4. The old rabbit burrow-field mouse-tick-rickettsia ecosystem and the rabbit link in Mediterranean tick typhus transmission to man and dog. This link was possibly broken by myxomatosis virus.

antibiotic ice). As a consequence, fish spoilage was retarded sufficiently so that herring and other fish formerly gutted promptly at sea were now gutted ashore after their landing. Under those circumstances, when the infectious larvae of *Anisakis*, normally present only in the gut of the fish, discovered that their host was dead, they reacted to their situation and burrowed frenetically into the dead fish's musculature and other tissues. From these sites, they could be ingested by consumers of raw or lightly pickled fish snacks. This new disease is now recognized in the United States.

FISHES AND FLUKES. Finally, the case of fishes and their fluke parasites is an instructive one.[13] In nature, about 90% of a large number of monogeneid fluke parasites of marine fishes are observed to be strictly host specific. However, freshwater monogenea are less host specific than their close marine relatives; and, in fresh water, populations of fishes of different species are often found *ecologically* more proximate to each other. However, the rather startling aspect is that the apparent host specificity of the marine monogenea virtually disappears when many different species of marine fish are placed in the same aquarium tank. Observations were made in the New York Aquarium, for example, that *Epidella melleni*, an apparently host-specific fluke in the ocean, readily parasitizes at least 41 different fish species of 15 different families when they are all confined within a single ecosystem! The host specificity—the niche relationships—of flukes and fishes thus appears to be purely ecological and does not reflect any innate biological characteristics of either the parasite or the host.

Mechanisms for escape of agents from their niches

In summary, a number of possible mechanisms have been suggested for extension of a parasite's "usual" host range, for an escape from its usual niche boundaries. Among these are: (1) introduction of a new host species into an ecosystem of which the infectious agent is a part; (2) introduction of an infected host species into a new ecosystem; (3) changes in the population dynamics of a usual host, a potentially new host, or an intermediary "transport" host; (4) ecological changes that bring two previously separated ecosystems into contact; (5) changes in the habits of a host, including its food habits; (6) technological changes brought about by man; and (7) mutation or genetic recombination of an agent (examples in Chapter 10).

SOME DIAGNOSTIC METHODS OF MEDICAL ECOLOGY

Use of specific ecological methods often is necessary in epidemiological work in order, for example, to gain access to and to study diseases in populations of wild reservoir hosts or vectors. It is beyond the scope of this book to do more than mention some of these methods.[14]

ANIMAL CAPTURE. To study diseases in a wild animal population, it is necessary to have access to a sample of the population. Available capture methods for such samples vary considerably depending upon whether the species of interest are deer, foxes, bats, birds, fish, mosquitoes, or ticks. A choice of methods also may be determined by whether one wants to be able to release the animals unharmed.

In general, techniques for capturing wild animals include use of various kinds of nets, traps, pitfalls, or watertraps; snares or hooks; sticky surfaces, attractants, or baits; and syringe guns.

Nets in common use include suspended nets that drop on an animal or group of animals or that are fired over groups of animals by cannons, drag or sweep nets or seines, purse-string nets, or stretched nets in which animals become entangled (such as mist nets for birds and gill nets for fish). Common traps include funnel traps, which have a large opening into which the animal can easily find its way, but a small and inaccessible exit. Shelter traps and others often are rigged so that an open door shuts after the animal enters. Snap or jaw traps injure or kill the trapped animal, possibly a disadvantage. For systematic trapping, as for population estimates, traps often are laid out in grids with uniform distances between, depending again upon the species.

Most traps are baited or contain some other attractant. Sticky surfaces are primarily useful for catching flying animals, such as insects or birds. Sticky surfaces may be baited to attract the animals or merely be their usual roosting surfaces.

Various baits or attractants are used, again depending upon the species of interest. Common baits include attractive and often odoriferous foods, reusable wicks soaked in animal fats or other substances, carrion, dung, light, sound and carbon dioxide, as well as various kinds of artificial lures and decoys.

A particular boon to work with wild mammals was the development of the compressed-air or charge-powered syringe gun and of proper drugs and doses for safely immobilizing a great variety of large species.

PREDATOR, PREY, HOST, AND PARASITE IDENTIFICATION. A *sine qua non* of wildlife epidemiology is the correct identification of animal species. This labeling often requires preparation and preservation of suitable specimens plus the consulting services of a specialist taxonomist. It cannot be overstressed that much time-consuming epidemiological work has been at least partially invalidated by inadequate attention to this important area.

For studies in which animal capture is necessary, there should also be an effort to coordinate one's own needs with those of other investigators or, preferably, with on-going studies of wildlife biology. Not only is this coordination economic of the animal populations involved; it may also inject into one's own study many additional data of value plus the services or knowledge of experts in related fields.

Species identification is an area of particular importance in working out niche relationships of vertebrate host species and vector species, species possibly useful for biological control and for other purposes. Special methods for animal identification include examination of stomach contents of predators and blood sucking vectors (e.g., for hair, bones, and other recognizable parts of animals; and for blood meals identifiable by precipitin tests[15]), as well as examination of their fecal pellets (e.g., for rodent skulls in pellets of birds of prey). Many specific techniques have been described; for example, stomach contents of birds have been examined using zooplankton counting devices.

MARKING OF ANIMALS. Such marking is necessary in many types of epidemiological studies. It may be initiated for the purpose of (1) subsequently identifying an individual animal; (2) identifying a particular animal population; (3) tracing back an animal through its successive stages of handling, ownership, or other experiences; (4) estimating the size of animal populations by the method of capture-mark-release-recapture; (5) determining the movement patterns or the range of an animal; or (6) identifying associated specimens such as serum, feces, and stomach contents. This subject will be considered here with respect to wild reservoir hosts and vectors and further in Chapter 14 with reference to domestic animals.

Considerations involved in selecting the most appropriate marking method vary depending on the purpose of the study. In general, however, the method chosen should not affect either the behavior or life expectancy of the marked animal.

Methods in common usage include (1) marking animals with paints or solutions of dyes (including reflective and fluorescent materials); (2) dusting with powdered dyes (including fluorescent dyes); (3) internal marking by injecting dyes or a radioactive label; (4) feeding dyes or label to mark feces or urine; (5) using various kinds of tags or labels (often sticky-backed, colored, fluorescent and/or numerically coded materials) attached to the animal's body proper or haircoat (including clips or tags inserted through, say, the ears); (6) amputating or notching a part of the body (sometimes in a coded pattern); (7) attaching collars, chains, or bands (often numerically and/or color coded); (8) tattooing; (9) hot or cold branding; or (10) implanting subcutaneous electronic transmitters or transponders.

DETERMINATION OF RANGES AND MOVEMENT PATTERNS OF RESERVOIRS AND VECTORS. These aspects are often important in medical ecological studies. Figure 4-5, for example, shows movement patterns of *Meriones meridianus*, a jird reservoir of several zoonotic infections, within a biotope mosaic. Methods used for these purposes include capturing, marking, releasing, and recapturing; detecting marked feces or urine; attaching radio-pulse transmitters; tracking by radar for birds; and aerial surveying for large game.

USE OF SENTINEL ANIMALS. These are individuals of a species that is susceptible to a given infectious agent (or some nonliving agent) and are deliberately exposed to risk of infection (or other hazard) in order to detect or quantitate the presence of the agent in a particular environment. In veterinary medicine, it has become a common practice in disease eradication efforts to introduce a small number of sentinel animals onto a farm from which an infection presumably has been eliminated by measures such as depopulation and environmental disinfection. If these animals do not become infected, then normal repopulation is permitted.[16]

Sentinel animals have also been used as living bait to collect disease vectors, to make quantitative estimates of intensity of vector-borne infections, or, sometimes, to ascertain host preferences of vectors. Constantine used sentinel animals in bat caves to first demonstrate that rabies virus could be transmitted under such conditions by the air-borne route.[17]

A number of these concepts and diagnostic methods of medical ecology can be illustrated by describing a biologically complex infection, western equine encephalomyelitis (WE).

Western equine encephalomyelitis

This metazoonotic, arthropod-borne viral infection is present throughout much of the United States and Canada.[18] During some summers, it occurs epidemically as a serious symptomatic infection of horses and people; otherwise, it exists endemically as an inapparent infection in wild birds and mosquitoes and possibly in other reservoir hosts.

The disease associated with the virus was first seen in horses during periodic large-scale epidemics in the American Middle West beginning about 1912. Most of these summer epidemics were observed in years of unusually heavy rainfall, but some also occurred with greater regularity in the vicinity of swampy areas. With the development of major irrigation projects in the West about 1919, WE became a more frequent and even an annual problem in horses there. In some areas, it soon assumed sufficient proportions to encourage farmers to replace horses by tractors.

The responsible virus was isolated from the brain of a horse during an unusually severe epidemic in the Central Valley of California in the summer of 1930. In 1933, it was first shown that mosquitoes were

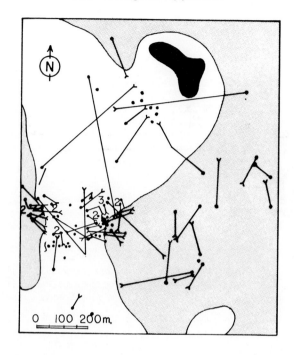

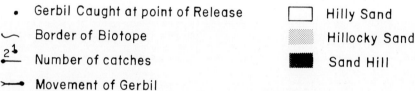

- Gerbil Caught at point of Release
- Border of Biotope
- 2¹ Number of catches
- Movement of Gerbil

☐ Hilly Sand
▒ Hillocky Sand
■ Sand Hill

Fig. 4–5. Movement of banded southern jirds (*Meriones meridianus*) released at banding point in different biotypes in Volta-Ural desert (redrawn from Naumov, N.P. 1972. *The Ecology of Animals*. University of Illinois Press, Urbana; after Fenyuk and Demayashev, 1936).

capable of transmitting this virus; subsequently, *Culex tarsalis* was identified as the most important mosquito vector of WE during epidemics in western North America, and *Culiseta melanura* in the eastern part of the continent. The viruses of WE and eastern equine encephalomyelitis were also differentiated in 1933. In 1938, both viruses were isolated from the brains of human beings who had died of encephalomyelitis during equine outbreaks. The eastern virus was isolated from wild birds in 1938, and in 1941 WE virus was obtained from a prairie chicken. An increase in frequency of human infections was noted during this period, with 2823 cases of encephalitis reported in five upper midwestern states and an adjoining Canadian province in the summer of 1941 alone. Serological evidence for WE virus infection in rodents was obtained for the first time in 1941; and virus isolations from sick and paralyzed ground and tree squirrels were made in California in 1956.

The consensus is that, originally, marsh-dwelling mosquitoes and birds, probably mostly blackbirds and swallows, comprised part of a balanced biotic community that, in its reed and rush marshland biotope, formed the type reservoir ecosystem, or

natural focus, of WE virus infection. Human population build-up of these areas in the 1800s resulted in subsequent alterations of this climax through drainage, irrigation, and cultivation. As a consequence, aberrant hosts for mosquitoes and virus intruded upon the restricted margins of the WE ecosystem at places where it interfaced with the cultivated tracts. At the same time, this restriction of their natural habitat forced some of the reservoir bird populations to divert their feeding to irrigated croplands and increasingly available stores of cultivated grains, that is, into the expanding man-horse-cultivation ecosystem. Thus, WE virus was afforded possibilities to escape its usual niche boundaries.

The complex natural history of WE virus in its normal hosts and habitat underlies the occurrence of this severe epidemic disease of horses and people. It has challenged the ingenuity of epidemiologists, and required the widest variety of investigative techniques and approaches, including virological and serological methods, a variety of entomological and zoological techniques, clinical and pathological observations, and measurements of climate (Fig. 4–6). The following example indicates some of the specific methods

The Ecological Approach

Variables   Methods of measurement

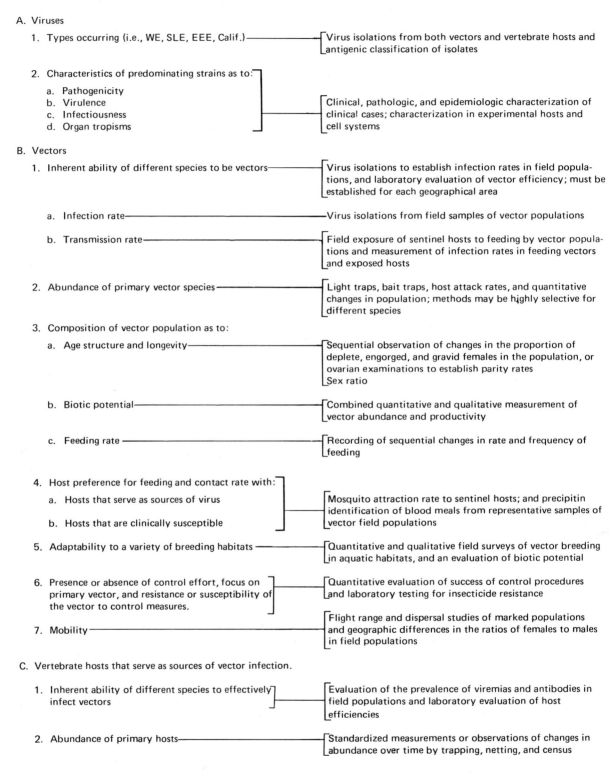

A. Viruses

  1. Types occurring (i.e., WE, SLE, EEE, Calif.) ——————— Virus isolations from both vectors and vertebrate hosts and antigenic classification of isolates

  2. Characteristics of predominating strains as to:

    a. Pathogenicity
    b. Virulence
    c. Infectiousness
    d. Organ tropisms

Clinical, pathologic, and epidemiologic characterization of clinical cases; characterization in experimental hosts and cell systems

B. Vectors

  1. Inherent ability of different species to be vectors ——————— Virus isolations to establish infection rates in field populations, and laboratory evaluation of vector efficiency; must be established for each geographical area

    a. Infection rate ——————————————————— Virus isolations from field samples of vector populations

    b. Transmission rate ———————— Field exposure of sentinel hosts to feeding by vector populations and measurement of infection rates in feeding vectors and exposed hosts

  2. Abundance of primary vector species ———————— Light traps, bait traps, host attack rates, and quantitative changes in population; methods may be highly selective for different species

  3. Composition of vector population as to:

    a. Age structure and longevity ———————— Sequential observation of changes in the proportion of deplete, engorged, and gravid females in the population, or ovarian examinations to establish parity rates
Sex ratio

    b. Biotic potential ———————————— Combined quantitative and qualitative measurement of vector abundance and productivity

    c. Feeding rate ———————————————— Recording of sequential changes in rate and frequency of feeding

  4. Host preference for feeding and contact rate with:

    a. Hosts that serve as sources of virus

    b. Hosts that are clinically susceptible

Mosquito attraction rate to sentinel hosts; and precipitin identification of blood meals from representative samples of vector field populations

  5. Adaptability to a variety of breeding habitats ———————— Quantitative and qualitative field surveys of vector breeding in aquatic habitats, and an evaluation of biotic potential

  6. Presence or absence of control effort, focus on primary vector, and resistance or susceptibility of the vector to control measures. ———— Quantitative evaluation of success of control procedures and laboratory testing for insecticide resistance

  7. Mobility ——————————————————— Flight range and dispersal studies of marked populations and geographic differences in the ratios of females to males in field populations

C. Vertebrate hosts that serve as sources of vector infection.

  1. Inherent ability of different species to effectively infect vectors ———— Evaluation of the prevalence of viremias and antibodies in field populations and laboratory evaluation of host efficiencies

  2. Abundance of primary hosts ———————— Standardized measurements or observations of changes in abundance over time by trapping, netting, and census

Fig. 4–6. Ecological factors in occurrence of epidemics of mosquito-born arbovirus encephalitis in North America (from Reeves, W.C. 1967. Factors that influence the probability of epidemics of western equine, St. Louis and California encephalitis in California. Vector News 14:13).

Fig. 4–6. Ecological factors in occurrence of epidemics of mosquito-born arbovirus encephalitis in North America (from Reeves, W.C. 1967. Factors that influence the probability of epidemics of western equine, St. Louis and California encephalitis in California. Vector News 14:13). (Continued)

3. Composition of host population as to:

    a. Age structure————————————— Physical examination to determine characteristics of size, sexual maturity, plumage, etc.

    b. Immunity status————————————— Serologic survey by HAI, neutralization, and/or CF tests of representative samples stratified as to age, sex, and geographic location

    c. Biotic potential————————————— Biologic observations of seasonal changes in abundance and age structure of population

    d. Attractiveness to vectors————————— Observations of vector attack and precipitin tests on engorged vector populations

    e. Occurrence of insusceptible hosts that may detract vectors and block transmission cycles ————— Correlations of antibody prevalence and knowledge of refractory status in vertebrate populations with vector activity

4. Habitats utilized

    a. Proximity to human populations————————— Observation and transect surveys

D. Human population

1. Abundance——————————————————— Census

2. Composition of population as to:

    a. Age and length of residence as related to clinical susceptibility ——— Epidemiologic evaluation of the age or length of residence, distribution of clinical cases, and age or residence adjusted rates

    b. Immunity status - natural or artificial————————— Serologic survey by HAI, neutralization, and/or CF of cross-section samples of total population

3. Vector exposure rate

    a. Habits
    b. Occupation
    c. Recreation
    d. Attractiveness to vectors
    e. Housing
    f. Encroachment on natural foci of infection

    Individual histories of vector attack
    Field observations of vector attack on humans
    Epidemiologic analyses of case distributions in population
    Epidemiologic analyses of antibody distribution in population
    Observation of standards of housing of cases and noncases

E. Environment

1. Temperature————————————————— U.S. Weather Bureau and special measurement in specific locations

    a. Influence on vector longevity————————— Correlation with changes in age structure of vector population

    b. Influence on frequency of vector refeeding————— Observation on changes in the physiological age structure of vector population and proportion of blood fed, gravid, and deplete specimens in the population

    c. Influence on extrinsic incubation of virus————— Correlation with changes in infection and transmission rates in vector populations and controlled laboratory experiments

    d. Influence on host exposure————————— Correlation with changes in vector population and vector attack rate on vertebrate hosts

2. Humidity

    a. Influence on vector longevity————————— As for temperature

3. Water — variations in excesses or deficiencies

    a. Vector breeding sources————————— Field survey and mapping on quantitative and qualitative bases

    b. Vertebrate host — nutritional————————— Observational

Fig. 4–6. Ecological factors in occurrence of epidemics of mosquito-born arbovirus encephalitis in North America (from Reeves, W.C. 1967. Factors that influence the probability of epidemics of western equine, St. Louis and California encephalitis in California. Vector News 14:13). (Continued)

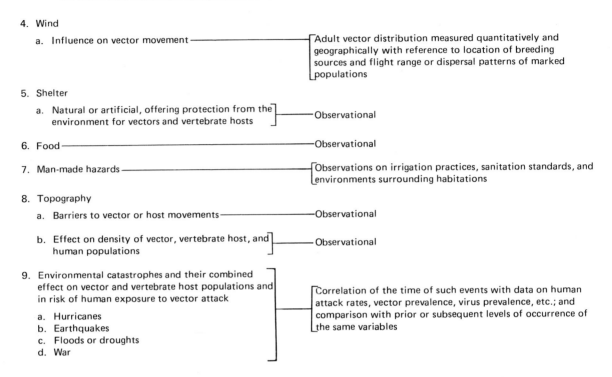

4. Wind
    a. Influence on vector movement ——————— Adult vector distribution measured quantitatively and geographically with reference to location of breeding sources and flight range or dispersal patterns of marked populations

5. Shelter
    a. Natural or artificial, offering protection from the environment for vectors and vertebrate hosts —— Observational

6. Food ————————————————————— Observational

7. Man-made hazards ——————————————— Observations on irrigation practices, sanitation standards, and environments surrounding habitations

8. Topography
    a. Barriers to vector or host movements ——————— Observational
    b. Effect on density of vector, vertebrate host, and human populations —— Observational

9. Environmental catastrophes and their combined effect on vector and vertebrate host populations and in risk of human exposure to vector attack
    a. Hurricanes
    b. Earthquakes
    c. Floods or droughts
    d. War
    —— Correlation of the time of such events with data on human attack rates, vector prevalence, virus prevalence, etc.; and comparison with prior or subsequent levels of occurrence of the same variables

being applied in one long-term study of the epidemiology of WE infection in Kern County in the southern part of the irrigated Central Valley of California.[19]

In this effort, mosquitoes, wild birds, and wild rodents are captured periodically. For census purposes, mosquitoes are trapped routinely in different localities with New Jersey light traps. Where virus isolations are to be attempted from mosquitoes, chick-baited and CO_2-baited funnel traps are also used at the same sites. Supplemental aspirator collections of mosquitoes are made in shelters. Virus infection rates are calculated per 1000 mosquitoes, and virus transmission rates to chicks also per 1000 mosquitoes. Census data for mosquitoes are calculated as average numbers caught per trap-night; and the number of mosquitoes and the date are recorded for different areas for the highest trap-night in stated time intervals.

Birds are collected in grain-baited ground traps and with Japanese mist nets strung in fly-paths. These birds are identified, bled, banded, and released. Recapture rates are calculated for census estimates. In addition, a bird census is made during the nesting season at selected sites. Virus isolations and viremia rates are determined, as well as rates for serologically positive birds.

Rodents are trapped in one large grid area and also in other selected areas using lines of Sherman traps at 8-meter intervals. Wire box traps are used for large rodents. Lagomorphs are shot. Recapture rates and population estimates are calculated, as are virus isolation and seropositive rates.

All of these captured animals are identified according to species, and the feeding hosts of vectors determined by examining blood meals in vectors by the precipitin test. Closely related mosquito hosts (e.g., hares and rabbits) are differentiated using a microcomplement fixation test for blood.

Studies are also carried out on flight ranges of potential vectors and on other appropriate aspects of vector biology. For the former, live-trapped mosquitoes and laboratory-reared mosquitoes are identified with different-colored dusts and released at predetermined points. Recoveries are made in light traps at varying distances from the release sites. Other flight habits are studied using truck-mounted funnel traps to collect mosquitoes at different time intervals throughout the night and day. Correlations with the census data are calculated for humidity, moonlight, and other environmental factors.

Also of interest are the rates of egg production in female mosquitoes that have not taken a blood meal (i.e., their autogenous rates). *Culex tarsalis* aspirated from shelters are dissected and classified as engorged (i.e., with any blood), gravid (i.e., without blood but with eggs), and deplete (i.e., with neither). For gravid mosquitoes, the ovaries are also dissected and the egg stage determined using the Christopher scale.

Flocks of sentinel chickens are established at selected sites. Each bird is bled monthly and its immunological conversion rate calculated. Serological tests also are performed on all clinically suspect horses. These same procedures are applied to all human cases from the study area; and, in addition, paired serum samples are examined serologically for special groups of school children. Virus isolations are attempted from poikilothermic vertebrates.

All of these animal data are related, where possible, to observations on patterns of vegetation cover and land use, as well as to observations on climate. These latter include such measurements as mountain snowpack, precipitation total, average precipitation departure from normal, water flow rate in the Kern River,

extent of flooding, daily minimum and maximum temperature, average of day's temperature departure from normal, days above 100°F., and humidity. The complexity of such multifaceted studies should be apparent.

In studying the epidemiology of a particular infection such as WE, specific problems may assume great importance. One such problem for WE has been the nature of the virus' year-round reservoirs, or its overwintering mechanism, in temperate areas. This subject has been investigated extensively for WE, but without a consensus. The currently considered mechanisms by which this infection may persist from one summer epidemic period to the next are shown diagrammatically in Figure 4–7.

Transovarian transmission of WE virus in its usual mosquito hosts seems not to occur; and, although the virus has been isolated from some wild-caught *C. tarsalis* every month of the year in California and Colorado, the infrequency of isolations during the

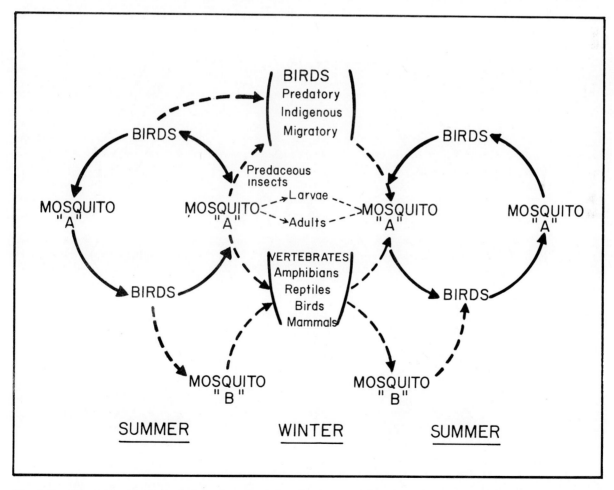

Fig. 4–7. Some hypothetical chains of transmission in the overwintering of arboviruses (redrawn from Hess, A.D., and Hayes, R.O. 1967. Seasonal dynamics of western encephalitis virus. Am. J. Med. Sci. 253:333).

winter months suggests its improbability as the usual overwintering mechanism. Most of these few over-wintering adults seem not to have taken a blood meal. Blood-feeding by mosquitoes also occurs at a very low rate during the winter months.

Reintroduction of virus by migrating birds is another possibility, but data on actual WE introductions from South America are lacking. Some evidence exists that virus may be maintained locally in chronically infected nonmigrating birds. Infection of rodents in endemic areas has been suggested as a conceivable mechanism, and WE virus has been isolated from both rodents and lagomorphs in the United States and Canada during the winter time. Rodent infections during the summer seem to occur largely as a "spill-over," as do horse and human infections, and they are thought generally to be symptomatic. Poikilothermic vertebrates also have been examined to some extent; and there are reports

from Utah and Saskatchewan of WE virus isolations from snakes (including newborn snakes) and frogs. The question of winter reservoirs is not a simple one; and further study in a variety of locales will probably be required to answer it fully.

These virtually endless epidemiological possibilities posed by ecologically complex diseases in nature may be illustrated further by reference to what is unquestionably the most complicated infectious cycle yet described. The complexities of salmon poisoning disease of dogs (Fig. 4–8) clearly indicate the constant need for epidemiologists to consider all possibilities and the fullest range of explanations for their observations.

Salmon poisoning disease of dogs

This disease was described in dogs in western Oregon and adjacent areas of northwestern California and southwestern Washington at the time the first

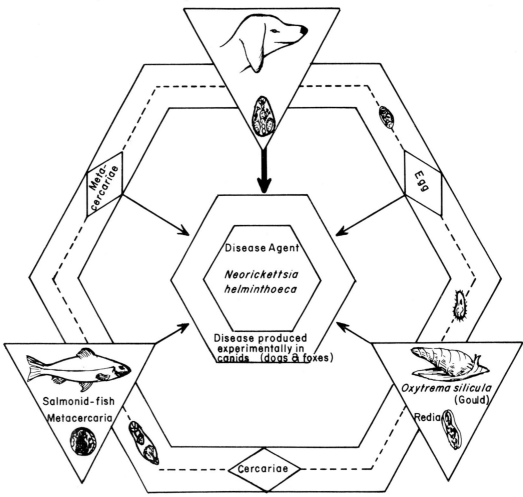

Fig. 4–8. Transmission cycle of *Nanophyetus salmincola* showing that disease agent (*Neorickettsia helminthoeca*) in infectious state for canids is present in all stages of trematode vector (redrawn from Knapp, S.E., and Millemann, R.E. 1970. Salmon Poisoning Diseases. *In* Infectious Diseases of Wild Mammals. Davis, J.W., Karstad, L.H., and Trainer, D.O. (Eds.). Iowa State University Press, Ames).

European settlers arrived. The report in 1853-55 of a survey crew for a railroad from the Mississippi River to the Pacific suggested that the disease might be a form of canine distemper. However, its association with eating raw salmon had been noted as early as 1849; and early explorers also reported that, while wild canids such as coyotes and wolves were prevalent in eastern Oregon, both species were oddly absent west of the Cascade Range.

The onset of this disease in individual dogs is marked by a sudden complete loss of appetite accompanied by a temperature rise to anywhere from 39.5 to 42°C. The animal becomes lassitudinous by the second day and develops great thirst. Vomiting usually follows drinking. On the third or fourth day, the body temperature begins to fall, and a purulent ocular discharge may be noted. Initial constipation leads to soft stools containing mucus, followed by bloody diarrhea. Dehydration and loss of weight are appreciable. Death or beginning recovery usually occurs about 10 days to two weeks following onset of symptoms. Pathologic changes include intestinal mucosal lesions, edema and hyperplasia of lymphoid tissues, and sometimes meningitic or encephalo-meningitic lesions.

The studies that led to understanding of the intriguing epidemiological intricacies of salmon poisoning disease were begun by D.R. Donham, in association with B.T. Simms and colleagues, in 1924, and were carried out over the next five or six years. They are an epidemiological classic. The key initial observation was that of Donham, who noted the presence of small intestinal trematodes in all dogs dying of salmon poisoning disease. Encysted metacercariae of this fluke, now known as *Nanophyetus salmincola*, were subsequently found in Oregon salmon and trout; and the disease was produced in dogs by feeding them this parasite dissected from infected fish.

However, despite this demonstration of the causative role of a fluke, Simms and Donham were not prepared—on the basis of the major symptoms, the acute systemic course of the disease, and the development of marked immunity in recovered animals—to ascribe the etiology of clinical salmon poisoning disease to the fluke *per se*. On the other hand, they found that, although the disease could also be produced experimentally by injecting ground-up flukes and metacercariae intraperitoneally into dogs, all their attempts to identify or isolate a bacterium or other microbial agent were unsuccessful. They concluded that the specific pathogen was an unknown infectious microorganism for which the fluke served as the vector.[20]

This initial group of workers also confirmed the unusually restricted geographic distribution of the clinical disease; and they and Cram showed that the adult fluke, *Nanophyetus salmincola*, occurred naturally in other local fish-eating carnivores such as coyotes, bobcats, raccoons, and mink. They found, too, that the first intermediate host of the vector fluke was a freshwater snail, *Oxytrema silicula*, and that the snail's distribution was limited to that of the clinical disease in dogs, and further that this snail's range explained the peculiar and restricted geographic localization of salmon poisoning disease.

The second intermediate host of the vector fluke was found to be any of a considerable variety of Salmonidae that spawn in the rivers and streams of the endemic area. However, Simms and Donham failed to find metacercariae in these fish caught in the open sea; therefore, they did not believe that the fluke infection in fish survived their prolonged life in the marine environment.

Subsequently, other workers have filled in the following additional details about the epidemiology of salmon poisoning disease.[21] The specific infectious agent is now known to be a rickettsia, *Neorickettsia helminthoeca*; and, as mentioned earlier, its discovery was responsible for modification of the accepted definition of rickettsiae from "arthropod-transmitted" to "invertebrate-transmitted" microorganisms. Now it has been demonstrated not only in dogs and in the adult flukes, but also in the eggs, snail liver stages (sporocysts and rediae), and metacercariae of the fluke.

In addition to Salmonid fish, naturally infected second intermediate hosts of the vector fluke include several other fish, as well as the Pacific giant salamander, *Dicamptodon ensatus*. Metacercariae of the vector fluke and the rickettsial agent do survive in fish in a marine ecosystem for up to three years; and dogs that eat fish returning from their long voyage at sea develop the disease. A number of fish-eating mammals and even some birds naturally harbor the adult fluke; but raccoons are the only noncanids that, in experiments, have developed even mild signs (fever) of the rickettsial infection.

Interestingly, in Siberia, man and other animals are infected with adults of *Nanophyetus schikhobalowi*, thought to be a synonym of *N. salmincola*; but salmon poisoning disease has not been reported. In an experimental infection in the United States, a human volunteer was successfully infected with *N. salmincola*, containing *N. helminthoeca*. The fluke developed to maturity and produced eggs, but there were no signs or symptoms of the rickettsial infection.

In summary, salmon poisoning disease is now known to be a rickettsial disease limited to canids. The vector is a parasitic trematode, which matures in a variety of mammals and birds, has one particular freshwater snail as its first intermediate host, and has various fish and a salamander as possible second intermediate hosts. The rickettsia passes transovarially and transstadially through the egg, free-swimming miracidium, sporocyst, redia, free-swimming cercaria, and metacercaria. Some species of second intermediate hosts of the infected vector migrate from fresh water to the open sea for a period of several years, returning to fresh water again to spawn and serve as the immediate source of infection for susceptible dogs. The geographically restricting link in this complicated cycle is the snail. The various statistical probabilities represented in the transmission of a minimal infective dose of these rickettsiae from one infected dog to another susceptible dog virtually defy comprehension.[22]

In this last example of the ecological complexity of some infections, further evidence is presented to convince students of diseases that they must keep a completely open mind to *all* new possibilities about "well-known" diseases.

Vesicular exanthema of swine and marine animals

In 1971, about 500 dead sea lions (*Zalophus californianus*) were found along California beaches. Investigation of this epidemic attributed these losses to leptospirosis. Further investigations of abortions in sea lions on off-shore islands resulted in isolation of a virus from sea lions and northern fur seals (*Callorhinus ursinus*), designated San Miguel Sea Lion Virus. Further virus isolations were made from seals in the seal-breeding Pribilof Islands in the Bering Sea. Its subsequent characterization indicates that this virus is indistinguishable from and probably a variant of that of vesicular exanthema of swine, the only infection thought to have been eradicated globally through man's efforts. The new isolate produces typical vesicular exanthema in exposed swine; and it has been speculated that the peculiarly erratic epidemiological history of vesicular exanthema in California between 1932 and 1952 resulted from sea lion carcasses fed to swine or even from presence of this virus in marine food scraps from seafood restaurants, a common denominator on the hog ranches in the first three California outbreaks in 1932.

To recapitulate briefly the 1932-1959 history of this infection,[23] vesicular exanthema was an unknown disease until April 22, 1932, when the owner of a garbage-feeding hog ranch in Orange County, California, informed the Los Angeles County Livestock Department of the widespread occurrence of lameness among the 3600 hogs on his ranch. Upon investigation, Department veterinarians found that lame hogs were distributed in practically every pen and that four affected animals had died. The condition was characterized by swollen joints, tenderness of foot pads, and ruptured vesicles on the feet. Because of the close resemblance of this condition to foot-and-mouth disease, the premises were imme-

diately quarantined and the Chief of the U.S. Bureau of Animal Industry notified.

During the next two weeks the same condition was observed in 37 other swine herds in three California counties, all within a radius of 50 miles. In order to confirm the suspected diagnosis, cattle, horses, guinea pigs, and swine were all inoculated with vesicle material, but only the inoculated swine became ill. Because the inoculated horses failed to show signs of infection, vesicular stomatitis was ruled out as a possible diagnosis, and the condition was tentatively diagnosed as an atypical form of foot-and-mouth disease. Although all four of the inoculated species are ordinarily susceptible to foot-and-mouth disease virus, public announcement of a foot-and-mouth disease outbreak was made on April 28.

Eradication measures were promptly initiated. In all, 18,799 cloven-hoofed animals were slaughtered, and all infected premises were thoroughly disinfected before restocking was permitted. The cost of this operation was about $280,000. No further cases were seen until about one year later when another outbreak of vesicular disease occurred in swine in San Diego County, about 100 miles south of the previous year's epidemic. Again, inoculated cattle, horses, and guinea pigs failed to become infected. Samples of the virus were sent to Washington and to Germany; on the basis of studies there, it was concluded that the infective agent differed from any of the known strains of foot-and-mouth disease virus. Dr. Jacob Traum proposed the name "vesicular exanthema" to designate the new disease.

For various politico-economic reasons, a program of eradication by slaughter was not instituted. Although infected premises were all strictly quarantined and every effort made to prevent the infection from spreading, a severe outbreak occurred in June, 1934, on a garbage-feeding ranch about 500 miles to the north of San Diego in San Jose, California. Extensive investigation revealed no contact between this ranch and the previously infected premises. Despite further efforts to confine it, the infection popped up again during the next three months on 27 other ranches in five counties of central California and on four ranches 400 miles to the south.

Although sporadic outbreaks of vesicular exanthema continued in California swine through 1935 and 1936, the infection seemingly disappeared in 1937, only to appear again in December, 1939. At that time it spread rapidly through the garbage-feeding ranches in northern California. Within six months about one-fourth of the state's swine population was involved.

Widespread outbreaks continued thereafter; but for over 20 years they were all confined within the state of California. During that period two unsuccessful efforts were made to eradicate the infection by slaughter. In addition, since all outbreaks were associated with garbage-feeding, a bill was presented to the California state legislature in 1941 to require cooking of all garbage fed to swine. It failed to pass.

From 1941 until 1952, the infection remained confined to California except for outbreaks in butcher hogs in the port of Honolulu in December, 1946, and November, 1947. These were discovered in quarantine and the infected animals returned to San Francisco. On June 11, 1952, however, the infection was diagnosed in a group of pigs owned by a biological manufacturing company in Grand Island, Nebraska. The infection was found to have originated among swine from Cheyenne, Wyoming, which were fed raw garbage from transcontinental trains coming from San Francisco. Other hogs from this exposed population had already been shipped from Cheyenne to several stockyards and distribution centers before this discovery was made; and, by July 11, infected pigs had been reported in 14 states from New Jersey to Alabama, Texas, and Washington.

Under a B.A.I. order issued in Washington on July 29, 1952, the state of California and counties in a number of other states were quarantined. From them, all interstate traffic in swine was halted except under special permit for immediate slaughter and processing. On July 31, this quarantine was extended to 19 states.

The infection continued to spread and in August the U.S. Secretary of Agriculture declared a national emergency in order to provide federal support to efforts to eradicate the infection by slaughter. Over 100,000 hogs in 22 states were killed and buried or slaughtered and processed at a cost of more than $3 million dollars. Although efforts were made to encourage the cooking of garbage fed to swine, the measures employed were insufficient to stop the further spread of the disease; and, by September, 1953, infected swine had been reported in 42 states and the District of Columbia.

Under B.A.I. order 308 of June 30, 1953, all swine fed raw garbage and all products of garbage-fed swine were placed under federal interstate quarantine. With out-of-state markets for garbage-fed swine closed, one state legislature after another quickly passed the necessary legislation to require garbage cooking. The technical and regulatory machinery was quickly set up to assure compliance. By September, 1953, 46 states had enacted such laws; and the last two states to comply, New Jersey and Connecticut, finally succumbed in 1958 and 1960.

By 1955, however, new epizootics had already ceased to occur; and, with the exception of continually infected premises in New Jersey through 1956, the disease was being brought under effective control. A second occurrence of the disease outside the continental United States took place in 1955 in swine in Hrafnarfjord, Iceland. This outbreak among swine that had been fed garbage from an American military base was quickly stamped out. On January 1, 1958, no cases were known to exist in the United States or elsewhere; and on October 22, 1959, the U.S. Secretary of Agriculture announced that vesicular exanthema had been eradicated.

The possibility now exists that vesicular exanthema was caused by a virus adapted to marine mammals and subsequently introduced into a domestic terrestrial species. The implications to livestock and human health generally of present knowledge of vesicular exanthema and salmon poisoning disease—with intriguing possibilities that marine animals, including poikilotherms, could be involved in a *number* of infectious cycles that also involve terrestrial species—is very interesting epidemiologically though frightening medically.

METHODS DEVELOPED BY MEDICAL ECOLOGISTS FOR DIRECTED ACTIONS AGAINST DISEASES

The general concepts of disease prevention, control, and eradication were discussed in Chapter 3. In addition to the specific methods for combatting herd disease considered in that chapter, several other methods became available with the discovery of the epidemiological roles of reservoir hosts and of vectors and with accumulated knowledge of parasitism in general. These advances include the essentially ecological methods of *vector control, reservoir control, disease control in the reservoir,* and *biological control.*

Vector control

Recognition of invertebrate carriers of vertebrate diseases immediately suggested a novel alternative method to combat such infections. Not only might measures be directed toward the infection in the vertebrate host itself or toward its physical environment, but also a third possibility existed. The first person to recognize the possible vulnerability of this phase of a parasite's transmission cycle was Cooper Curtice of the U.S. Bureau of Animal Industry. He proposed that bovine piroplasmosis, for which there was no available drug or vaccine, be attacked through its single-host tick vector, *Boophilus annulatus.* Beginning in 1906, Curtice designed and directed a vector control program against this disease in North Carolina. It was an unqualified success.[24] Subsequently, development of larvicides and, later, residual adulticides enabled this same approach to be applied to control of flying vectors of infections, such as urban yellow fever, malaria, trypanosomiasis, and the viral encephalitides, as well as to the nonflying vectors of typhus fever and other diseases.

As with control measures directed toward the physical environment of a population, some vector control measures can be carried out without handling or doing anything to the susceptible or affected animal population directly. This type of control is often an advantage.

Disease control in the reservoir host

If the animal species of greatest concern does not itself serve as a reservoir of a particular infection to which it is susceptible, then there is another control alternative, namely, disease control *in* the reservoir host. This approach has been directed most often and most successfully to the control of human infections with various zoonotic organisms. The first such large-scale efforts were begun in the United States against glanders in horses in 1888 and tuberculosis in cattle in 1906. This latter program was extended to a national scale in 1917.

Subsequently, similar measures were undertaken in the United States and other countries against brucellosis and other zoonoses. Most of these infections constituted important economic problems in the food animal species itself, in addition to their public health importance.

Following World War II, this approach was also successfully focused upon human rabies in the United States where canine infections were prevented through a mass immunization campaign involving cooperative clinics run by private veterinary practitioners. Dogs acted as the principal transmitting link between the wild reservoir hosts of rabies virus and man.

These types of zoonoses control efforts, resulting in the virtual disappearance of human diseases such as nonpulmonary tuberculosis and glanders from a number of countries and marked reductions in the incidence of infections such as human brucellosis and rabies, have been among the most important legacies of veterinary medicine to human health. A related veterinary approach to prevention of human diseases has been the exclusion of infected animals as human food. Beginning about 1868, this method was successfully applied in Europe against trichinosis.

Reservoir control

The approach outlined previously has been practically limited to infections with their reservoirs in domestic animal species. Wild animal reservoirs present the additional complications of accessibility and approach. Depopulation of wild vertebrate reservoir hosts has been a method resorted to with some success, particularly when the reservoir was recognized as a species with little or no value. Thus, rat control by trapping and poisoning has been an important feature, for example, of efforts against urban plague. Occasionally, valuable wild species have had to be decimated to combat particularly important diseases.

A novel method using this approach has been applied recently against vampire bat reservoirs of rabies in Latin America. Anticoagulants mixed with petroleum jelly are applied to the backs of captured bats, which are then released. When these return to their colonies, they are groomed by many individual bats, each of which usually ingests enough of the anticoagulant to kill it. This highly effective approach takes unusual advantage of knowledge of the reservoir host's physiology and behavior.

Biological control

This control method depends upon making use of natural enemies of parasites, vectors, or vertebrate reservoirs. It was first applied successfully in the field of entomology, and overlaps several of the disease control approaches already discussed in this chapter and in Chapter 3. It is a rational, applied ecological approach designed to make use of natural predators and parasites to control unwanted species. Although inherently attractive, it has seldom if ever been applied with any practical success to control of vertebrate diseases, but it has been used against various pest species *per se*. One such special use, that of myxomatosis virus against rabbit pests in Australia, is well known.

Disease pressure and predator pressure on a reservoir or vector species may be interrelated in epidemiologically important ways, as suggested from the interesting data on hare and vole populations shown in Figure 4–9 and Table 4–3.

A related idea of interfering with the reproductive cycle of parasitic or vector arthropods was developed as a measure to combat screwworm disease of cattle and other livestock. Here, male flies raised in large numbers in captivity are sterilized by radiation and then released into the environment. By this approach, screwworms have been eliminated from most of their host range in the United States. Research on this technique and similar use of chemosterilants and pheromones is now being focused upon other insects of medical importance.

The wide range of potentially useful ecological concepts and methods available to the epidemiologist can be no more than touched upon in this chapter. Much ecological research today involves quantitative studies that make use of some of the mathematical concepts of design and analysis introduced in the following chapter. In many epidemiological studies today, these sometimes separate schools of former years are melded.

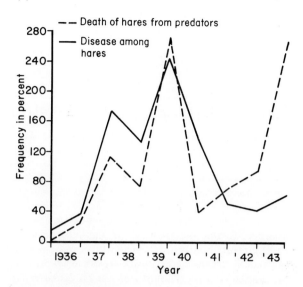

Fig. 4–9. Frequency of successful predation on vary-ing hares (*Lepus timidus*) in relation to fre-quency of hare diseases in northern and eastern regions of European USSR (re-drawn from Naumov, N.P. 1972. *The Ecol-ogy of Animals*. University of Illinois Press, Urbana).

Table 4–3.   Condition of Common Voles Caught in Belovega Virgin Forest by Hawks Versus Condition of Population as a Whole (modified from Naumov, N. P. 1972. *Ecology of Animals*. University of Illinois Press, Urbana; after Folitarek, 1948)

State	Caught by hawks (%)	Natural population (%)
Infected with parasitic worms	34.5	17.1
Internal organs congested	2.2	–
Pathological changes in liver	20.7	7.9
Pathological changes in spleen	56.3	30.3

Chapter 5

THE MATHEMATICAL APPROACH

THE newest school of epidemiology is the biostatistical or mathematical. Its development, mostly in the past 30 years, has been spurred by frustratingly slow progress in identifying the causes of a large number of human degenerative diseases. However, its applications already are far wider; and, to veterinarians, it offers useful techniques for many aspects of public and private practice.

A mathematical approach to epidemiology provides students of disease with several broad classes of investigative procedures. These include methods for (1) designing and conducting studies; (2) developing and presenting data; and (3) analyzing data to make comparisons, determine associations, interpret results, and draw inferences or conclusions. Since many of these techniques also are applicable to veterinary research generally, *every* practitioner of veterinary medicine needs to understand at least enough statistics to be able to interpret papers that appear in veterinary and other medical journals. Beyond that level, most veterinary practitioners will have many occasions to use mathematical tools to help them understand the causes and behavior of diseases or to attempt their control. For most such efforts, veterinarians will also want to know when to seek the assistance of a biostatistician.

METHODS FOR DESIGNING AND CONDUCTING EPIDEMIOLOGICAL STUDIES

Epidemiology, even in its practice applications, is essentially an investigative or research discipline. Epidemiological investigations are conducted in diverse ways, a number of which are illustrated throughout this book. An awareness of this diversity and of the different designs that are useful for epidemiological studies is a prerequisite to selecting and evaluating appropriate statistical procedures for practice purposes.

Descriptive studies

As indicated in Chapter 1, descriptive studies are carried out in epidemiology to indicate what is happening, i.e., to describe the state of nature in some place and at some point or interval of time. On the one hand, such studies may call attention to an unusual finding or an interesting group of animals; more often, they provide data about phenomena that were not well described previously. Examples would include the initial identification of chlamydial polyarthritis in a foal, the prevalence of complement fixing antibodies to *Anaplasma marginale* in hunter-killed deer from a 5000-acre area of the coastal mountains of California, or the description of an outbreak of trichinosis in a cattery. Results of such descriptive studies show the existence, distribution, or other characteristics of selected phenomena; but no comparative analyses are attempted. Frequently, however, they stimulate subsequent analytic research.

Analytical studies

The principal ingredient lacking in most descriptive studies but basic to epidemiological studies to be subjected to mathematical analysis is *comparison*. The design of such analytical studies can be outlined in the question: What *group* of individuals has received what *maneuver* to achieve what *response*? In this context, the word maneuver refers to the principal factor whose effects are to be noted. The maneuver may be a suspected determinant of disease (e.g., a weather variable, a nutrient, a socioeconomic condition, or a concurrent disease), a mode of therapy, or some other factor. For example, "leg weakness" of turkeys may be studied to see whether it is caused by deficiency of a dietary factor, prevented or exacerbated by antibiotic therapy, or alleviated by a particular change in housing, caging, or rearing practices. It should be noted that the maneuver can be the result of self-selection (e.g., by the animal patient or by the owner), or the result of preplanned assignment. This outline of *group*, *maneuver*, and *response*, which is a generalization of population, determinant, and disease, has been used in discussing the elements of study design in the sections that follow.[1]

In a clinical trial or other prospective epidemiological *experiment* involving a series or population sample of animals, the investigator chooses and assigns the maneuvers to which each experimental subject is exposed. Clinical trials, as the name implies, are planned tests of intervention in a disease process involving therapeutic or prophylactic maneuvers. Other types of field experiments include studies performed to explain causal or other biological mechanisms in groups of animals, to test veterinary services delivery, and the like. Such field experiments require at least two groups of animals for, as already stated, the essence of all such experimentation lies in comparison. In any good experiment, every effort is made to ensure that, prior to any maneuver, all groups to be compared will be as nearly alike as possible.

In contrast, in a retrospective study, the maneuvers under study were self-selected by the animal (or were assigned by someone else, usually an animal attendant, the animal's owner, or a veterinarian). Self-selection may include diverse notions. An animal may choose to eat or not eat the feed supplement that later was found to contain the organism responsible for its intestinal illness or death. The hired hand may feed all the chickens on the north tier from sacks two and three, and those on the south tier from sacks one and four, in spite of the specific directions to mix all feeds and feed this ration to all birds on all tiers. Finally, self-selection may involve the housing location of an animal or the use to which it (the house *or* the animal) is put.

Retrospective observational studies also may have etiologic, therapeutic, or other objectives. Etiologic or diagnostic observational studies are conducted to ascertain possible associations of disease and suspected causal determinants, and, like experiments, are quintessentially comparative. Therapeutic surveys are sometimes performed to collect results from use of drugs or other factors that have been assigned *ad hoc* for prophylactic or remedial purposes. Other types of retrospective studies of particular interest to epidemiologists may include such things as comparisons of neonatal mortality rates among dairy calves on farms of different sizes, comparisons of the same rates among calves on the same group of farms at different temporal eras, or the detection of risk factors or prognostic indicators associated with different mortality levels in the groups under investigation.

Statistics play a major role in the types of comparison studies described. Thus, any discussion of the elements of epidemiological research design includes statistical concepts and/or terminology and pertains equally to prospective studies or retrospective studies (see also Chapters 11 and 12). This discussion is organized with respect to the *group-maneuver-response* triad of research design.

Groups

The groups one forms in conducting epidemiological studies depend on (1) admission criteria, (2) allocation, (3) stratification, (4) chronologic tactics, and (5) various sources of bias. Naturally, each of these factors should be considered in detail *before* groups are formed, as well as when one interprets the results of the completed research. Later on, critical readers will note resemblances between admission criteria/allocation, allocation/stratification, and chronological tactics in forming groups and factors, dosage, and timing in maneuvers. These similarities are not entirely fortuitous, but serve to emphasize the principle that, under practical circumstances, no aspect of study design and performance should be considered without reference to other aspects.

The target population, or population at risk, is, by definition, the population of interest, which by the very nature of many epidemiological studies cannot be studied in its entirety. The group(s) studied may be samples from this target population. If so, they must be statistically acceptable samples. The *admission criteria* must specify the particular conditions of age, climate, disease, or other relevant factors (including such things as costs, availability, response, and measurement) by which subjects (e.g., animals, herds, geographic entities) are included in the groups under investigation. The relationship of these groups to the target population should be detailed.

Allocation refers to the formation of the groups relative to how the maneuvers are assigned. Allocation may be the result of self-selection, clinical judgment, randomization, or other activities. The type of allocation may be related to the type of study being conducted, e.g., some form of ramdomization in prospective experimentation, or some form of self-selection in retrospective studies. Problems in allocation are discussed further under the section on bias.

Attempts to increase precision in studies, by avoiding or reducing bias through reducing the degree of heterogeneity in the groups being compared, are referred to collectively as *stratification*. If the epidemiologist has sufficient knowledge of the population at risk, he may be able to divide it into well-defined subgroups or strata, and then draw a probability sample from each stratum. In epidemiological research, stratification sometimes takes the form of medical studies of pure-disease groups, using limited numbers of such groups. The comparison of results in a study employing stratification may be carried out in matched pairs or in subgroups of these homogeneous strata. Strata may also be selected prognostically, defining them as groups having distinctively different degrees of risk for the particular outcome event of interest, e.g., newly diagnosed cases of bovine leukemia (recent onset) versus newly diagnosed cases of bovine leukemia (delayed recognition).

Chronological tactics require decisions concerning whether the study will be conducted longitudinally or cross-sectionally. The purpose of longitudinal studies is to determine the association, if any, between an antecedent condition or event and a subsequent effect. Longitudinal studies may be conducted prospectively (using cohort groups, Chapter 12) or retrospectively (using case-control groups, Chapter 11). Cross-sectional studies are used to examine for associations between two or more entities noted concomitantly, one such example being a study of the relation of serum cholesterol and hematocrit in a group of canine patients with anemia. An additional, and obvious, chronological tactic is to decide what duration of study will be used, e.g., how long cohorts are to be followed or how far into the past one will search for the suspected antecedent condition or event.

Sources of bias in groups are manifold, but may be broadly classified as selection bias or chronological bias. *Selection bias* occurs most commonly in the mental transfer of an individual from the general population to the target or risk population to a particular group actually under investigation. In forming these latter groups, one must decide whether to select them by random samples as opposed to convenience samples, volunteer samples, pure-disease samples, or compliance samples. Following are examples of selection bias.

(1) Animal patients brought to the Veterinary Medical Teaching Hospital of the University of California (e.g., many referral patients attracted by clinical specialists) may not be at all representative of patients brought to private clinical facilities, which, in turn, may not resemble potential patients that never or seldom are seen by the veterinary practitioners.

(2) Dogs brought to one hospital in Yolo County during 1970 may have been of different breed-sex-age backgrounds than those licensed in Yolo County that year, and also may have differed from the actual dog population of Yolo County in 1970.

(3) Animal patients that are volunteered for a study by their owners may differ in many ways from the general animal population.

(4) The use of a pure-disease group of patients, excluding patients with co-morbid diseases, may produce a group that does not properly represent the disease as usually seen.

(5) People (owners of animals) able to comply with complex experimental protocols may differ from the noncompliers, who are omitted from epidemiological studies. Selection bias can be produced easily when maneuvers are self-selected or judgmentally assigned rather than randomly allocated.

Chronological bias, on the other hand, may be due to (1) the effect of dropouts or other losses from cohort studies, (2) the effect of losses of original cohort from the survivors studied in cross-sectional and retrospective studies, or (3) longitudinal cross-sections. These latter studies are cross-sections taken at different points in time, giving the illusion of a cohort follow-up study. For example, in certain cross-sectional studies, a particular type of heart disease in dogs may be found to have a much higher prevalence among patients with recurrences of a well-known infection than among patients that were initially free of it. However, in cohort studies, it may be found that recurrent attacks of this infection are particularly likely to develop in dogs that have already acquired the special type of heart disease in their first attack.

SAMPLING. The sampling of target populations to form study groups is often a necessity in veterinary studies or may be desirable for reasons of cost or for other reasons. Although the general subject of sampling is considered in elementary statistics courses, its epidemiological importance recommends specific consideration here, particularly with respect to alternative approaches to sampling and methods for determination of sample size.

As stated earlier, a useful, but not all-inclusive, distinction in kinds of epidemiological investigations is that of experiments versus observational studies or studies using extant data. As epidemiologists constantly study samples of larger populations, they may deliberately draw a sample from such a larger population. In conducting observational studies, they examine the state of nature as it exists, and look for meaningful associations or differences. In experiments, on the other hand, they control events and populations under investigation. Epidemiological investigations may often incorporate both approaches to solving real problems in veterinary medicine. Then, the relevance of the terms "experiment" and "observation" lies in the sources of error in these epidemiological studies.

Internal validity in an experimental study can usually be improved by strictly controlling the factors in that experiment. Unfortunately, strictly controlled experiments may tend to be artificial and thereby decrease the likelihood that the results obtained can be generalized to the real, less-controlled world. Observational surveys, on the other hand, may provide eminently generalizable results; but the design of some surveys may be so uncontrolled that innumerable alternative interpretations of the results can be made.

The design of research, or the *research protocol*, is the plan the epidemiologist will follow to collect the appropriate data and to control as many sources of error as possible. The epidemiologist's primary interest lies in the *variation* in the variable(s) being measured, as he attempts to understand how the various elements being studied contribute to that variation. The epidemiologist also tries to eliminate or control variation due to extraneous or confounding factors.

Randomization, one of the usual techniques for controlling extraneous variation, plays an important role in experiments as well as in observational surveys. For example, in therapeutic experiments, randomly assigning individuals to treatment groups is an attempt to have the groups be as similar as possible, except for the single factor of treatment. Failing to randomize produces unknown bias in samples and is a leading source of error in epidemiological research. The principles of randomization apply throughout all aspects of research, e.g., assigning experimental subjects to treatment groups, assigning observers to evaluate the outcome of experimental treatments, assigning days for taking certain measurements on the experimental subjects, and determining any other factors in the study design that could conceivably affect the outcome.

It will be useful to consider randomization further relative to sampling surveys, keeping in mind that an outbreak investigation, in some aspects, may resemble a sample survey. In sample surveys, epidemiologists intentionally examine less-than-all of a population of interest; yet, in such sampling, they introduce sampling error. However, by careful study of this smaller sample, they can often attain great precision by careful attention to each datum collected.

Random sampling is a procedure for selecting individuals from the population in such a way that each individual has a known chance of being selected in the sample. If each individual, as well as each combination of individuals, has an equal chance of being selected, the scheme is known as *simple random sampling*. It should be noted that simple random sampling is not a technique for controlling all aspects of the factors under study; it simply controls bias in the way individuals are selected. Random sampling numbers (tables of random digits) provide a basic process for simple random sampling.

If groups within the population under study are known to vary widely in their relevant characteristics, random sampling schemes other than simple random sampling should be used. In one such procedure, the population is first divided into these relevant groups, or *strata*, and an appropriate random sample is drawn from each stratum. Such *stratified random sampling* can be used to assure that the sample contains representatives from each of the strata. This stratification is dependent upon the variation within strata being less than that within the entire population. Otherwise, there is no reason for stratification prior to sampling.

Other kinds of subdivisions also can occur. Suppose the epidemiologist is interested in knowing the number of admissions for fractures of the leg (or legs) in all canine patients entering veterinary hospitals in a given month in Washington, Oregon, and California. It would be difficult to sample the population of patients directly. However, it would be a simple matter to list the counties of the three-state area, and draw a random sample of counties. Within this sample of counties, one could form a list of animal hospitals and draw a random sample from this list. Such a procedure is known as *sampling by stages*. It should be kept in mind that the canine populations (or human populations) would not be the same for all counties in the example cited. Sampling the counties with probabilities of selection being proportional to their resident populations would be a reasonable strategy. In the absence of reliable data on canine populations, the human population at the last decennial census might be used as a reasonable alternative for identifying selection probabilities. However, in so doing, the epidemiologist may be guilty of the substitution fallacy mentioned elsewhere.

To illustrate two-stage sampling, suppose that there are seven counties (Allegan, Bravo, Chippewa, Delta, Eureka, Foster, and Granite) with populations of 1, 6, 3, 4, 2, 1, and 4 tens of thousands of dogs, respectively, and one wants to sample two counties. First, assign 1, 2, 3, . . . 21 to these tens of thousands of dogs, giving 1 to Allegan, the next 6 (2, 3, . . . 7) to Bravo, etc.:

County	A	B	C	D	E	F	G
Size	1	6	3	4	2	1	4
Tags	1	2,3,4 5,6,7	8,9 10	11,12 13,14	15,16	17	18,19 20,21

Now select two numbers randomly from 1, 2, . . . 21, taking as the counties those for which the randomly chosen numbers were tags. If the randomly chosen numbers were 4 and 17, choose Bravo and Foster counties. (If the two numbers chosen had been tags for the same county, choose additional numbers until one is a tag for a different county than any county already chosen.) The second sampling stage now consists of listing the animal hospitals in Bravo and Foster counties, and randomly sampling from this list.

The procedure described for two-stage random sampling can be extended to multistage sampling. Furthermore, in sampling by stages, it may be appropriate to introduce stratification at one or more stages. For example, in the situation just given, one might consider stratification of animal hospitals (e.g., companion animal, mixed practice, or feline specialty).

There are numerous varieties of random sampling. For example, a sample that systematically draws every sixth individual on a list after a random start (i.e., toss of a fair die) is a random sample since each individual on the list has an equal chance of being selected. Unfortunately, such *systematic* samples may be biased, as might occur if there is some periodicity in the listing.

In the same way, a sample of cattle from a large beef herd that included every fourth male and every third female (based on ear tags or other identifying numbers) would be a random sample. However, systematically choosing every third female (and every fourth male) herded through a chute would be likely to produce a biased sample because of the social distance among (pecking order of) different cattle.

Nonresponse is one of the most frustrating problems in random sampling. For example, in sampling dairy heifers, some will be unidentifiable because they have lost their ear tags; or, in sampling beef cattle on a range, some may not be rounded up in time for sampling. In other instances, animal owners may refuse to let their animals be included in the study; some animals may be too ill to be included; or, in using clinical files for a sampling study, the critical data may not have been recorded in some clinical case histories. At least some of the nonresponders, whatever the reason for their absence or nonresponse, are likely to differ in relevant ways from the responders, thereby biasing the sample. For this reason, every effort should be made to keep down the proportion of nonresponders. The epidemiologist can sometimes hold down the proportion of nonresponse among animal owners by keeping questionnaires short and simple. Moreover, it is usually helpful to detail the purpose of the study to the owner, and to provide the interested owner with a summary of results at the conclusion of the study.

The random sampling procedures discussed have one additional advantage; namely, the results from the sample can be extended to the population. The construction of confidence intervals for means, proportions, and differences in means or proportions of samples are discussed after this short sample exercise.

Problem 4. Randomization in experimentation

Suppose you asked an animal health assistant to form three randomized groups of 20 chicks each, from a shipment of 60 one-day-old chicks of the same breed and source.

Should he:

(1) pick up 20 chicks to form the first group, place the next 20 in the second, and use the remaining 20 to form the third group?

(2) assign the first chick he picks up to group A, the second to group B, the third to C, the fourth to A, etc.?

(3) use another strategy? (If so, describe it.)

Explain why you made your choice.

Estimation of population characteristics by sampling

A sample of a population can be used to estimate certain characteristics of the population, such as mean values or the variance of these values.

ESTIMATING THE MEAN OF THE POPULATION. The method used for estimating the mean of a population depends upon the type of sample taken.

Simple random sample. The sample mean $\bar{x} = \dfrac{\Sigma x_i}{n}$ is an unbiased estimate of the mean of the population from which the sample was drawn. If a sample consists of the five numbers, say, the weights in kilograms of five animals, 3.1, 2.7, 8.3, 7.8, and 4.1, then the sample mean weight is

$$\bar{x} = \frac{3.1+2.7+8.3+7.8+4.1}{5} = \frac{26.0}{5} = 5.2.$$

Stratified sample. Suppose there are k strata, and random samples of $n_1, n_2, \ldots, n_k$ have been selected from the strata that contained $N_1, N_2, \ldots, N_k$ individuals, respectively. If $\bar{x}_1, \bar{x}_2, \ldots, \bar{x}_k$ denote the sample means within the k strata, then an estimate of the population mean is

$$\hat{m} = \frac{N_1}{N}\bar{x}_1 + \frac{N_2}{N}\bar{x}_2 + \ldots + \frac{N_k}{N}\bar{x}_k = \Sigma\left(\frac{N_i}{N}\right)\bar{x}_i,$$

where $N = \Sigma N_i$, the total population size.

Consider two strata, having 64 and 36 individuals, respectively, from which are drawn samples of size 3 and 2. If these data are (3.1, 2.7, 4.1) and (8.3, 7.8), then the sample means within strata are

$$\bar{x}_1 = \frac{3.1+2.7+4.1}{3} = \frac{9.9}{3} = 3.3 \text{ and } \bar{x}_2 = \frac{8.3+7.8}{2} = 8.05.$$

The population mean is estimated as

$$\hat{m} = \frac{64}{100}(3.3) + \frac{36}{100}(8.05) = \frac{501}{100} = 5.01.$$

Two-stage sample. Suppose the k first-stage units are samples with probability proportional to size of unit, and samples of size n are chosen from each of these k units. Let $\bar{x}_1, \bar{x}_2, \ldots, \bar{x}_k$ be the sample means in the k units chosen. Then, the population mean is estimated as

$$\hat{m} = \frac{\bar{x}_1 + \bar{x}_2 + \ldots \bar{x}_k}{k} = \frac{1}{k}\Sigma\bar{x}_i.$$

ESTIMATING POPULATION VARIANCE. Similarly, the variance of a population may be estimated according to these different sampling procedures.

Simple random sample. In sampling from an infinite population, the sample variance

$$s^2 = \frac{\Sigma(x-\bar{x})^2}{n-1} = \frac{n\Sigma x^2 - (\Sigma x)^2}{n(n-1)}$$

is an unbiased estimate of σ^2, the population variance.

For the previous data,

$$s^2 = \frac{5\left\{(3.1)^2 + (2.7)^2 + \ldots + (4.1)^2\right\} - (26)^2}{5(4)}$$

$$= \frac{817.20 - 676}{20} = 7.06.$$

The square root of s^2 is the sample standard deviation.

A precautionary note is in order. Suppose, in sampling from a *finite* population, one denotes by f the sampling fraction $\frac{n}{N}$. Then, use the finite population correlation $(1-f)$ in estimating the variance:
Estimate of variance $= (1-f)s^2$.

For inferences to the finite population, use the estimated variance of the sample mean, given by

$$\text{Var}(\bar{x}) = (1-f)\frac{s^2}{n}.$$

It should be noted further that, if the sampling fraction is small, say less than 10%, the finite population correction may be relatively unimportant.

Stratified sample. Again, suppose random samples of $n_1, n_2, \ldots n_k$ are drawn from population strata containing $N_1, N_2, \ldots N_k$ individuals, respectively, with sampling fractions $f_1 = n_1/N_1$, $f_2 = n_2/N_2, \ldots f_k = n_k/N_k$. The variance estimates in the k strata are s_1^2, $s_2^2, \ldots s_k^2$, where

$$s_i^2 = \frac{\displaystyle\sum_{j}^{n_i} (x_{ij} - \bar{x})^2}{n_i - 1}$$

The overall estimated variance of the mean m, used for inferences, is

$$\text{Var}(\hat{m}) = \left(\frac{N_1}{N}\right)^2 (1-f_1)\frac{s_1^2}{n_1} + \left(\frac{N_2}{N}\right)^2 (1-f_2)\frac{s_2^2}{n_2} + \ldots$$

$$+ \left(\frac{N_k}{N}\right)^2 (1-f_k)\frac{s_k^2}{n_k} = \Sigma\left(\frac{N_i}{N}\right)^2 (1-f_i)\frac{s_i^2}{n_i}$$

Two-stage sample. With k samples chosen, as was done for the mean of a two-stage sample, the estimated variance of m is

$$\text{Var}(\hat{m}) = \frac{\Sigma(\bar{x}_i - \hat{m})^2}{k(k-1)} = \frac{1}{k^2(k-1)}\left(k\Sigma\bar{x}_i^2 - (\Sigma\bar{x}_i)^2\right).$$

ESTIMATING A PROPORTION (PERCENTAGE RATE): BINOMIAL DISTRIBUTION. If a population consists of items belonging to two mutually exclusive cate-

gories, for example, sick and not sick, it is said to be a *binomial* population. In such a population, one can assign a value of 1 to all items having the trait (e.g., sick) and 0 to all those not having the trait (e.g., not sick). Then, the population mean (μ) is simply the proportion (π) having the trait.

Suppose a random sample of size n is drawn from such a binomial population; then p, the proportion of sampled items having the trait, is an unbiased estimate of π.

The sampling distribution of p is approximately normal, with variance $\sigma_p{}^2 = \frac{(\pi)(1-\pi)}{n}$. However, when π is near zero or unity, the sampling distribution of p is no longer approximately normal unless n is large. A commonsense rule, then, is to avoid the normal approximation unless both np and n(1-p) exceed 5. Tables giving exact binomial probabilities for small values of n are available in many statistical texts. Larger, more extensive tables of the binomial distribution are also available.[2]

CONFIDENCE INTERVALS. Confidence intervals are constructed by building an interval around the best available point estimate (sample mean, sample proportion, or differences between means or proportions). In constructing confidence intervals, one uses data from the sample to make inferences about some characteristic(s) of the *population* from which the sample was drawn.

Confidence interval for a population mean. To construct a confidence interval for the *mean*, one calculates a point estimate $(\bar{x})$, uses the variance of $\bar{x}$ $(\sigma_{\bar{x}}^2$, or its estimate $s_{\bar{x}}^2)$, and designates the confidence level (commonly 95%, 99%, or 90%). The construction of a 95% confidence interval for the mean is illustrated here based on the simple random sample given previously, with $\bar{x} = 5.20$, and $s_{\bar{x}}^2 = \frac{7.06}{5}$. From tables of the t-distribution, one finds $t_{(4)} = 2.78$ for n-1 = 4 degrees of freedom.

The 95% confidence limits are

$$\left(5.20 \pm (2.78)\sqrt{\frac{7.06}{5}}\right) = (5.20 \pm (3.30)) = (1.90, 8.50).$$

It should be noted that the population mean may or may not be contained in the interval (1.90, 8.50). The 95% confidence means that, if we had chosen an infinite number of random samples of size 5 from this population, and constructed intervals for each of these samples, 95% of the confidence intervals would actually contain the population mean.

Confidence interval for population proportion. One can construct confidence intervals for a *proportion* in the same way. Suppose, in a sample of 100 animals, 36 animals have the characteristic of interest, say, a particular disease. A 99% confidence interval would be

$$p \pm z \sqrt{\frac{p(1-p)}{n}}, \text{ or}$$

$$0.36 \pm (2.58) \sqrt{\frac{(0.36)(0.64)}{100}} = 0.36 \pm 0.12$$

$$= (0.24, 0.48), \text{ or from } 24 \text{ to } 48\%.$$

Confidence interval for difference between population means. Confidence intervals for *difference between means* have the same form:

$$(\bar{x} - \bar{y}) \pm t_{(n_x + n_y - 2)} \sqrt{s^2 (\bar{x} - \bar{y})}.$$

Confidence intervals for differences between population proportions. Confidence intervals for *differences between proportions* also have the same form:

$$(p_1 - p_2) \pm z \sqrt{\frac{p_1(1-p_1)}{n_1} + \frac{p_2(1-p_2)}{n_2}}$$

For example, suppose 16 animals have the trait of interest in a random sample of size 25, and 36 of 100 have the trait in another sample. A 95% confidence interval for the difference in proportions would be

$$(0.64 - 0.36) \pm 1.96 \sqrt{\frac{(0.64)(0.36)}{25} + \frac{(0.36)(0.64)}{100}}$$

$$(0.28 \pm 0.21) = (0.07, 0.49), \text{ or from } 7 \text{ to } 49\%.$$

Sample size determination

One frequently asked question is: What size must the sample be to give a reliable result? Although there is seldom a simple answer, discussion of some specific examples may be instructive.

MINIMUM SAMPLE SIZE FOR DEMONSTRATING AN EXTREME OUTCOME. Suppose a disease of cattle has a known case fatality rate of 10% in the absence of treatment. What number of patients would be required to demonstrate the efficacy of a completely curative treatment?

Choosing $\alpha = 0.05$ as the significance level, and using the known rates

$$\text{probability of fatality} = 0.1$$

$$\text{so that probability of recovery} = 0.9$$

Set

$$(0.9)^n \leqslant \alpha, \text{ and solve for } n,$$

$$n \geqslant 29.$$

On the other hand, if we had chosen $\alpha = 0.01$,

$$(0.9)^n \leqslant 0.01 \text{ would yield}$$

$$n \geqslant 44.$$

ESTIMATING MEAN WITH SPECIFIED DEGREE OF PRECISION. Use the formula

$$n = \frac{\sigma^2 z^2}{d^2}$$

where σ^2 is the variance, and z is obtained from the standard normal distribution, with common choices for z being $z = 1.96$ for 95% confidence level or $z = 2.58$ for 99% confidence level. The value $d = (\bar{x} - \mu)$ is the maximum acceptable difference between an observed sample mean and the true but unknown population mean.

Suppose there is a need to estimate the average pulse rate in resting, nontranquilized dogs, prior to a clinical trial on the effects of several tranquilizers. It has been decided that this average must be known within two pulses per minute, and it is known that the variance of this pulse rate is from 16 to 25. How large a sample should be used?

It has been specified that $d = 2$, $\hat{\sigma}^2 \doteq 20$ (i.e., choosing an approximation for the values in the range of 16 to 25). After choosing the probability level, say 95%, calculate

$$n = \frac{(20)(1.96)^2}{4} \doteq 20.$$

Had the choice been $\hat{\sigma}^2 = 25$, the result would be $n \doteq 24$, so the pulse-rate information desired, with the specified precision, and at the requested confidence level is attainable by examining less than 25 dogs.

ESTIMATING DIFFERENCE BETWEEN TWO PROPORTIONS. A comparison of two proportions can be made easily using a 2×2 table of frequencies and applying the chi-square test for independence. The principle can be reversed to estimate desired sample sizes.

Suppose that one wants to estimate the prevalence of a certain condition that occurs in sheep in northern California and one also wants to compare the effect, if any, of the locale on which the sheep are pastured during summer. Preliminary studies on sheep indicate that the condition is prevalent in 6 to 10% of adult ewes (>2 yrs of age), and some clinical evidence indicates that the difference between 6 and 10% prevalence has biological (reproductive) significance. Further preliminary studies suggest that the use of certain mountain pastures may predispose ewes to this condition. How many ewes should be pastured on mountain pastures and on other range lands?

Suppose one agrees first to use the same numbers of ewes in each of the two groups, and further agrees that the difference he wants to detect is the difference between 10 and 6%. Finally, one decides to work at the 5% significance level. Arranging the foregoing information in the usual 2×2 array produces:

		Comparison group	Mountain group	Totals
Trait	+	0.06n	0.10n	0.16n
	−	0.94n	0.90n	1.84n
	Totals	n	n	2n

For the 5% level of significance, and for one degree of freedom, the critical value of χ^2 is 3.84. Recalling that the chi-square formula for a 2×2 table is

$$\chi^2 = \frac{(ad-bc)^2 n}{(a+b)(c+d)(a+c)(b+d)}$$

the result is

$$\frac{[(0.06n)(0.90n)-(0.10n)(0.94n)]^2(2n)}{(0.16n)(1.84n)(n)(n)} \geq 3.84.$$

Solving, n ≥ 354.
(Somebody's going to be *busy* examining sheep when they come back from summer pastures!)

The preceding discussion of sample sizes has been based largely on the notion of statistical significance (or confidence level). However, the design of an adequate epidemiological study should take into account Type II error (the error one commits by accepting the null hypothesis when the alternative hypothesis is true) as well as Type I error (the error one commits by rejecting the null hypothesis when the null hypothesis is actually true). We control for Type I error by setting the probability of making this error. This probability is referred to as the level of significance.

Rather than a lengthy treatise on statistical sampling theory, a few examples have been cited. When dealing with more difficult sampling problems, one can seek further help from resident statisticians or statistical textbooks.

Maneuvers

The *maneuvers* one conducts will be related to the types of comparison one wishes to make, and the evaluation of the effects of these maneuvers must take into account possible sources of bias in conducting the maneuvers. The familiar situation of the prospective clinical trial will be used as a type example for discussion of these general elements.

Types of comparisons commonly include *factors*, *dosage*, and *timing*. Comparisons of factors may be choices between geographic areas or other environmental factors (e.g., urban versus rural residence of

dog owners), between host factors (e.g., breeds, ages, sexes), between type of treatment (new treatment versus no treatment, placebo, old treatment, or other new treatment), or between other variables implied by the term "factor." Comparisons of dosage include an obvious reference to level of medication (high dose versus low dose versus other arrangements), but may also include *levels* of other factors (e.g, urban versus suburban versus rural). Comparisons involving timing may include concurrent observations by way of parallel or cross-over groups,[3] use of historical controls, or a form of dosage comparison, e.g., length of residence in an area served by a particular veterinary service. Distinctions between factors, dosage, and timing may not always be clear; but the three terms are useful in describing strategies for designing epidemiological studies.

There are manifold sources of bias in the conduct of these maneuvers including, in particular, inequities due to (1) performance or experience, (2) compliance or availability, and (3) ancillary maneuvers. Some examples of each of these sources of bias are, respectively:

(1a) Results from a radical operation done by a skillful surgeon are compared with a simple operation done by an inexperienced surgeon.

(1b) An analytical survey compares a veterinary service in two regions in Nigeria. In one region, the interviewers are fluent in the various dialects spoken; in the other, some interviewers are only passably conversant in these dialects.

(1c and 2a) A retrospective study compares the effectiveness of spay clinics in two counties of California. In one county (human population 50,000), there are four licensed practicing veterinarians; in the other (population 100,000), there are 40 licensed practicing veterinarians.

(2b) Drugs A and B have the same pharmaceutical effectiveness if taken by patients, but drug A is grossly unpalatable and is avoided, making it seem ineffective.

(3a) A retrospective study concerns the use of a veterinary service. All selected animal owners resident within 5 miles of City A are visited in person, with up to six return visits if necessary; all selected owners residing 5 to 50 miles from City A are contacted by mail questionnaire, with up to six return mailings if necessary.

(3b) A radical operation plus special care in a recovery room is compared with a simple operation without use of a recovery room.

Many examples other than clinical trials or surveys could be cited, but only the following additional example has been chosen. Decide how one could introduce each general source of bias (1d, 2c, and 3c) when a survey is made of the use of a veterinary service. A systematic sample is based on listings in the telephone directory (third name in first column, sixth name in second column, etc., on each page of the directory) for each of two geographic areas.

Responses

Response is a general term used to encompass any and all variables that characterize the baseline state (that preceding the maneuver), the subsequent state (that following the maneuver), and the transition between the two states. The baseline state *per se* may be the objective of study in descriptive studies, and is the point of departure in studies subjected to mathematical analysis. The experimental approach, one of the strongest weapons in the epidemiologist's investigative arsenal, is concerned with all three aspects of response.

In observing the response, a variety of procedures can be used to improve objectivity and to assess accuracy, reproducibility, and data-acquisition techniques. To improve objectivity, a common device is to use double-blind techniques, where neither the animal's caretaker nor the investigator is aware of which maneuver the subject receives.

Sources of bias in measuring response variables are related to perception, observation, validity, and detection. Perception and observation errors commonly occur when the subject's caretaker or the investigator (i.e., the observer) is aware of the identity of the maneuvers being compared. Double-blind techniques were developed to control or reduce these types of errors. Validity may be compromised by the "substitution game," in which an easily measured variable (e.g., the size of pupil) is substituted for the variable that is more important but also more difficult to measure (e.g., psychological distress). An example of this risk is given elsewhere in the use of gamma globulin level as an indicator of Aleutian disease in mink.

Detection errors, on the other hand, may be due to inequalities in intensity of procedures used to detect target events. For example, more frequent use of veterinary services is made by owners of purebred dogs than by owners of mixed or unknown breeds; thus, one could gain a mistaken impression of a target event by a simple comparison of purebred and nonpurebred dogs.

Finally, in choosing the expression of observation (i.e., the response), careful consideration must be given to the choice of the dependent and the independent variables, the former being outcome or effect measures, and the latter being input or cause variables. In observational studies, the distinction between cause and effect is often less than clear, and probably should be avoided in favor of independent-dependent-codependent terminologies. (See also the terminology in Chapter 13 with respect to multiple regression.)

Next, we will consider in more detail a few important areas of study design and conduct with respect to the research instruments used to measure responses.

MEASUREMENT AND ASSESSMENT. Measurement and assessment are activities for creating and evaluating the "instruments" used to provide research data. For different purposes, these data-creating instruments might include such things as a serological test measuring a particular type of antibody against *Toxoplasma gondii*, a spectrophotometer measuring serum calcium, a veterinarian auscultating a heart, or a questionnaire indicating a veterinary service user's degree of satisfaction with the health care provided.

In a particular research effort, methodologic research on the instruments chosen and their characteristics should precede subsequent experiments or other studies that make use of these instruments. For example, the validity of questionnaires and of specific questions within the questionnaire should be tested with pilot studies before conducting an actual survey. The scientific value of research data depends on the quality-control procedures and processes by which the reliability of the instruments used is established and maintained. Without such quality-control processes, evaluations of the results of research efforts become problems in "salvage statistics," and no amount of statistical salvage will correct an inappropriate instrument.

One form of evaluation is concerned with the instrument's inherent performance on a particular "specimen," and questions such as the following are examined: What is the result if three different technicians in the same laboratory do the test? What is the result if the same technician does the test three times on the same specimen? What is the result when other laboratories test the same specimen? Is the interview too long (e.g., does the subject tire)? Is the interview too brief? Does the interviewee really understand what was asked in Question #17? Would this grader give the same rating for identical responses by three different animal owners? Would three different graders give the same rating to the response by this animal owner?

A second type of evaluation is concerned with the external connotation or validity of the data. A key question to be asked here is "Does the 'instrument' measure what it purports to measure?" as, for example, "Does a test for immunoglobulin levels in mink really measure the presence or absence of Aleutian disease?"

Two specific measures that epidemiologists often use when referring to the external connotations of data obtained from a particular research instrument are sensitivity and specificity.

Test sensitivity and specificity. Diagnostic or screening tests seldom measure exactly what they are purported to measure. For example, tuberculin tests yield "positives" as a result of an animal's exposure to *M. tuberculosis, M. avium,* and several other organisms; but the test result may be "negative" during the early stages of the infection. Such false negatives, as well as other false positives, can be troublesome in prevalence surveys as well as in disease diagnosis *per se.*

The performance characteristics of various diagnostic tools or instruments are conveniently described in terms of sensitivity and specificity. *Sensitivity* is the probability of a diagnostic test correctly identifying as positive those animals that truly are positive, and *specificity* is the probability of identifying as negative those individuals that truly lack the characteristic of interest. Sensitivity and specificity are illustrated in the following chart as N++/N.+ and N--/N.-, respectively. The ratio N+-/N.- is the probability of a false positive, and N-+/N.+ is the probability of a false negative. It is desirable that the probabilities of false positives and false negatives be small, although cost, ease of application of the test, and other factors may be highly relevant.

True state of nature
(population)

		+	-	
	+	N++	N+-	N+.
Test result	-	N-+	N--	N-.
		N.+	N.-	N. . = population size

In practice, the probabilities of misclassifications may be estimated from surveys. Suppose a special survey of a random sample from the target population gave the following frequencies:

True state of
nature (sample)

		+	-
	+	a	b
Test result	-	c	d

The probability of a false negative would be estimated as c/(a+c), and the probability of a false positive as b/(b+d), both shown graphically in Figure 5-1. The sampling errors of these estimates can be obtained from standard binomial expressions.

It may also be useful to examine a sample ratio $\frac{a}{a+b}$ as an estimate of the universe ratio $\frac{N++}{N+.}$, i.e., the proportion of test-positives that are truly positive. This proportion $(\frac{N++}{N+.})$ has sometimes been called the "diagnosability" of the test. Similarly, $\frac{d}{c+d}$ may be a useful approximation of $\frac{N--}{N-.}$, the proportion of test negatives that are truly negatives. The diagnosability of a test is not static, and can vary greatly depending upon the prevalence (or incidence) of the disease being studied.

PROBABILITY. The preceding notion of probability can be defined in various ways, but one useful simplistic form is p = s/(s+f), where s = the number of observed successful outcomes of a random experiment, and f = the number of failures. Probability is measured by a number between 0 (the probability of the impossible event) and 1 (the probability of the sure event). For example, in a herd of 100 cattle, 40 of which are less than four years of age, the probability of randomly choosing one animal less than four years of age (in a single draw) would be 40/100 or 0.4. Another simplistic yet useful definition is based on the notion of relative frequencies. For example, observing the sex of successive live human births, the probability of a male birth is slightly over one-half.

In discussing sensitivity and specificity of diagnostic tests, it was noted that an observed ratio c/(a+c) was an estimate of the probability of a false negative. The extent to which the ratio c/(a+c) is a "good" estimate depends on a number of factors, including the size of the sample (a+c, and a+b+c+d), the care and thought that went into the design of the study from which the result c/(a+c) was derived, and the "risk" in using the ratio c/(a+c) as an estimate of the true but unknown probability of a false negative. Rather than using the single value (point estimate) c/(a+c), a range of values

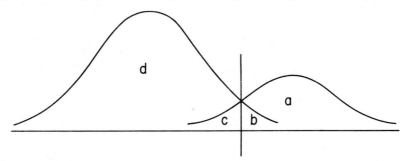

Fig. 5-1. Test results on subpopulations of animals (diseased and not diseased): *a,* diseased animals that test positively; *b,* nondiseased animals that test positively; *c,* diseased animals that test negatively; and *d,* nondiseased animals that test negatively.

or an interval estimate may be specified. Standard statistical texts provide more details on the construction of such confidence intervals (discussed briefly earlier in this chapter).

One broader view of probability interprets it as a measure of one's belief in a proposition (subjective probability). Under this view, direct statements can be made about the probability that a specific scientific hypothesis is true. The problem is the subjectiveness of the probabilities.

The following epidemiological situations illustrate the concepts of probability and of test sensitivity and specificity.

Probability of failing to detect Mycoplasma-infected chicken flock using given screening test.[4] Suppose a poultry practitioner wishes to carry out a diagnostic test of known sensitivity and specificity for *Mycoplasma gallisepticum* in a flock of chickens. He wants to know the probability of failing to detect infection in this flock, that is, the probability of obtaining a false negative flock. The flock is considered infected if it contains at least one infected bird. H is taken to be the total number of birds in the flock, which contains r infected birds and H-r uninfected birds. The diagnostic test T is conducted on a random sample of the flock of size n. The possible test results are T+ and T-, and s_e and s_p denote the sensitivity and specificity, respectively, of the test. A tested bird that actually is infected is designated G+ and one not infected G-.

Therefore, $s_e = P(T+|G+)$ is the sensitivity of the test. The probability of a false negative is $1-s_e = P(T-|G+)$. Similarly, $s_p = P(T-|G-)$, and the probability of a false positive is $1-s_p = P(T+|G-)$.

The prevalence of *M. gallisepticum* is $\frac{r}{H}$, which also is the probability of drawing an infected bird in a single drawing. From these variables, it is possible mathematically to construct the graphs shown in Figures 5-2 and 5-3. Actual prevalence rates of 0.1 and 0.001, test sensitivities of 0.9 and 1.0, and test specificities of 0.9 and 1.0 are indicated. Using these graphs, the probability of a false negative flock may be obtained, given these variables.

Probability that brucellosis test-positive animal actually is infected.[5] Suppose a governmental veterinarian is responsible for "down the road" testing of dairy cattle for brucellosis and for local implementation of an eradication program. He tests 10,000 dairy cattle annually and wants to know what proportion of animals that are test-positive (T+) are actually infected (D+) with *Brucella*, that is P(D+|T+), or the diagnosability of the test.

Let us assume that he is using a test that is 95% sensitive P(T+|D+) and 97% specific P(T-|D-) and that at the time he first tested this population in

Fig. 5-2. Graph for determining probability of false-negative flock given test sensitivity, specificity, and actual prevalence rate: n = flock size, sp = specificity of test, r/H = prevalence. Specificity for this graph is .9. See also Figure 5-3 (from Adler, H.E., and Wiggins, A.D. 1973. Interpretation of serological tests for *Mycoplasma gallisepticum*. World Poul. Sci. J. 29:345).

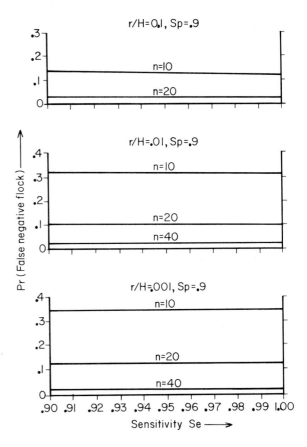

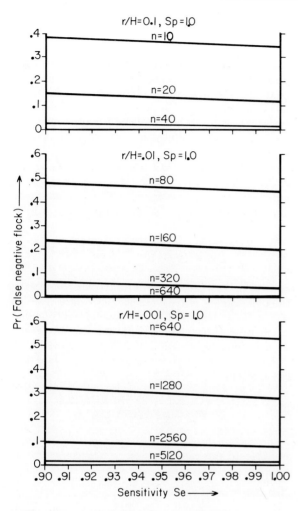

Fig. 5–3. Graph based on test specificity of 1.0. See legend for Figure 5-2.

1960, the actual prevalence of infection was 15% P(D+). This situation could be expressed as:

	D+	D–	
T+	1,425	255	1,680
T–	75	8,245	8,320
	1,500	8,500	10,000

Using Bayes' Rule, namely

$$P(D+|T+) = \frac{P(D+)P(T+|D+)}{[P(D+)P(T+|D+)] + [P(D-)P(T+|D-)]}$$

the official can calculate the diagnosability

$$P(D+|T+) = \frac{(0.15)(0.95)}{(0.15)(0.95) + (0.85)(0.03)} = 0.8482.$$

The result shows that even given a test with this high specificity, only 85% of the 1680 cattle with positive tests, or 1425 cattle, are actually infected with *Brucella*. (If the actual initial prevalence of

infection was 0.5, substitution of those data would have yielded a calculated diagnosability of 97%).

Why does one not use $\frac{1425}{1680}$ directly to get 0.848? The answer is that one does not usually know how many animals are in the D+T+ category, 1425 in this example, so he must use the *marginal* data to estimate the diagnosability of the test.

Now consider several similar questions one might encounter during a control program of this type.

Problem 5. Determining the number of false positive reactors.[5]

Suppose that you are assigned to retest the dairy cattle population of the county mentioned previously. The year is 1965, and the actual prevalence of *Brucella* infection is down to 0.01 (say, the total population is again 10,000). What proportion of test-positive (T+) animals now are infected with *Brucella*?

Suppose the test you actually had available for use was a standard brucellosis agglutination test that is said to have a sensitivity of only 52% and a specificity of 89%.[6] What proportion of your test-positive cattle now would actually be infected, assuming again an actual prevalence of 1% among 10,000 cattle?

Assuming prompt removal of all reactors, no additions to the population, and no further transmission in the interval, you retest three months later; then, given the same assumptions, you screen the population a third time three months after that. What percentage of diseased animals have you removed by these three test rounds in succession?

Following these three successive testings, what is the number of healthy cattle you have branded as reactors and sent to slaughter from the initial 10,000 animals?

Now suppose you *also* had available a complement fixation test for brucellosis, and this test had a sensitivity of 98% and a specificity of 84%. Using these two available tests in *any combination of ways*, and again assuming no transmission or replacement of cattle during the interval, show what would be the expected differences in percentage of infected cattle removed and number of healthy cattle sent to slaughter by your different approaches.

APPROXIMATION OF REAL PREVALENCE FROM TEST RESULT DATA. As noted, a common problem not always considered fully in disease control programs is the importance of test *specificity* to the surveillance or mass case finding of diseases of low prevalence, a situation that arises as successful control programs progress. In the beginning of such a program, when prevalence of the disease is high, prime interest is in having a *sensitive* screening test that will locate as many of the affected animals as possible. As prevalence declines, however, even with a test of fairly high specificity, the vast majority of animals with positive tests will be false positives. This result partly accounts, for example, for the commonness of "no visible lesion" reactors in the terminal stages of a tuberculosis eradication campaign.

To illustrate this situation again, suppose that the real prevalence of bovine tuberculosis is 0.001, the hypothetical tuberculin test being used has a sensitivity of 99% and a specificity of 95%, and 100,000 cattle are being tested. These data could be expressed in a fourfold table:

	D+	D−	
T+	99	4,995	5,094
T−	1	94,905	94,906
	100	99,900	100,000

The apparent prevalence on the basis of test results is 5094/100,000 or 0.05094. However, of the 5094 positive reactors, 4995 will be false positives. This result may not only be economically consequential if these reactors are sent to premature slaughter, but it will also play havoc with assessment of progress of the control effort.

To help solve the latter of these two problems, the following method has been described. It can be used to calculate real prevalence from test results in such situations.[7] With knowledge[4] of the sensitivity (s_e) and specificity (s_p) of the test used, the real prevalence (RP) can be calculated from the apparent, or test, prevalence (AP) by the following formula:

$$RP = \frac{AP + s_p - 1}{s_p + s_e - 1}$$

Substituting the previous tuberculin test data:

$$RP = \frac{0.05094 + 0.95 - 1}{0.95 + 0.99 - 1} = \frac{0.00094}{0.94} = 0.001$$

which is the real prevalence of tuberculosis among the 100,000 cattle tested. Marchevsky[7] also gives a graphic solution to this problem and points out that this method of calculation of real prevalence is *invalid* in the unlikely situation that the sensitivity and specificity of the test are complementary values (i.e., $s_p + s_e = 1$).

DEVELOPING AND PRESENTING EPIDEMIOLOGICAL DATA

The second broad class of mathematical methods available to the epidemiologist concerns data *per se* and their presentation.

Characteristics of data

In expressing the response to a study instrument, whether it be a diagnostic test, laboratory procedure, questionnaire, or other method, there are generally a number of variables for indicating principal responses. The unit of expression for observations may be, for example, animals, people, events, concentrations, political areas, climatological regions, as well as modes of activity or transport. The statistical tools and procedures used for depicting and reporting responses may depend on the nature of the expression of the observations. Therefore, a simple taxonomy is useful in choosing among scales and criteria for individual measurements. In this taxonomy, categorical (qualitative) data are distinguished from dimensional (quantitative) data.

Categorical data may be nominal (i.e., "named," for example, breed, sex, location) or ordinal (i.e., "ordered," for example, improved versus not improved; larva versus subadult versus adult). As the name implies, categorical data are sometimes difficult to quantify, but dichotomies (dead versus alive; male versus female) are commonly assigned numerical scores (e.g., 0 versus 1).

Dimensional or quantitative data may occur as discrete counts or as continuous (measurement) data. Discrete counts may be, for example, number of survivors out of 100 animals tested, numbers of "responders" out of 12 test animals at each of 10 levels of treatment, or numbers of tuberculosis-test positive cattle passing through a certain screening procedure. Measurement data occur as titer, blood pressure, weight, and age (which often may be discretized to full years). In fact, due to the crudeness of our customary measuring devices, much of the measurement type of data is discretized, e.g., weight to nearest kilogram and titer to reciprocal of greatest twofold dilution in which the reaction is noted.

The arrangement of numerical data is called a distribution or series. Epidemiologically useful data may be arranged according to magnitude, time of occurrence, or geographical location. The resulting series is called, respectively, a frequency distribution (discussed here), a time series (discussed in Chapter 6), or a spatial distribution (discussed in Chapter 7).

CHARACTERISTICS OF A DISTRIBUTION. Whether organizing data for additional analysis or for presentation to a reading or listening audience, one can characterize them in certain ways. Two standard types of characteristics are measures of *location* and measures of *dispersion*. With quantitative data, common measures of location are those indicating central tendency such as the mean, the median, or the mode. With qualitative data, percentiles are usually used for designating location (or its qualitative analog). For example, suppose a sample of persons in the health professions contained three physicians, two veterinarians, two Ph.D.'s, one dentist, and two nurses. It would be illogical to try to calculate an average health professional, but to say that 20% were veterinarians would be a meaningful statement about the sample. On the other hand, to say that the average health professional in the sample was about 42 years old could also be a meaningful statement.

Measurements of dispersion as applied to quantitative data include variance, standard deviation, coefficient of variation, and range. With qualitative data, percentile-ranges are commonly used to designate dispersion.

Data reduction

If a collection of data is worth eventual analysis, it is worth the best form of analysis, that is, the form that allows the maximal amount of information to be extracted from the data. As noted earlier, a variety of statistical tools exist, and the appropriateness of each for a particular use depends upon, among other things, the *type* of data being analyzed. Some of these tools will be described relative to the types of data one might be interested in collecting.

One of the tasks that epidemiologists do most often is to enumerate events such as illnesses or deaths and display them in a fashion that may indicate a pattern of occurrence. For example, they are given the 1972 mortality records of a "backyard" broiler producer (Table 5–1). Do these data suggest anything? Do they lack anything they would need to know?

Such data are called "dangling numerators," and they are used more commonly in the medical literature than they should be (for example, in Table 3–7 on hog cholera diagnosis). What obviously is lacking are the denominator populations (populations at risk) to which these data relate. When these populations are supplied for the preceding data (Table 5–2), any suggestions that may have been made by the incomplete data in Table 5–1 are not valid.

The foregoing is the reason why enumerated epidemiological data are so commonly summarized as proportions, particularly as percentages or other *rates*. As the name implies, a proportion is a number of the form a/(a+b), where the numerator (a) is also part of the denominator. A simple example would be an expression of the number of cattle slaughtered in 1971 in an abattoir relative to the number of animals of all species, e.g., 10,821/14,622 = 0.740. The same notion can be expressed as a percentage (10,821/14,622) $\times$ 100 = 74.0%. Implicit in this example is the notion of time, and the result should be stated as 74.0% per year (or 74.0% in the year 1971).

Epidemiological rates are commonly expressed per 100 (percentages), per 1000, per 10,000, per million, or per some other convenient index (generally some power of 10):

$$\text{Rate} = \frac{\left(\begin{array}{c}\text{No. individuals having the characteristic}\\ \text{during the time interval of observation}\end{array}\right)}{\left(\begin{array}{c}\text{No. individuals at risk of}\\ \text{having or getting the}\\ \text{characteristic during the}\\ \text{interval of observation}\end{array}\right) \times \left(\begin{array}{c}\text{Length of the}\\ \text{interval of}\\ \text{observation}\end{array}\right)} \times 10^{a}$$

Table 5–1. Number of Deaths in Birds Less than Nine Weeks of Age, by Month of Death, B and D Broiler Farm, 1972.

	Jan.	Feb.	Mar.	Apr.	May	June	July	Aug.	Sept.	Oct.	Nov.	Dec.
No. deaths	32	41	26	35	34	60	192	216	102	40	31	35

Table 5-2.   Number of Deaths, Population of Birds, and Death Rates by Month, in Birds Less than
                  Nine Weeks of Age, B and D Broiler Farm, 1972

	Jan.	Feb.	Mar.	Apr.	May	June	July	Aug.	Sept.	Oct.	Nov.	Dec.
No. deaths	32	41	26	38	34	60	192	216	102	40	31	35
Population of birds	1000	1000	1000	1000	1000	2000	6000	6000	2000	1000	1000	1000
Death rates per month per 1000	32	41	26	38	34	30	32	36	51	40	31	35

Expressing epidemiological data as rates

Some commonly used epidemiological rates, morbidity prevalence and incidence, were introduced in Chapter 2. The two essential features of such a rate are that the numerator ("haves") is included in the denominator ("haves and have-nots") and a time duration is specified. The denominator is generally the number of individuals present at the midpoint of the interval of observation when the investigator is working with large dynamic populations (e.g., number of dogs licensed in Ingham County during a three-year period, persons resident in Sacramento County, number of ewes in a very large flock in Nevada). Sometimes, however, the midpoint population is not a good approximation of the average population during the time interval and some other average is preferred. An example might be the number of cattle in a particular large feedlot, where such factors as sales prices, feed prices, or availability of replacement cattle would be strong influences on the numbers of cattle maintained on the lot at any time. In these cases, daily (weekly) losses and daily (weekly) population figures should be used for daily (weekly) incidence rates.

VITAL STATISTICS RATES. Rates *per se* are important in many areas of veterinary medicine other than epidemiology. In addition to the usual laboratory use of the term (e.g., amount of material liberated per unit weight or volume of biological material; weight gain per laboratory animal per unit of time), certain other standard terms have been developed for rates relative to frequency data. Those that are of particular value to the epidemiologist include various types of reproductive rates and death rates. Some of these commonly used vital statistics rates are given in Table 5-3. Birth rates, death rates, and similar vital statistics are incidence rates of those events in the same sense as morbidity incidence rates (as noted in Chapter 2).

MORBIDITY RATES. Other types of rates commonly used by epidemiologists include such things as attack rates, incidence rates, and prevalence rates. Frequently, in reporting such rates in the literature,

no mention is made of the time factor or period of observation, when, in fact, time is a crucial factor in all such measures.

As indicated in Chapter 2, the incidence rate is defined as the number of new cases of an illness (or a particular diagnosis) arising in a population in a given interval of time. In contrast, the instantaneous or point prevalence rate refers to the number of illnesses existing at a specified point of time, and is related to the number of individuals exposed to risk at that time.

In using incidence, prevalence, or other measures of morbidity, it is necessary to specify whether one is measuring numbers of individual animals sick or numbers of "spells of illness." With infectious diseases that produce lifelong immunity following recovery, these numbers will not differ; but with others, such as common respiratory or intestinal infections, some individual animals may suffer several episodes of illness in periods of observations as short as a few months. A similar problem arises with respect to readmissions data from hospitals.

In obtaining prevalence data in practice, a "point" of time is never precisely that, since a tuberculin test survey of one cattle herd may take several hours to complete, and that of a county's cattle population three weeks. For epidemiological purposes, these times are usually considered "points." In the case of chronic infections of low incidence, errors that result are usually small. However, if the observation period for the cross-sectional survey is unduly prolonged, it becomes, in a sense, the cross-sectional longitudinal type of study already mentioned. In such cases, alternative possibilities for expression exist, and care must be exercised in data interpretation.

Prevalence data collected over a period of time are often expressed in veterinary medicine as an *accumulated prevalence rate*. This rate is something of a "bastard" in that it represents the accumulation of a series of point prevalence data for a stated time period. For example, Market Cattle Identification Program data for bovine brucellosis in California yield a daily series of prevalence data for cattle slaughtered on that particular day. To obtain sufficient data or to

Table 5–3.   Some Commonly Used Vital Statistics Rates and Ratios (All Indices Refer to a *Defined Population* of Animals *Observed for One Year** Unless Otherwise Stated)

Name of rate or ratio and definition	Remarks
No-return rate at n days: $\dfrac{\text{No. animals bred that have not come back in heat in } n \text{ days after breeding}}{\text{No. animals bred}} \times 10^a$	Used by breeders as an approximation of pregnancy rate
Pregnancy rate at N days: $\dfrac{\text{No. animals pregnant at } N \text{ days after breeding}}{\text{No. animals bred}} \times 10^a$	Sometimes referred to incorrectly as conception rate
Crude live birth rate: $\dfrac{\text{No. live births occurring}}{\text{Avg. population}} \times 10^a$	Not strictly a measure of risk; useful as measure of population increment due to natural causes
General fertility rate: $\dfrac{\text{No. live births}}{\text{Avg. no. female animals of reproductive age}} \times 10^a$	The reproductive age will depend on the particular species of interest
Crude death rate: $\dfrac{\text{No. deaths occurring}}{\text{Avg. population}} \times 10^a$	
Age-specific death rate: $\dfrac{\text{No. deaths among animals in a specified age group}}{\text{Avg. no. in the specified age group}} \times 10^a$	Breed-specific, or sex-specific rates would be defined similarly
†Calf (lamb, piglet, puppy, etc.) mortality rate: $\dfrac{\text{No. deaths under a specified age } N}{\text{No. live births}} \times 10^a$	Not all young animals dying in one calendar year were born in the same calendar year; i.e., denominator of rate does not completely include numerator. Also, the specified age may vary among species and will depend in part on the normal life span of the species; in man the equivalent is the infant mortality rate.
†Neonatal (calf, lamb, etc.) mortality rate: $\dfrac{\text{No. deaths under a specified age } n}{\text{No. live births}} \times 10^a$	See preceding note. For man the neonatal period includes the first 28 days of life.
Fetal death rate (also called stillbirth rate): $\dfrac{\text{No. fetal deaths}}{\text{No. live births plus fetal deaths}} \times 10^a$	For man, WHO subdivides fetal deaths as follows: Early — Under 20 weeks Intermediate — 20–27 weeks Late — 28 weeks and over WHO uses late fetal deaths to compute fetal death rate
Fetal death ratio (also called stillbirth ratio): $\dfrac{\text{No. fetal deaths}}{\text{No. live births}} \times 10^a$	Note that this is not a rate; in epidemiology a ratio is usually a proportion in which the numerator is not included in the denominator
Maternal mortality ratio: $\dfrac{\text{No. deaths in dams from puerperal causes}}{\text{No. live births}} \times 10^a$	While this is the current U.S. definition applied to man, some states use live births plus fetal deaths in the denominator. Modifications of this ratio are required when used for species in which multiple births are frequent
Cause-specific death rate: $\dfrac{\text{No. deaths from a specified cause}}{\text{Avg. population}} \times 10^a$	
Proportional mortality rate: $\dfrac{\text{No. deaths from a specified cause}}{\text{Total no. deaths}} \times 10^a$	See comments in text relating to Table 5–4.
Case fatality rate: $\dfrac{\text{No. deaths from a specified cause}}{\text{Total no. cases of the same disease}} \times 10^a$	In chronic disease, all of the numerator animals may not be included in the denominator

*All rates could use other specified time periods.
†Note: Agreement on the desirable time intervals for each species has not been reached in veterinary medicine.

get data that may be at all representative, the data collection period is usually several months or longer, and the results are accumulated accordingly. Such rates can be misleading in situations where the incidence of the disease, composition of the population, or the sampling procedure is undergoing change.

These rates are the only ones that are obtainable in some circumstances, but they should be scrutinized closely before conclusions are based upon them.

In longitudinal studies, incidence rates are of special value, while only prevalence rates can be obtained from cross-sectional studies. The respective uses of these two approaches in epidemiological surveillance programs have been discussed in Chapter 3.

RELATIONSHIPS BETWEEN INCIDENCE AND PREVALENCE. It should be noted that the *duration* of an illness affects the relationship between its incidence and its prevalence. For chronic diseases, mastitis for example, cross-sectional prevalence surveys detect not only cases of disease acquired fairly recently but also cases of relatively long duration, some of which may have been acquired in time intervals prior to those used for calculating a current incidence rate. Thus, the prevalence of a disease varies as the product of its incidence and duration.

For various reasons, either the incidence data or the prevalence data may be impossible to secure. Therefore, it is useful to know that, under certain prescribed conditions, one may be calculated from the other.

CALCULATING INCIDENCE RATES FROM REPEATED PREVALENCE MEASUREMENTS. In some situations, such as efforts to control infectious diseases, it is important to determine as quickly as possible whether transmission of an agent is being interfered with and whether the risk of acquiring the infection, that is, the incidence rate, is being reduced. For chronic insidious diseases in which prevalence rates, but not incidence rates, can be determined, as is often the case, this lack may present a problem. For example, say that a mollusciciding program has been initiated to control fascioliasis in a population of sheep and one needs to know whether the incidence of infection is being reduced as a result. The incidence of new infections usually cannot be determined directly for such an infection, but its prevalence can be determined by a stool survey for ova. By repeating a series of cross-sectional surveys for this *entire* sheep population, one may not see any decrease in prevalence for a long time after transmission has been interrupted because of the chronic nature of the infection, with long persistence of test-positive stools.

What can be done in such circumstances is to *estimate* the incidence of infection for a given period by carrying out two successive prevalence surveys on a *cohort of young lambs* being born into this population and, therefore, initially free of infection. To express these incidence rate estimates (IR) for a one-year period, Hairston has given a formula for their easy calculation:[8]

$$IR = 1 - x^{12/y}.$$

Here x = the proportion of the newborn cohort

negative on the first cross-sectional examination and still negative on the second. For an incidence rate expressed as a one-year incidence, y = the number of months between prevalence surveys; $x^{12/y}$, therefore, is the probability of remaining uninfected and $1-x^{12/y}$ the probability of infection or the incidence. For example, if 20 lambs are negative on the first examination and 18 of this cohort are still negative on the examination two months later,

$$IR = 1 - \left(\frac{18}{20}\right)^{12/2} \text{ or } 1 - (0.9)^6 = 1 - 0.53$$

$$= 0.47 = 47\% \text{ per year.}$$

To ascertain whether fluke transmission was being interrupted, pairs of such prevalence surveys would need to be made, one before the attempt to control and *another* after initiation of control, making note of any chronological bias introduced in the process.

Problem of proportional morbidity or mortality rates

One of the most common errors seen in the medical literature is conclusions about diseases based upon *proportional* morbidity or mortality rates. This subject was touched upon already, but is sufficiently important to elaborate at this point. This problem occurs most frequently when attempts are made to analyze collections of clinical or postmortem data from hospitals or laboratories. Consider this example.

SQUAMOUS CELL CARCINOMA OF CATTLE. Suppose Dr. A is the veterinarian responsible for a large Hereford herd in Arizona. He maintains complete illness and autopsy records on all animals that become ill or die. In a year-end study of these clinic and pathology records for 1974, he finds that a total of 1200 animals had become ill during the year. Among them were records for 40 cases of ocular squamous cell carcinoma (S.C.C.) and eight for malignant lymphoma (M.L.). In 1973, he had had 30 S.C.C. cases and seven M.L. cases among a total of 1100 ill animals. For 1972, these figures had been 25 S.C.C. cases and nine M.L. cases in a total of 1400 sick cattle. From these data, he calculated a so-called incidence for S.C.C. of 3.3% (40/1200) for 1974, 2.7% (30/1100) for 1973, and 1.8% (25/1400) for 1972. From these three years' data, he concluded that the "incidence" of S.C.C. was increasing in this herd.

What errors has he committed?

In the first place, this type of rate is not an incidence rate but a *proportional morbidity rate*. It says that, *of the animals in this population that became sick* during a given year, such and such a proportion had S.C.C. The incidence rate for S.C.C., on the other hand, would state that, out of the total population of cattle at risk in this herd for the year, such and such a proportion developed S.C.C. during the year. From the data of these three years, all one can conclude is that the *proportion of diagnoses* for S.C.C. has increased. There is no way to determine from such data whether the incidence of the disease has been altered.

Proportional mortality rates from autopsy records are misapplied similarly as a substitute for cause-specific or other mortality rates. In the example shown in Table 5–4 for human cirrhosis deaths in the United States, the changes in cause-specific death rates for cirrhosis and the proportional mortality rates for cirrhosis between 1900 and 1966 are compared.

What do these data mean? Simply that for the U.S. human male population in 1956, the risk of dying of cirrhosis was 14% less than it had been in 1900. However, *had a male died in 1956,* the chances were 57% greater that he would have died of cirrhosis than *had he died in 1900.* However, some pathologists had concluded erroneously from analyses of different subseries of such data on human deaths that the death rate for cirrhosis had risen in the United States during the first half of the 20th century. The reason for the opposite pattern of change shown for these two rates in Table 5–4 is related to the effect of an overall decrease in the human *crude* death rate for the United States during that 56-year period.

The next example also illustrates a type of proportional rate.

EPILEPSY IN DOGS. Clinicians in a veterinary school saw a total of 125 cases of canine epilepsy in a 10-year period. One clinician thinks it would be useful to write up for the literature a clinical summary of these hypothetical cases, the characteristics of the patients, and the methods used to treat them. He notes, for example, that 25 of these patients were breed X, 28 breed Y, and the remainder all other breeds (no one breed accounting for more than six patients).

The clinician calculated that 20% of canine epilepsy cases in his series were breed X and 22% breed Y. However, the error in such reports comes when the author concludes, as sometimes is done, that canine epilepsy *occurs most frequently* in breed X and breed Y dogs. No such evidence is given by these data. The *most* that this clinician could state from his series would be the *possibility* of a breed predisposition for canine epilepsy, and he could conclude that breeds X

and Y possibly show such a predisposition. To conclude anything further, the veterinarian would have had to show (1) that his series of 125 epilepsy cases were representative (i.e., an acceptable sample) of the *total* number of epilepsy cases occurring in the community population of dogs from which this veterinary school clinic drew its patients and (2) that the breed *distribution* among the epilepsy patients differed in a statistically significant way from the breed distribution in this same general community population of dogs.

Other rates and ratios reflecting population health status

The epidemiologist in veterinary medicine often has data available for calculation of other health indices not generally obtainable for human populations. These data include such indices as egg production and hatchability rates, milk production rates, fecundity rates, other reproduction or production rates, and feed conversion rates, some of which are very sensitive indices of health (see Table 5–3). Insufficient use has been made of such valuable measures in the practice of preventive veterinary medicine.

Other rates of particular epidemiological value include the *case fatality rate* and the *secondary attack rate*. The *case fatality rate* (C.F.R.) is defined as:

$$C.F.R. = \frac{\text{No. deaths from a specific cause in a given time period}}{\text{No. cases of the same disease occurring in the same time period}} \times \text{time}$$

This rate is used to measure the seriousness of a disease, which, for infections, may reflect the relative resistance of a population of hosts or the virulence of a population of infectious agents, or both. It could also reflect the availability of veterinary care. It should also be noted that the C.F.R. may lack clear meaning in chronic diseases where many of the deaths in the measurement period represent cases of the disease acquired *prior* to the measurement period. A common error in the literature is not to distinguish between case-fatality rates and death rates *per se* (see Table 5–3).

The *secondary attack rate* was defined in Chapter 3. It is a measure of communicability of infections, chiefly those transmitted by direct physical contact

Table 5–4.   Mortality Data for Cirrhosis of Liver in Man in United States (U. S. Public Health Service)

	1900	1956	Change (%)
Cause-specific mortality rate per 100,000	12.5	10.7	-14
Proportional mortality rate (%)	0.7	1.1	+57

or air-borne droplets within a defined population during an outbreak.

SPECIAL INCIDENCE RATIOS. In epidemiology, a ratio is the relationship between a numerator and a denominator in which the former is not included in the latter. An example is a stillbirth ratio. Often in veterinary medicine, applicable population denominators are not available for disease incidence numerator data. For example, the number of new cases of rabies detected in skunks or foxes may be known, but not the animal populations, so these data cannot be correlated. In the case of the zoonoses, such data still may be expressed sometimes in epidemiologically useful forms. An example is the zoonosis incidence ratio (Z.I.R.),[9] which is defined as follows:

$$\text{Z.I.R.} = \frac{\begin{array}{c}\text{No. new cases of a zoonotic disease in an} \\ \textit{animal} \text{ reservoir species in a given} \\ \text{geographic area in a stated time period}\end{array}}{\begin{array}{c}\text{Avg. human population in the same} \\ \text{area during the same period}\end{array} \times \text{time}}$$

This ratio gives an indication of the *risk* of human infection with a zoonosis acquired by man only from animals. This ratio is much more valuable for that purpose than is a human incidence rate *per se*.

Of similar comparative value with respect to disease control, particularly in wild animal reservoir species, may be the *area incidence ratio* (A.I.R.),[9] defined as follows:

$$\text{A.I.R.} = \frac{\begin{array}{c}\text{No. new cases of a disease in an animal} \\ \text{population in a given time period}\end{array}}{\begin{array}{c}\text{Unit geographic area in which the} \\ \text{observations are made}\end{array} \times \text{time}}$$

These two ratios have been used in studying the recent westward advance of rabies in Europe. However, caution must be exercised in attempting to use such ratios. With the latter, for example, a common source of error might be that one geographic area was under closer surveillance than another.

RATES SPECIALLY APPLICABLE TO VECTORS. Some of the many special types of rates applicable to epidemiological studies of vector species were indicated in Figure 4–6 and elsewhere in Chapter 4.

Rate adjustment or standardization

In comparing death or morbidity rates, or in using them as a measure of the success of some health-related maneuver, it is important to remember that such rates usually are affected considerably by the age distribution of the population concerned. Furthermore, sex, breed, and other factors may influence death or morbidity rates. Consequently, the only really satisfactory way to compare rates is to examine, and compare, rates that are as specific as possible, such as age-sex-breed specific rates. In the words of one pioneering medical statistician, *"no single figure, however derived, can ever fully replace [specific rates] and succinctly summarize the contrasts."*[10]

On the other hand, rates that are very specific may be based on relatively small numbers of individuals at risk, making these rates imprecise and unreliable. Furthermore, it is natural to desire a single mortality or morbidity rate that summarizes findings of a large complex collection of data. For these reasons, procedures have been developed for adjusting, or standardizing, rates. Two such procedures are illustrated using the hypothetical data of Table 5–5.

Superficially, it appears from that table that farm Y's herd is more severely affected than farm X's. However, considering a standardized population, for example, the pooled numbers of animals in both herds, and applying the age-breed specific rates in each herd to the standardized population, one obtains the age-breed adjusted rates shown in Table 5–5. Examination of these age-breed specific rates indicates no difference between these farms with respect to the rates. It is also clear that the age specific rates for breed B are lower than those for breed A.

An easier way to adjust for age, breed, or sex differences is to take the simple arithmetic averages of the rates on each farm. This method is equivalent to using a standard population consisting of equal numbers of individuals in each age (or, for example, age-breed, age-sex) category. The result is called the *equivalent average death rate* (E.A.D.R., or equivalent average morbidity rate if some measures of illness are to be compared). For both farms in the example, E.A.D.R. = 0.16 = 160 deaths per 1000 cattle per calendar interval.

The choice of a standard population is relatively unimportant if the age specific (age-sex specific, age-breed specific) rates in one group are consistently less than those in the other, or if the age specific rates are the same in both groups. On the other hand, if the rates for younger animals on one farm (group) indicate favorable survivorship conditions, but rates for older animals indicate more favorable survivorship on the other farm (group), either group can be made to appear to have lower age adjusted mortality rates. If a standard population is chosen so that it contains a large proportion of young animals, the farm having the lower rates in young animals will have the lower standardized mortality rate. If a standard population contains a large proportion of older animals, the group having lower age specific rates among older animals will have a low age-adjusted mortality rate. For these reasons, age adjustment or standardization usually provides little information beyond that obtained by direct, simple comparison of age specific (age-breed specific) rates.

Table 5–5. Population and "Deaths"* by Age and Breed, in Two Herds of Cattle (Hypothetical Data), per Some Calendar Interval

Age	Breed	Farm X Pop.	Farm X Deaths	Farm Y Pop.	Farm Y Deaths
< 1 year	Breed A	50	10	60	12
	Breed B	60	10	50	8
1 to 3 years	Breed A	150	10	250	17
	Breed B	300	15	200	10
> 3 years	Breed A	400	100	800	200
	Breed B	700	140	300	60
		1660	285†	1660	307†

*"Deaths" refer to loss of life or removal of cows from the milk string due to mastitis and other causes.

†Crude death rates:

Farm X: $\frac{285}{1660}$ = 171.7 per 1000 cattle per calendar interval

Farm Y: $\frac{307}{1660}$ = 184.9 per 1000 cattle per calendar interval

Age-breed adjustment:

Age	Breed	Std. population (Farm X + Farm Y)	Age-breed specific-rates* Farm X	Age-breed specific-rates* Farm Y	Expected deaths per std. population Farm X	Expected deaths per std. population Farm Y
< 1 year	Breed A	110	0.20	0.20	22	22
	Breed B	110	0.17	0.17	19	19
1 to 3 years	Breed A	400	0.07	0.07	28	28
	Breed B	500	0.05	0.05	25	25
> 3 years	Breed A	1200	0.25	0.25	300	300
	Breed B	1000	0.20	0.20	200	200
		3320			594†	594†

*Equivalent average death rate:

$$\frac{0.20 + 0.17 + 0.07 + 0.05 + 0.25 + 0.20}{6} \times 1000 = 160 \text{ per 1000 cattle per calendar interval}$$

†Age-breed adjusted rates for the two farms are identical: $\frac{594}{3320} \times 1000 = 178.9$ per 1000 cattle per calendar interval

Ratio of rates

It is often convenient and instructive in epidemiology to express the ratio of two rates; for example, if farm A had a calf neonatal mortality rate of 15%, and farm B's was 18%, the ratio of farm A's to farm B's rate is 15/18 = 0.833. Two ratios, *relative risk* and *odds ratio*, are commonly used in this manner. These two measures can be illustrated with the example shown in Table 5–6.

The *relative risk* (farm A relative to farm B) of calf neonatal mortality is

$$\frac{180}{1200} \div \frac{108}{600} = 0.833 \text{ as noted.}$$

The odds ratio, $\frac{180}{1020} \div \frac{108}{492} = 0.804$ in this example, is sometimes used as an approximation of the relative risk. If the rates to be compared are the same, then it makes little difference whether one uses the odds ratio or relative risk. On the other hand, "risk" of the event of interest (calf neonatal mortality in the example) is specified in the rates, so that the odds

Table 5–6.   Hypothetical Neonatal Mortality Data for Calves Born on Two Farms in Same Year

	No. calves		No. born alive
	Dying within 28 days of birth	Surviving more than 28 days	
Farm A	180	1020	1200
Farm B	108	492	600
Total	288	1512	1800

ratio can at best be only an approximation of the true relative risk.

Additional specific details on the use of relative risk and odds ratio as epidemiological tools are given in Chapter 11 on retrospective case-control studies.

Life table or actuarial methods

The life table, developed in its modern form by an astronomer, is another basic tool of vital statistics. It is an important analytical instrument, and is also a useful way to summarize and display results of some epidemiological investigations. There are two ways in which a life table can be constructed from mortality data for a large population. The two forms are called the *current* life table and the *cohort* or *generation* life table.

The current life table is, in a certain sense, a cross-sectional life table, conveniently summarizing current mortality experiences for the various age groups in the population without describing the actual mortality experience of any group. The current life table, therefore, describes the survival experience of a *hypothetical* group of individuals, based on observations in a particular population at some particular time. The cohort life table describes the actual survival experience of a group (cohort) of individuals born at the same time. The basic element of the life table is the probability of dying between one age and the next. Once these values are known, the life table can be constructed quite easily.

The life table can be used in a variety of situations. For example, a life table could be constructed for a large herd of breeder animals, where "life" refers to reproductive life in some way, and "birth" to the attainment of sexual maturity.

DESCRIPTION OF CURRENT LIFE TABLE. There are usually seven columns in a current life table. However, some of these columns are useful only for computations, and do not always appear in published life tables.

Column 1 indicates the age interval, (x, x+1). Each interval in this column is defined by two exact ages stated.

Column 2 represents the proportion dying in interval (x, x+1), q_x. Each q_x is an estimate of the probability that an individual alive at the exact age x will die during the interval (x, x+1). Figures in this column, derived from the corresponding age specific death rates of the current population, are the basic quantities from which figures in other columns of the table are computed. To avoid decimals, they are often expressed as the number of deaths per 1000 population.

Column 3 reports the number alive at age x, ℓ_x. The first number in this column, ℓ_0, is the arbitrary radix, while the successive figures represent the numbers of survivors at exact ages out of a cohort of ℓ_0 individuals born alive. Thus, the figures in this column have meaning only in conjunction with the radix ℓ_0. For this reason, they are often referred to as the life table survivors; and the radix is usually assigned a convenient number, such as 100,000.

Column 4 tabulates the number dying in interval (x, x+1), d_x; and the figures in this column are also dependent upon the radix ℓ_0. For each age interval (x, x+1), d_x is merely the number of life table deaths.

The figures in the ℓ_x and d_x columns are computed from the observed values of $q_0, q_1, \ldots q_w$ and the radix ℓ_0 by using the relations

$$d_x = \ell_x q_x, \qquad x = 0, 1, \ldots, w, \qquad (1)$$

and

$$\ell_{x+1} = \ell_x - d_x, \qquad x = 0, 1, \ldots, w-1. \qquad (2)$$

Starting with the first age interval, equation (1) is used for x = 0 to obtain the number d_0 dying in the interval; and equation (2) is used for x = 0 to obtain the number ℓ_1 surviving to the end of the interval. With ℓ_1 individuals alive at the exact age 1, the relations (1) and (2) are used again for x = 1 to obtain the corresponding figures for the second interval. By repeated application of (1) and (2), the figures in columns 3 and 4 are easily calculated.

Each of the d_x individuals who die during the interval (x, x+1) has lived x complete years plus some fraction of the year (x, x+1). The average of the fractions, denoted by a_x, will be called the fraction of last year of life for age x. Based on the available data for humans, the fraction a_x may be assumed to be 0.5 for x $\geq$ 5; and for the first five years of life, $a_0 = 0.10$, $a_1 = 0.43$, $a_2 = 0.45$, $a_3 = 0.47$, and $a_4 = 0.49$. In constructing life tables for wildlife or domestic animal species, in the absence of other data, it often is assumed that $a_x = 0.5$ for all ages x.

Column 5 is the number of years lived in interval $(x, x+1)$, L_x. Each member of the cohort who survives the $(x, x+1)$ year contributes one year to L_x, while each member who dies during the year $(x, x+1)$ contributes, on the average, a fraction a_x of a year. Thus,

$$L_x = 1(\ell_x - d_x) + a_x d_x, \quad x = 0, 1, \ldots, w-1, \quad (3)$$

where the term $1(\ell_x - d_x)$ is the number of years lived in the interval $(x, x+1)$ by the $(\ell_x - d_x)$ survivors, and the term $a_x d_x$ is the number of years lived in $(x, x+1)$ by the d_x individuals who die during the interval. When a_x is assumed to be 0.5,

$$L_x = \ell_x - 0.5 d_x = \frac{\ell_x + \ell_{x+1}}{2} \quad (4)$$

Column 6 records the total number of years lived beyond age x, T_x. This total is equal to the sum of the number of years lived by the radix in each age interval beginning with age x, or

$$T_x = L_x + L_{x+1} + \ldots + L_w, \quad x = 0, 1, \ldots, w. \quad (5)$$

The relationship

$$T_x = L_x + T_{x+1} \quad (6)$$

is useful for rapid calculation of the figures for Column 6.

Column 7, the expectation of life at age x, $\mathring{e}_x$, is the average number of years to be lived by all individuals now aged x. Since the total number of years of life remaining to the ℓ_x individuals is T_x,

$$\mathring{e}_x = \frac{T_x}{\ell_x}, \quad x = 0, 1, \ldots, w. \quad (7)$$

Each $\mathring{e}_x$ summarizes the mortality experience of individuals beyond age x in the current population under consideration, making this column the most important in the life table. Further, it is the only column in the table other than q_x that is meaningful without referring to the radix ℓ_0. As a rule, the expectation of life $\mathring{e}_x$ decreases as the age x increases, with the single exception of the first year of life, because of high mortality during that year. In the 1960 California human population, for example, the expectation of life at birth was $\mathring{e}_x = 70.58$ years, whereas at age one, $\mathring{e}_1 = 71.30$. This means that, having survived the mortiferous first year, one has a greater expectation of life at age one.

The symbol w refers to the beginning of the last age interval in a life table. Typical values for w are 85, 95,

and 100 for the human life table. In order for the life table to cover the life span of every individual in a population, the last age interval is often an "open" interval, such as 85 and over, 95 and over, or 100 and over.

Cohort life tables have general applicability in population follow-up or cohort studies, and a salient feature in such tables is the proportion surviving to each successive age. For example, in epidemiological studies of human cancer, 10-year, 5-year, and 3-year survivorship rates have been used. The uses and analysis of cohort life tables are detailed in Chapter 12.

For obvious reasons, the current life table has not been used widely in veterinary medicine, except with respect to wildlife. Nevertheless, life tables for animals have been prepared for a number of species, including horses. Although livestock do not normally survive to ages where deaths would occur mainly as a result of "natural causes," life tables can be useful in studies of livestock, by defining "life" as productive life (such as dairy cattle in the milk string, or reproductively active animals in a breeder herd or flock). Some good sources of data for construction of life tables exist for various animal species, e.g., in stud books (horses), in breeder farm records (e.g., cattle), and in brooder flock genetic records (chickens).

Construction of a current life table will be illustrated by using available data from 608 Dall Mountain Sheep.[11] Two features should be noted; first, the radix is chosen to be 1000 (approximating the size of the sample from which the data arose). Second, in the absence of any prior estimates of a_0, the data for first year survivorship were recorded by half years (Table 5–7).

The data from the 608 sheep indicated that about 5.4% should die within six months of birth ($0.054 \times 2 = 0.108$ per year). Similarly, of the animals alive at six months of age, about 15.3% died before reaching one year of age ($0.153 \times 2 = 0.306$ per year). The remainder of the q_x column has been prepared from the mortality experience of the 608 sheep observed by finding sheep skulls and determining their age.

By applying the rule $d_x = \ell_x q_x$, one finds that $d_0 = \frac{108}{2} = 54$ because the interval covers only six months. By using the relationship $\ell_{x+1} = \ell_x - d_x$, one finds that $\ell_1 = 801$. Applying these relationships repeatedly, it is easy to calculate the numbers surviving (ℓ_x) and the numbers dying (d_x). The number of years lived in the interval, L_x, is also calculated easily by repeated use of the relationship $L_x = (\ell_x + \ell_{x+1}) \div 2$. However, the first two intervals are of only six months duration. Consequently,

$$L_0 = \left(\frac{1000+946}{2}\right) \times 1/2 \text{ yr} = 486.5 \text{ yr, and}$$

The Mathematical Approach

Table 5–7.   Life Table for Dall Mountain Sheep (*Ovis d. dalli*).*

Age (x, x+1)	Proportion dying in interval (q_x)	No. alive at age x (ℓ_x)	No. dying in interval (d_x)	No. years lived in interval (L_x)	Total years lived beyond age x (T_x)	Expectation of life at age x ($\overset{o}{e}_x$)
[0–0.5]	[0.108] †	1000	54	486.5	7081.8	7.08
[0.5–1]	[0.306]	946	145	436.8	6595.3	6.97
1–2	0.015	801	12	795.0	6158.5	7.69
2–3	0.016	789	13	782.5	5363.5	6.80
3–4	0.015	776	12	770.0	4581.0	5.90
4–5	0.039	764	30	749.0	3811.0	4.99
5–6	0.063	734	46	711.0	3062.0	4.17
6–7	0.070	688	48	664.0	2351.0	3.42
7–8	0.108	640	69	605.5	1687.0	2.64
8–9	0.231	571	132	505.0	1081.5	1.89
9–10	0.426	439	187	345.5	576.5	1.31
10–11	0.619	252	156	174.0	231.0	0.92
11–12	0.937	96	90	51.0	57.0	0.59
12–13	0.500	6	3	4.5	6.0	1.00
13–14	1.00	3	3	1.5	1.5	0.50

*After Deevey (1947)[11]; data on 608 sheep, from Murie (1944)
†Proportions are expressed per year.

$$L_1 = \left(\frac{946+801}{2}\right) \times 1/2 \text{ yr} = 436.8.$$

Thereafter,

$$L_x = \left(\frac{\ell_x + \ell_{x+1}}{2}\right) \times 1 \text{ yr} = \left(\frac{\ell_x + \ell_{x+1}}{2}\right).$$

Having constructed the L_x column, T_x's are simply the accumulated sums of the L_x's, beginning at the uppermost age.

$$T_{13} = L_{13} = 1.5$$

$$T_{12} = T_{13} + L_{12} = 6.0$$

$$T_x = T_{x+1} + L_x$$

The length of the interval is no longer relevant for the calculations.

The columns for d_x, L_x, and T_x are sometimes omitted from published life tables, but are necessary elements in calculation of the expectation of life $\overset{o}{e}_x = \frac{T_x}{\ell_x}$.

The remaining calculation is again straightforward. For example,

$$e_0 = \frac{7081.8}{1000} = 7.08 \text{ years}, \quad e_{0.5} = \frac{6595.3}{946} = 6.97,$$

$$\text{and } e_1 = \frac{6158.5}{801} = 7.69 \text{ years}.$$

Expressing epidemiological data in tables and graphs

A properly constructed, adequately labeled table or graph can be read and understood without consulting its accompanying text. On the other hand, poorly constructed tables and graphs may confuse the meaning of a text that is otherwise understandable. Reading and interpreting tables and graphs, as in writing and reading textual materials, requires special skill and care.

The objectives of most data collection procedures in epidemiology, as in other activities, are to obtain numerical measurements of one type or another, and to apply them to the solution of problems. These measurements are commonly presented in tabular or graphic form; the former for presenting greater detail, the latter for rapid review but less detail.

When a mass of data is to be presented in tabular form, there is always a problem of dividing the data into categories, that is, of classifying the data. Occasionally, obvious categories exist. In classifying 20,000 cattle surveyed for the presence of antibodies to *Anaplasma marginale*, it might be natural to use breed and/or sex categories. A convenient method for determining the maximal number of categories is given in Sturges' rule:

$$\text{No. of categories} = 1 + 3.3 \log N,$$

where N = number of individuals in the set of data collected. For the anaplasmosis example,

$$\text{No. of categories} = 1 + 3.3 \log (20,000)$$
$$= 1 + (3.3)(4.3)$$
$$= 1 + 14.19 \sim 15 \text{ categories}.$$

Thus, detailed tables for these data should not have more than 15 categories. For sex (2 categories) and breed (7 categories), a two-way table categorizing sex and breed distributions has 14 categories, and is not excessively "busy"[12] for most readers. On the other hand, to present the distribution of results by age, one would be well advised to limit the number of age categories, or to prepare sex specific tables.

Aside from a guideline on the approximate number of categories for particular tabular presentation, some general rules should be observed in establishing these categories. The two essential requirements of any set of categories are that they should be *exhaustive* (or inclusive) and mutually *exclusive*; that is, every observation should fit into some category, and no observation should belong in more than one category or interval. With qualitative data, forming exclusive categories is essentially a problem of precise definition. For example, in describing the calf-raising facilities for dairies as being adequate or not adequate, the term "adequate" must be defined carefully before the categories are used to collect or report data.

In some cases, the definition of a category may be an objective one, but often it will be at least partially subjective. The inconsistency that may be inherent in subjective definitions does not imply that they are bad or that they have no practical merit. In fact, in defining the criteria on purely objective grounds, the criteria may be incomplete. For example, in attempting to describe an adequate calf-rearing facility on only objective grounds, it is fairly likely that the description would be incomplete, i.e., that some dairy in the area of study would defy categorization. Naturally, the researcher would make some *subjective* assignment to a category, perhaps footnoting the fact that the dairy defied objective categorization and describing some of the salient characteristics of the facility.

Quantitative measures may be discrete or continuous variables. Discrete variables (counting results) are easily categorized; e.g., number of visits to a veter-

inarian during the past year could be zero, one, two, three, four or more, or unknown, yielding five exclusive and inclusive categories. With continuous variables, the measure can never be made with complete precision. The measure of a continuous variable is made with reference to a scale of measurement, and there are limits to the number of divisions that can be made on any scale, e.g., pounds, ounces, miles, yards, kilometers, meters, and centimeters. These physical limitations then "discretize" our continuous variables, and certain customs have arisen relative to discretizing our measurements; for instance, age is commonly expressed as last completed year, month, or week. Weights and heights are expressed to the nearest unit such as pound, gram, inch, or centimeter. In constructing categories, the customs for using continuous variables should generally be followed.

In one common type of table, the data are categorized with respect to a single variable, the body of the table consisting of the frequencies with which individuals fall into each category. In another commonly used form, tabulation is structured with respect to relative frequencies (frequency ÷ total number in all categories), or percentages.

Finally, the title of a properly constructed table usually gives (1) the nature of the data, (2) the variables used for classifying the data, and (3) the place and time period to which the data apply.

In brief, tables should be self-explanatory, and all units should be stated for each numerical variable. The title should be concise, yet fully descriptive, providing information on "what, how classified, where, and when," relative to the body of data presented. Footnotes may be used to provide information not included in the title or body, but generally they should be few in number. The style, format, and ruling of a table should follow (1) the style of a particular journal to which the report is to be submitted, or (2) the style of other publications in the subject matter area if the report is not to be submitted for publication. A table should be as simple as is practicable for transmitting and exhibiting the desired information.

Graphs may be used to transmit the same types of data presented in tables, but with less detail. In drawing graphs, equal intervals in terms of the original units should appear as equal intervals of length on the axes. The many varieties include bar graphs, component bar graphs, line graphs (including frequency polygons), and others (population pyramids, scatter diagrams, pie graphs).

General principles for constructing graphs are similar to those for constructing tables. Graphs should be fully self-explanatory without reference to the accompanying text. If necessary, footnotes can provide supplementary information or detail, or specify the source of the data being graphed. The vertical (dependent variable) and horizontal (independent variable) scales should be clearly labeled, with units specified. A graph should be simple, giving an overview or general summary of findings rather than a detailed picture of the data. Generally with regard to format, style, and title, the principles for construction of tables also apply to graphs. In graphs and in tables, values that are to be compared should be adjacent or as nearly so as possible.

The next problem involves constructing a graph from disease data and applying epidemiological reasoning in an attempt to understand these data.

Problem 6. Trends in diagnosis of bovine cancer.

Table 5–8 was compiled from a number of annual reports of the Meat Inspection Division of the U.S. Department of Agriculture.

(1) Comment on the suitability of this form of data expression for epidemiological purposes.

(2) Plot on a graph the yearly rates for postmortem diagnoses of malignant lymphoma, sarcoma, epithelioma, and carcinoma for 1946–1974.

(3) What do these graphs show? Offer explanations for apparent trends indicated.

(4) Discuss possible epidemiological implications

Table 5–8.   Diagnoses of Neoplasms Resulting in Carcass Condemnations of Cattle in United States (from Statistical Summary, U.S.D.A., Federal Meat Inspection, 1946–1974)

Year	Total cattle subjected to postmortem inspections	No. cattle carcasses condemned for			
		Carcinoma	Epithelioma	Malignant lymphoma	Sarcoma
1946	12,581,268	879	1923	1429	656
1947	14,093,769	1022	1842	1393	625
1948	14,248,351	1275	1748	1341	745
1949	13,182,962	1227	1652	1191	681
1950	13,115,889	1593	2161	1213	714
1951	12,570,825	1643	1762	1166	784
1952	12,136,210	1532	2513	1180	887
1953	15,204,998	1533	2895	1517	540
1954	18,475,936	1768	3215	2123	533
1955	18,725,455	1645	2889	2679	516
1956	19,676,898	1602	2922	2998	411
1957	20,142,195	1508	3314	3418	309
1958	18,579,099	1531	2687	3277	312
1959	17,320,716	1275	2305	3151	304
1960	18,454,319	1254	3127	3124	324
1961	19,861,644	1703	3202	3736	304
1962	20,158,743	1854	3963	3786	276
1963	20,859,520	2203	4028	3559	228
1964	23,200,954	2107	4721	3946	256
1965	25,803,948	2796	5816	4616	275
1966	27,373,829	2680	5225	4892	241
1967	27,859,980	2175	4622	4867	178
1968	28,140,097	2709	5429	4886	167
1969	30,176,248	2561	6103	4831	225
1970	30,893,547	2867	7593	5726	250
1971	31,144,262	2202	9901	4765	160
1972	31,843,375	2353	14,835	5423	202
1973	31,723,265	2724	16,615	5676	166
1974	31,123,776	2892	18,310	4669	328

of the fluctuation, by year, of cattle *examined* postmortem, taking into consideration any explanations for these fluctuations.

(5) What do these data tell us about these diseases in the general population of cattle in the United States?

(6) Plot on the same graph the total numbers of cattle inspected postmortem each year.

(7) Does there appear to be any relationship between the number of cattle examined and the condemnation rates for any of the tumors? Examine this relationship by plotting (for each type of tumor) another graph showing the number of carcasses condemned against number of cattle inspected.

Using regression methods (discussed later in this chapter), analyze these data and calculate the regression coefficients.

(8) If there were high correlations, what factor(s) might explain them?

(9) Can you think of other possibly obtainable animal statistics that might indirectly relate to the mean annual slaughter age of cattle in the United States?

(10) Obtain from the library one or more of the following annual U.S. statistics for each year between 1946 and 1974: adult beef cattle on farms, adult dairy cattle on farms, consumers' price index, average retail price of beef. Examine these data and your condemnation rates by regression methods.

Handling of data[13]

Basic to the analysis of any quantity of epidemiologic data is the use of some type of punched card or other system for mechanically or electronically handling and sorting suitably coded data. For relatively small quantities, various types of hand-punched marginal punched cards are available, the most common being either a 5 X 8-inch card with holes numbered consecutively or a four-digit system, both sorted by knitting needles. For large quantities of data, IBM cards are in most general use. The two most common types are mark-sensing cards (on which graphite pencil marks are read electronically) and punched cards. Such cards may be machine sorted and serve as a common data source for computer analysis.

There are other systems for handling moderate quantities of data, say, clinical data representing less than 1000 accessions per year. The Termatrex Data Retrieval System is used for case retrieval and epidemiologic analysis in at least one American veterinary school, as well as in a number of diagnostic laboratories and zoologic gardens. This system is based on a color-number coded card file in which (for clinical record use, as an example) each card represents a diagnostic term or descriptor variable such as age, sex, breed, geographic origin, month, year, or hospital service. Holes are punched in the appropriate cards at a specific grid location

corresponding to the accession number (1 to 10,000). Retrieval is accomplished by using an illuminated reader to identify the grid locations of all punched holes in a card. Analysis is facilitated by an electronic scanner, which counts the entries on a given card or combination of cards. Combinations and permutations of variables on diagnostic terms are performed by overlaying cards. This system does not handle large volumes of quantitative data (e.g., white blood counts, serum protein values) as well as IBM-type card systems as it is limited to 1000 diagnostic terms and descriptive variables in its basic format.

ANALYZING DATA TO DETERMINE ASSOCIATIONS, MAKE COMPARISONS, INTERPRET RESULTS, AND DRAW CONCLUSIONS

The third important area in application of mathematics to epidemiological studies has to do with the analysis of data. The remainder of this chapter reviews and illustrates more of these analytical techniques, which are usually considered in a basic course in statistics. Some more advanced methods for epidemiological analysis are discussed in most of the following chapters, particularly in Chapters 11, 12, 13, 15, and 16.

Trends in proportions

Many problems for analysis in epidemiologic investigations can be reduced to the question, "Is there any association between these two factors?" If the answer is affirmative, a second natural question concerns the nature of that association. Simple illustrations of such analyses have already been given. In particular, epidemiologists are frequently interested in knowing whether the data they are collecting show linear trends, so the problem of linearity in proportions will be illustrated.

The numbers of strains of *Staphylococcus aureus* isolated from canine patients at a certain veterinary hospital between 1970 and 1974 are shown in Table 5–9. The strains isolated were tabulated relative to whether they were resistant or sensitive to a standard dose of penicillin. The proportion of resistant strains increased from 18.3 to 57.5%, and the increase appears to be important. It would be useful to know whether the trend was significant, and furthermore whether the increase was gradual or whether at least one sudden change may have occurred during the five year period.

The usual chi-square test for independence yields $\chi^2_{(4)} = 113.7$, which greatly exceeds the values in chi-square tables. The subsequent test for linear trend uses the test statistic

$$\chi^2_{(1)} = \frac{(\Sigma n_i)[(\Sigma n_i)(\Sigma r_i x_i)-(\Sigma r_i)(\Sigma n_i x_i)]^2}{(\Sigma r_i)(\Sigma n_i-\Sigma r_i)[(\Sigma n_i)(\Sigma n_i x_i^2)-(\Sigma n_i x_i)^2]}$$

The Mathematical Approach

Table 5-9.   Distributions of Strains of *Staphylococcus Aureus* Isolated from Canine Patients at XYZ Animal Hospital, by Resistance to Penicillin, 1970 to 1974.

Reaction to penicillin	Year					Total
	1970	1971	1972	1973	1974	
Resistant (r_i)	44	72	97	112	180	505
Sensitive	196	218	203	208	133	958
Total (n_i)	240	290	300	320	313	1463
Proportion resistant	0.183	0.248	0.323	0.350	0.575	
Score (x_i, $\Sigma x_i = 0$)	-2	-1	0	1	2	

Substituting numerical values from Table 5-9, $\chi^2_{(1)} = 99.6$, which greatly exceeds the critical chi-square value for even the $\alpha = 0.001$ level.

The difference between the two chi-square statistics provides another convenient chi-square statistic for testing departures from linearity of trend. In the example, this difference is

$$\chi^2_3 = 113.7 - 99.7 = 14.0.$$

This chi-square test statistic likewise indicates a significant departure from linearity ($14.0 > 11.3 = \chi^2_{3, 0.99}$. Several additional analytical strategies could be followed, including (1) transforming the data to look for further patterns, e.g., a possible sudden rise from 1973 to 1974; (2) removing an additional component from the "residual chi-square"; or (3) stopping, because of the overwhelming magnitude of the chi-square statistic for linear trend.

The previously outlined test for linearity of trend is an approximate chi-square procedure but should be a reasonable technique if most frequencies are at least 5 and if the totals, n_i, are at least approximately equal.

The chi-square technique also has epidemiological application in situations in which neither factor is "time." The following data are self-explanatory, and serve as an exercise in use of the approximate chi-square test for linearity of trend.

Problem 7. Relationship of eyelid pigmentation to ocular carcinoma in Hereford cattle

The distribution of "cancer-eye" in cattle in a Texas herd was tabulated by degree of pigmentation of the eyelid.

Is there a significant deviation from linearity?

Pigmentation of eyelid

	None	Partial	Heavy	
Animals with cancer	5	10	2	17
Animals without cancer	50	152	232	434
	55	162	234	451

Regression

Another statistical tool used in testing for possible association between two variables is regression. Regression analysis is usually applied to variables that are continuous. The input, or independent, variable (x) is assumed to be known exactly, and the problem is to compute how the output, or dependent, variable (y) is related to it.

The method will be illustrated using the following artificial data.

x	y	n=5	
3.0	2.3	$\Sigma x = 30.0$	$n\Sigma x^2 - (\Sigma x)^2 = 112.5$
4.5	4.7	$\Sigma y = 32.0$	$n\Sigma y^2 - (\Sigma y)^2 = 242.6$
6.0	5.2	$\Sigma x^2 = 202.50$	$n\Sigma xy - (\Sigma x)(\Sigma y) = 162.0$
7.5	8.7	$\Sigma y^2 = 253.32$	
9.0	11.1	$\Sigma xy = 224.40$	

A line, $y = A + Bx$, is fitted to these data using the method of least squares. The slope, B, of the line is estimated by

$$b = \frac{\Sigma(x - \bar{x})(y - \bar{y})}{\Sigma(x - \bar{x})^2} = \frac{n\Sigma xy - (\Sigma x)(\Sigma y)}{n\Sigma x^2 - (\Sigma x)^2} = \frac{162.00}{112.5} = 1.44.$$

The intercept, A, is estimated by

$$a = \bar{y} - b\bar{x} = \frac{32}{5} - 1.44\left(\frac{30}{5}\right) = -2.24.$$

For these data, the least squares line is

$$y = -2.24 + 1.44x.$$

In other words, for every unit change in the independent variable x, there should be about 1.44 units change in y. Furthermore, the line crosses the y-axis at -2.24.

To test whether the relationship between x and y is significant, one can test whether the observed value of b differs significantly from zero. Performing the test makes use of the variation in y about the least squares line as well as the variation in x. The measure of the former $s_{(y\cdot x)}$ is called the *standard error of estimate* and delineates the extent to which the observed values of y deviate from the y values estimated by the line. The definition of $s^2_{x\cdot y}$ is

$$s^2_{y\cdot x} = \frac{(n-1)}{(n-2)}(s^2_y - b^2 s^2_x),$$

which is easier to calculate using

$$s^2_{y\cdot x} = \frac{[n\Sigma x^2 - (\Sigma x)^2][n\Sigma y^2 - (\Sigma y)^2] -}{(n-2)(n)[n\Sigma x^2 - (\Sigma x)^2]}$$

$$\frac{[n\Sigma xy - (\Sigma x)(\Sigma y)]^2}{(n-2)(n)[n\Sigma x^2 - (\Sigma x)^2]}$$

$$= \frac{1048.5}{1687.5} = 0.6213.$$

In the usual way, we obtain

$$s^2_x = \frac{\Sigma(x-\bar{x})^2}{n-1} = \frac{n\Sigma x^2 - (\Sigma x)^2}{n(n-1)} = 5.625.$$

It is now possible to calculate the significance of the regression coefficient using a t-test. The test statistic, t_B, follows the t-distribution with n−2 degrees of freedom.[14]

$$t_B = \frac{(b-B)s_x\sqrt{n-1}}{s_{y\cdot x}} = \frac{(1.44-0)(2.372)(2)}{(0.788)} = 8.67.$$

The tables of the t-distribution show that the critical value of t, for three degrees of freedom at the 5% level of significance, for a two-tailed test is $t_c = 3.18$.

Since $|8.67| > 3.18$, the null hypothesis can be rejected, so there is a significant relationship between the variables x and y. Stated in still another way, when the estimated regression coefficient b differs significantly from zero, by knowing something about x, one can say something meaningful about y.

TRENDS IN RATES. A situation that occurs repeatedly in epidemiological studies is the examination of a series of rates for possible trends. Regression analysis is especially useful in such situations, but should be applied cautiously for the following reasons:

(1) An underlying assumption in regression is that there is constant variation in y about the regression line; that is, the conditional distribution of y given x is independent of x. Therefore, in using regression analysis on rates, one should pay particular attention to the magnitude of the rates as well as the numbers of individuals at risk of being affected.[15]

(2) Extrapolation of regression lines outside the control area can be misleading. This difficulty, or precaution, is not peculiar only to regression with

rates. Any cyclic pattern having periods greater than the interval used for analysis will destroy any "trends" discerned with regression analysis.

(3) It is assumed that x, the independent variable, is known exactly; yet, with rates expressed per year, the cases occur throughout the year. In spite of this difficulty, it may be informative to use *time* as the predictor or input variable in regression of rates on years. It should be noted that there are regression techniques for circumstances where both x and y variables are subject to error. These techniques, described in several intermediate-level statistical texts, are outside the scope of this text.

Problem 8. Incidence of clinical diagnoses of toxicosis caused by industrial pollutant ABC in cattle.

Given the following series of incidence rates, for clinically detectable poisoning of cattle with an industrial pollutant ABC, test for significance of trend. The cattle population for the area studied has remained at about 2.5 to 3 million residents (per year) since 1960.

Year	Incidence per 10,000 cattle per year
1 (1963)	7.6
2	9.0
3	8.7
4	9.1
5	9.9
6	10.3
7	10.6
8	11.7
9	12.3
10	13.8
11	14.7
12 (1974)	14.9

Comparing several groups (one-way analysis of variance)

Many epidemiological investigations center on more than two groups. In order to be able to compare results from three or more groups, one-way analysis of variance may be an appropriate analytical tool. Before using any statistical tool, it is wise to consider the limitations of that tool and to compare its properties with other potentially useful tools. Analysis of variance has several underlying assumptions; e.g., (1) each group is a random sample from the corresponding populations; (2) samples are selected independently; (3) the variable being measured is normally distributed in each of the $k \geq 2$ populations; and (4) the variable being measured has the same variance in all the populations. Fortunately, the analysis-of-variance procedure is "robust," or relatively unaffected by modest violations of the underlying assumptions.

The analysis-of-variance procedure is based on a comparison of two variances. Suppose there are three groups, with variances s_A^2, s_B^2, s_C^2 in each group, with a pooled estimate of the (assumed) common variance $s_p^2 = w_A s_A^2 + w_B s_B^2 + w_C s_C^2$, where w's are "weights." These weights have the form $w_i = (n_i - 1)/(n_{i_A} + n_{i_B} + n_{i_C} - 3)$, where n_i = sample size for the ith group. Another estimate of the common variance can be made using the sample means $\overline{X}_A$, $\overline{X}_B$, $\overline{X}_C$. If all the samples have come from the same population (i.e., there is no difference among populations from which the samples are drawn), and if each sample is the same size (say n), then it should be clear that another estimate of σ^2 is given by $n s_{\overline{x}}^2$.

Forming the ratio of these two estimates $n s_{\overline{x}}^2 / s_p^2$ is a convenient test. If, in fact, there is little difference among group means, then the ratio should be approximately unity. On the other hand, if there is excessive variability among group means, this variability can be measured relative to the variability that is inherent within groups. Thus, if the calculated ratio of variances is "too large," a significant difference exists among groups. Unfortunately, a significant result in a one-way analysis of variance means only that at least one group differs from at least one other. Which particular groups may differ from others depends on subsequent analyses, such as Duncan's new multiple range test, Dunnett's t-test, and Scheffe's S-method.[16]

Table 5–10. Weight Gains (in Pounds) of Pigs Fed Prophylactic Doses of Two Different Broad Spectrum Antihelmintics (Groups A and B) and Animals Given Placebo (C) in Double-Blind Trial Over X Days (Calculations for One-Way Analysis of Variance).

The Data:

Group:	A	B	C	
	10	19	9	
	12	27	16	
	15	19	10	
	20	25	13	
	18		12	
	15			

H_0: No difference in means among groups

H_a: At least one group mean differs from at least one other

We are choosing the 5% level of significance (a = 0.05).

		A	B	C	Totals
Sums	$\sum_j x_{ij}$	90	90	60	240
Sums of squares	$\sum_j x_{ij}^2$	1418	2076	750	4244
Sample sizes	n_i	6	4	5	15
Sample means	$\overline{x}_i$	15.0	22.5	12.0	$\overline{x} = \dfrac{240}{15} = 16$

$$\frac{(\sum x)^2}{n_i} \qquad \frac{90^2}{6} = 1350 \; ; \; \frac{90^2}{4} = 2025 \; ; \; \frac{60^2}{5} = 720 \qquad \sum \frac{\left(\sum_j x_{ij}\right)^2}{n_i} = 4095$$

$$\text{Correction term} = c = \frac{\left(\sum_{ij} \sum x_{ij}\right)^2}{\sum_i n_i} = \frac{240^2}{15} = 3840$$

$$\text{Total sum of squares} = 4244 - c = 404$$

Analysis of variance:

Source of variation	Sum of squares	Degrees of freedom	Mean Square	F-ratio
Among groups (treatment)	4095 – c = 255	k – 1 = 2	$\dfrac{255}{2} = 127.5$	10.27
Within groups (residual)	Difference = 149	Difference = 12	$\dfrac{149}{12} = 12.42$	
Total	404	$\sum n_i - 1 = 14$		

These other procedures could be followed without first doing the analysis of variance. However, in first doing the one-way analysis of variance, two benefits accrue: (1) if no significant difference is indicated, there is not much point in using the "posterior" procedures, and (2) if a significant difference exists, the estimates of variance needed for Duncan's test (or others) are already calculated and available for application.

Although the discussion on formulation of the variance ratio was based on an assumption of equal numbers of observations in each group, the computational procedure does not require equal sample sizes. Before calculating, one should specify the level of significance at which he has chosen to work, and specify the null and alternative hypotheses. The analysis-of-variance procedure and its utility are illustrated for data from a prospective clinical trial in Table 5–10.

One compares the calculated F-ratio (10.27) against the tabled F for $\alpha=0.05$ with 2 and 12 degrees of freedom. The calculated value exceeds the tabled value (10.27 > 3.89), so the null hypothesis is rejected in favor of the alternative. The conclusion is that the means differ significantly.

There are other more general models for the analysis of variance, including two-way anova, factorial design, and nested models. They are outside the scope of this book, but interested readers will find them described in standard statistical textbooks. In using the analysis-of-variance techniques in epidemiological studies, the investigator should proceed with caution because violations of the underlying assumptions in anova, particularly those assumptions concerning independence, are likely to lead to fallacious conclusions when interpreting results of the analysis.

Other test statistics useful in analytical epidemiology are given in Table 5–11.

In summary, this chapter has introduced mathematical aspects of epidemiological study design, described the methods most used to present data derived from such studies and, finally, reviewed briefly some statistical tools commonly used for epidemiological analyses.

Table 5–11. Characteristics of Some Test Statistics Frequently Used in Analytical Epidemiology

Types of tests of hypotheses (1)	Hypothesis tested (null hypothesis) (2)	Alternative hypothesis (3)	Statistic used (4)	Distribution of the statistic under H_o (5)	Critical region (6)	Assumptions (7)
I. Tests of hypotheses concerning a single population mean						
a) When population variance σ^2 is known	$H_o:\ \mu = \mu_o$	$H_1:\ \mu > \mu_o$	$Z = \dfrac{X - \mu_o}{\sigma/\sqrt{n}}$	$N(0,1)$	$Z > Z_{1-\alpha}$	Independent observations (independence)
		$H_2:\ \mu < \mu_o$	Same	Same	$Z < Z_\alpha$	Same
		$H_3:\ \mu \neq \mu_o$	Same	Same	$Z > Z_{1-\frac{\alpha}{2}}$ $Z < Z_{\frac{\alpha}{2}}$	Same
b) When population variance σ^2 is unknown	$H_o:\ \mu = \mu_o$	$H_1:\ \mu > \mu_o$	$t = \dfrac{X - \mu_o}{s/\sqrt{n}}$	The t-distribution with $n-1$ degrees of freedom	$t > t_{1-\alpha}$	1) Independence 2) The random variable X has the normal distribution (normality assumption).
		$H_2:\ \mu < \mu_o$	Same	Same	$t < t_\alpha$	Same
		$H_3:\ \mu \neq \mu_o$	Same	Same	$t > t_{1-\frac{\alpha}{2}}$ $t < t_{\frac{\alpha}{2}}$	Same
II. Tests of hypotheses concerning the means of two populations						
a) When population variances σ_1^2 and σ_2^2 are known	$H_o:\ \mu_1 = \mu_2$ $(\mu_1 - \mu_2 = 0)$	$H_1:\ \mu_1 > \mu_2$ $(\mu_1 - \mu_2 > 0)$	$Z = \dfrac{(\bar{X}_1 - \bar{X}_2) - 0}{\sqrt{\dfrac{\sigma_1^2}{n_1} + \dfrac{\sigma_2^2}{n_2}}}$	$N(0,1)$	$Z > Z_{1-\alpha}$	Independence
		Note: If the two variances are equal, e.i., $\sigma_1^2 = \sigma_2^2 = \sigma^2$, then the statistic becomes $Z = \dfrac{(\bar{X}_1 - \bar{X}_2) - 0}{\sigma\sqrt{\dfrac{1}{n_1} + \dfrac{1}{n_2}}}$				
b) When population variances σ_1^2 and σ_2^2 are unknown	$H_o:\ \mu_1 = \mu_2$ $(\mu_1 - \mu_2 = 0)$	$H_1:\ \mu_1 > \mu_2$ $(\mu_1 - \mu_2 > 0)$	$t = \dfrac{(\bar{X}_1 - \bar{X}_2) - 0}{s_p\sqrt{\dfrac{1}{n_1} + \dfrac{1}{n_2}}}$ where s_p is the pooled sample std. deviation	The t-distribution with $n_1 + n_2 - 2$ degrees of freedom	$t > t_{1-\alpha}$	1) Independence 2) Normality 3) Equal variances
c) By means of pairing observations	$H_o:\ \mu_1 - \mu_2 = 0$ $(\mu_1 = \mu_2)$	$H_1:\ \mu_1 - \mu_2 > 0$ $(\mu_1 > \mu_2)$	$t = \dfrac{\bar{Y} - 0}{s_Y/\sqrt{n}}$ where $\bar{Y}$ and s_Y are the sample mean and sample std. deviation respectively, of $Y = X_1 - X_2$	The t-distribution with $n-1$ degrees of freedom	$t > t_{1-\alpha}$	1) Observations on Y are independent. 2) Distribution of Y is normal.

	Hypotheses	Test statistic	Distribution	Critical region	Assumptions
III. Tests of hypotheses concerning a single population proportion	$H_0: p = p_0$ $H_1: p > p_0$	$Z = \dfrac{\hat{p} - p_0}{\sqrt{\dfrac{p_0(1-p_0)}{n}}}$ where $\hat{p} = \dfrac{X}{n}$ is the sample proportion	$N(0,1)$	$Z > Z_{1-\alpha}$	1) Independence 2) Large sample
IV. Tests of hypotheses concerning the proportions of two populations	$H_0: p_1 = p_2$ $(p_1 - p_2 = 0)$ $H_1: p_1 > p_2$ $(p_1 - p_2 > 0)$	$Z = \dfrac{(\hat{p}_1 - \hat{p}_2) - 0}{\sqrt{\hat{p}(1-\hat{p})\left(\dfrac{1}{n_1} + \dfrac{1}{n_2}\right)}}$ where $\hat{p}_1 = \dfrac{x_1}{n_1}$, $\hat{p}_2 = \dfrac{x_2}{n_2}$ and $\hat{p} = \dfrac{x_1 + x_2}{n_1 + n_2}$	$N(0,1)$	$Z > Z_{1-\alpha}$	1) Independence 2) Large samples
V. Tests of hypotheses concerning a population variance	$H_0: \sigma^2 = \sigma_0^2$ $H_1: \sigma^2 > \sigma_0^2$	$\chi^2 = \dfrac{\sum (X_i - \bar{X})^2}{\sigma_0^2}$	The chi-square distribution with $n-1$ degrees of freedom	$\chi^2 > \chi^2_{1-\alpha}$	1) Independence 2) Normality
VI. Tests of hypotheses concerning the variances of two populations	$H_0: \sigma_1^2 = \sigma_2^2$ $(\sigma_1^2 / \sigma_2^2 = 1)$ $H_1: \sigma_1^2 > \sigma_2^2$ $(\sigma_1^2 / \sigma_2^2 > 1)$	$F_1 = \dfrac{s_1^2}{s_2^2}$	The F-distribution with (n_1-1) and (n_2-1) degrees of freedom	$F_1 > F_{1-\alpha}$	1) Independence 2) Normality
	$H_2: \sigma_1^2 \neq \sigma_2^2$ $(\sigma_1^2 / \sigma_2^2 > 1$ or $\sigma_2^2 / \sigma_1^2 > 1)$	$F_2 = \dfrac{s_1^2}{s_2^2}$ $F_2 = \dfrac{s_2^2}{s_1^2}$	F with (n_1-1) and (n_2-1) degrees of freedom F with (n_2-1) and (n_1-1) d.f.	$F_1 > F_{1-\alpha/2}$ $F_2 > F_{1-\alpha/2}$	Same
VII. The χ^2 tests a) Single classification	H_0 completely specifies the theoretical distribution of the random variable. H_1: the distribution specified under H_0 is not true.	$\chi^2 = \displaystyle\sum_{i=1}^{k} \dfrac{(f_i - F_i)^2}{F_i}$	χ^2 with $(k-1)$ degrees of freedom	$\chi^2 > \chi^2_{1-\alpha}$	1) Independence 2) Large sample
b) Two-way classification	H_0: the distributions of two random vars. are independent of each other. H_1: they are not independent.	$\chi^2 = \displaystyle\sum_{i=1}^{rc} \dfrac{(f_i - F_i)^2}{F_i}$	χ^2 with $(r-1) \times (c-1)$ degrees of freedom	$\chi^2 > \chi^2_{1-\alpha}$	Same
c) Test for goodness of fit	H_0: the distribution of the random variable belongs to a certain family of distributions. H_1: the distribution does not belong to this family.	$\chi^2 = \displaystyle\sum_{i=1}^{k} \dfrac{(f_i - F_i)^2}{F_i}$	χ^2 with $(k-1-a)$ degrees of freedom, where a is the number of parameters in the distribution	$\chi^2 > \chi^2_{1-\alpha}$	Same

Part 3

STUDY OF MULTIPLE VARIABLES

*"Know one disease completely
and you know all of medicine."*
—William Osler

Chapter 6

TEMPORAL DISTRIBUTIONS OF DISEASE EVENTS

DISEASE events in populations all take place in a continuum of time. Because time is easily quantifiable, either as calendar or absolute time, this variable provides a scale against which disease phenomena are often measured. All epidemiologically useful rates have a necessary time component, and other methods are available to help identify regular temporal patterns of disease events or their irregular clustering in time. Moreover, time considerations are usually involved in selecting the most appropriate study approach to particular disease phenomena and in understanding the meaning of data obtained through different study approaches.

CLUSTERING OF DISEASE EVENTS IN TIME

Hypotheses of determinants of diseases can sometimes be derived from observed clustering of epidemiologically important events along a time axis. Temporal clustering of outbreaks of Asian Newcastle disease after visits to poultry farms by commercial vaccination crews was observed in a study of the epidemic of that disease in California in 1971-73.[1] In another example, a clustering of onset of human poliomyelitis cases was observed among children 7 to 18 days after tonsillectomy, a period compatible with the incubation time of that disease.[2] Approaches to the recognition of clustering will be considered in the next chapter in connection with clustering in space.

EPIDEMIC CURVES AND OTHER TIME GRAPHS

Occurrences of disease events in populations often are presented graphically—as histograms or frequency polygons—using a coordinate system in which the ordinate represents the number of new cases in a given time interval (hours, days, weeks) and the abscissa represents time, either calendar time or absolute time measured from some preceding event.

Calendar time graphs for relatively short time intervals or for a specific population event are called *epidemic curves*, a subject already mentioned in Chapter 2. Epidemic curves thus are incidence curves; and they express increase and decrease of the number of new disease cases, as well as the rate (speed) of changes in disease occurrence (Fig. 6–1 to 6–3). In plotting epidemic curves, it is advisable to use the smallest time intervals that are practical for the

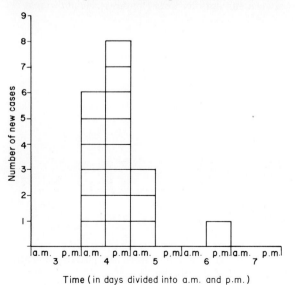

Fig. 6–1. Histogram of common source (point) epidemic of disease with short incubation period.

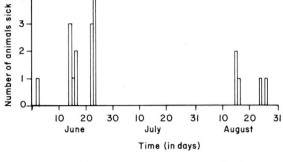

Fig. 6–2.   Histogram showing number of new cases per day during epidemic in cattle herd (see Problem 1, Chapter 2).

abscissa, since this procedure can reveal details that might be lost were longer time intervals used. Sometimes, especially in attempts to show disease trends over longer periods of time, prevalence rates also are used in time graphs, instead of using incidence data. Absolute time graphs are used to show clustering with respect to a preceding event.

Point epidemics

Pronounced clustering is observed in common source or point epidemics, which occur when a number of animals are exposed to a common event, such as an agent present in water or food or on fomites they share. A typical example of a food poisoning outbreak is the one detailed in Chapter 3. Just as the expression "point prevalence" is a relative term, "point epidemic," too, is relative; for not every animal eating a contaminated feed, for example, necessarily does so at *exactly* the same time. Each square in the epidemic curve histogram of a point epidemic (e.g., see Fig. 6–1) represents the onset of disease in one individual, and these onsets often are plotted for intervals as short as one hour. Sometimes the time covered by such point epidemic curves is shorter than the incubation period of the disease.

When, however, a contaminated feed, for example, is not eaten at approximately the same time, the situation could be a common source, multiple-event epidemic. Here the distribution of cases would be stretched out in time, or a number of point epidemics would appear when cases are plotted against calendar time. Such a situation could occur, for example, when grain treated with a mercurial fungicide is marketed as livestock feed or when contamination of feeds is accidental, as in the disease outbreak problem described in Chapter 3. However, if such data are plotted in absolute time, i.e., when time from consumption of the infective or toxic food until onset of disease is used for the abscissal scale, a single point epidemic will appear on the graph. The basic principles of investigation of common source epidemics were discussed under outbreak investigation in Chapter 3, and further information on methods for their analysis is considered in Chapter 11.

Propagated epidemics

In propagated epidemics, agents are transmitted directly or indirectly from infected hosts to other susceptible hosts. The rapidity of "build up" of a propagated epidemic depends on a variety of factors. Among these are (1) the mode of transmission of the agent, (2) the infectivity and the free-living longevity of the agent, (3) the direct or indirect social distance between susceptible hosts ("indirect social distance")

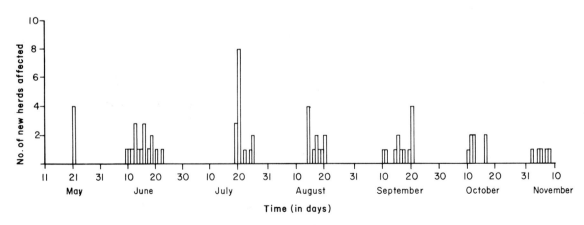

Fig. 6–3.   Histogram of epidemic affecting a number of cattle herds. It spread in a wave-like pattern, and the period between waves corresponded to the incubation period of the disease.

reflects such things as numbers of available vectors and extent of movement of fomites), (4) the length of the infectious organism's prepatent period, and (5) the proportions of susceptible or infective animals in the population. As a propagated epidemic continues, those individuals infected either die or recover (and often become immune), with the result that the supply of susceptibles is depleted. In consequence, the epidemic tapers off and finally stops. Epidemics among livestock generally taper off prematurely because of intervention (e.g., quarantine).

Figure 6–2 is a histogram representing the disease events described in the problem in a dairy herd considered in Chapter 2. This graph is clearly different from that for the point epidemic curve shown in Figure 6–1. Inspection of Figure 6–2, while considering facts discussed earlier, suggests either that this disease was a common source, multiple-event epidemic or that it spread by contact, and also suggests that its incubation time is one to two weeks. This latter is inferred from the observation that two weeks passed between the first case and the three cases on June 14-16 and that one week passed before the next cases appeared on June 22-24. There was also one week between the cases on August 15-17 and the cases on August 23-25.

Since veterinary studies in epidemiology often deal with the flock or herd as a primary unit rather than the individual animal, temporal patterns of disease may be plotted on a herd basis. This factor makes little difference with respect to the basic epidemiological approach. Figure 6–3 illustrates a cattle epidemic in a township containing a number of farms. In the graph, the ordinate represents the number of new *herds* affected. This infectious disease was assumed to be transmitted between adjacent farms by a biting fly, which acted as a short-range mechanical vector (it remained infective for about five minutes only). This particular epidemic curve seems to be composed of a number of point epidemics, and in a sense it is. The mean distance between peaks is 28 days, which agrees fairly well with the incubation time of the disease that was diagnosed. These features are obvious because the numbers of newly affected herds are plotted by day. If they had been plotted by month, such details would have been lost. This illustration shows again that care should be exercised in selecting the appropriate time scale in plotting epidemic curves.

In the examples given previously, the *number* of cases or herds were plotted. For other purposes, the *percent of cases* based on population at risk or on total population may be similarly plotted.

Mathematical models have been created to illustrate —and study—the process of spread with respect to time of infectious diseases. Modelling is described in Chapter 16.

DIURNAL AND OTHER SHORT-TERM PATTERNS

Disease incidence may fluctuate over very short periods of time for various reasons. For instance, livestock species follow different diurnal activity patterns, which may influence the risk of their acquiring particular diseases. Some of these patterns are man-influenced or man-determined to a great degree. Thus, the common practice of extending the hours of light for chickens may have direct disease-related effects upon the host and also may attract large numbers of certain vector insects to the chicken house. Many wild reservoir and vector species also show *photoperiodism* in habits and activity. Thus, *Culex tarsalis*, a mosquito vector of certain arboviruses, feeds at sunset, when it has easy access to roosting birds. *Haemagogus*, another mosquito vector of yellow fever, feeds in daylight on animals that rest then. Vampire bats, which transmit rabies, feed mainly at night. The infectious agent itself may be subject to such patterns. For example, filarial worms show circadian periodicities with respect to their appearance in the peripheral blood and, hence, their availability to vectors.

SEASONAL VARIATIONS

Seasonal variations in disease occurrence are those that show periodicities of one year. The reasons for some of these patterns are well known, at least superficially. For example, variation in incidence of vector-borne diseases throughout a year is related to different levels of activity of vectors such as mosquitoes or flies, which remain inactive in cold seasons. Another season-associated factor is the crowding that occurs when animals are housed in barns in the wintertime. Crowding not only facilitates direct and indirect contact but also may be associated with increased stress and changes in feed, both of which will also affect the host population. Parturient paresis follows calving, which in some places is also fairly closely associated with season. Other seasonal variations affect agents; for example, poisoning caused by toxic plants occurs only in their growing season, and sometimes only in a specific period of their growing season.

Some seasonal variations are fairly easy to explain, at least in a descriptive way; but detailed analysis is required to obtain more exact information about their etiological significance. Thus, seasonal variations in neonatal calf mortality have been observed for some time, and association with weather conditions has been hypothesized. However, it was found only recently that the weather conditions on the day of birth may have a significant effect on a calf's ability to survive its first month. Weather may exert a direct effect on the dam as well, since that study also found that daily weather condition is a determinant with respect to time of calving.[3] The exact underlying mechanisms for these phenomena are not known, but similar mechanisms may be behind the observations that parturient paresis occurs in association with weather conditions.

In the preceding examples, the eliciting factors have been external ones (e.g., temperature, light, rainfall) that happen to be associated with season. It is known too that biorhythms, or "internal clocks," operate in various organisms. They may have an effect on seasonal disease patterns independent of external stimuli. For instance, endogenous biorhythms determine hibernation in squirrels and time of emergence of flies from their pupal cases. These patterns would doubtlessly influence the reservoir or vector roles of such species. Annual rhythms, which are comparable in timing for populations in different geographic locations and dissimilar climates, may be dependent on such underlying endogenous rhythms; but this possibility has been little explored with respect to disease phenomena. Time series methods useful for the identification of such seasonal changes are considered at the end of this chapter.

CYCLIC PATTERNS

In epidemiology, cyclic patterns refer to the rise and wane of disease incidence with a fairly constant periodicity of several years—in contrast to seasonal variations, which show yearly cycles. Some cyclic patterns result from fluctuation in herd immunity. Among the better-known examples is human measles (in cities), which occurs with increased incidence in children at intervals slightly less than three years. Meningococcal infection in people also occurred in cycles of seven to nine years before the advent of sulfonamides and penicillin.

Many documented instances of cyclic variation are also known for animal diseases, but virtually all of these involve wild species and periodic population die-offs. Examples include the role of disease in population cycles of lemmings, varying or snowshoe hares in the Arctic, and squirrels in several parts of the United States. In most such instances, the specific diseases and infectious agents involved have not been adequately investigated. The truncated lives of most domesticated animals tend to disrupt recognizable cycles. The effect of herd immunity on cyclical patterns is discussed in Chapter 9.

SECULAR CHANGES

Changes in disease frequency that occur gradually over long periods of time are called secular changes or trends. In human studies in epidemiology, death certificates are the main source of information about secular changes. However, there are many difficulties in interpretation when death certificates are used for studies of trends. A somewhat similar source of information about secular changes is available to the veterinary epidemiologist—postmortem reports of causes for condemnation of carcasses in slaughterhouses. Table 6–1 shows computed accumulated prevalences of disease conditions found at postmortem examination of mature cattle in the United States in the period from 1925 to 1962. (Some of the raw data from which these figures were derived are given in Table 5–8.)

Several apparent trends are present. Diagnoses of tuberculosis have shown a continued decrease. Diagnoses of cysticercosis, echinococcosis, and sarcoma of cattle have also declined over the period of recording, while malignant lymphoma seems to have increased. Two diagnoses not displaying secular trends are carcinoma, which has remained relatively constant (or perhaps has shown some evidence for a cyclic change), and hyperkeratosis, which shows a rapid increase followed by almost complete disappearance over an eight-year period. Such changes are difficult to interpret, and only for the tuberculosis trend and the hyperkeratosis pattern have adequate explanations been found. Causes for the secular change in tuberculosis are obviously related to continued eradication efforts.

Speculation on the meaning of the cattle cancer statistics in Table 5–8 should help one realize that the most difficult aspects of interpreting apparent trends in such records as death certificates and condemnation statistics relate to possible changes in diagnosis, concepts, and terminology. Such changes can present apparent trends; and since it is difficult to evaluate procedures that were in use many years ago, the best chance of discovering such external factors is when they occur suddenly—with the result that a discontinuity or abrupt change occurs in an otherwise smooth trend curve. No such changes are discernible upon inspection of Table 6–1; but if a gradual change had taken place in terminology resulting in more cases of sarcoma being called malignant lymphoma (also called lymphosarcoma), the two apparently opposite trends for these diagnoses would tend to cancel each other. In other words, if the two diagnoses were combined into a sarcoma-malignant lymphoma category, the prevalence of this "entity" would remain approximately constant.

The only way to decide whether a gradual change in diagnosis has taken place would be to examine samples of tumor tissue stored in a tissue bank. However, with rare exceptions, such as the Veterinary Tumor Registry of the Armed Forces Institute of Pathology, such tissue banks have not been established. Even in that instance, the collecting procedure has not been a systematic one. *Hints* that real secular changes have occurred are evident if, for example, there are different trends for different breeds or if there are different trends for diseases that are similarly difficult to diagnose.

Table 6-1.   Mature Cattle Condemned at Postmortem Examination (per 100,000 Examined) in United States by Selected Causes, 1925-1962 (Rates Calculated from Data in the Annual Reports of the Meat Inspection Division, U.S. Department of Agriculture)

Year	Total cattle examined	Tuberculosis	Cysticercosis	Echinococcosis (livers)	Malignant lymphoma	Sarcoma	Carcinoma	Hyperkeratosis (chlorinated naphthalene poisoning)
1925	9,773,883	625.0	1.9	NR*	5.7	NR	NR	NR
1926	10,098,121	660.0	1.3	NR	6.8	NR	NR	NR
1946	12,581,268	13.4	1.6	NR	11.4	5.2	7.0	NR
1947	14,093,769	10.8	1.4	NR	9.9	4.4	7.3	NR
1949	13,182,962	10.4	1.4	NR	9.0	5.2	9.3	0.12
1950	13,115,889	8.7	0.8	20.7	9.3	5.4	12.1	0.24
1951	12,570,825	7.2	0.8	20.4	9.3	6.2	13.1	0.14
1952	12,136,210	6.6	0.9	20.6	9.7	7.3	12.6	0.02
1953	15,204,998	5.4	1.1	12.1	10.0	3.6	10.1	4.09
1954	18,475,936	4.2	0.9	14.7	11.5	2.9	9.6	0.05
1955	18,725,455	3.1	0.7	15.2	14.3	2.8	8.8	0.04
1956	19,679,898	2.4	0.7	12.5	15.2	2.1	8.1	0.02
1957	20,142,195	2.2	0.9	13.2	17.0	1.5	7.5	
1958	18,579,099	1.6	0.6	14.8	17.6	1.7	8.2	
1959	17,320,716	1.3	0.6	12.3	18.2	1.8	7.4	
1960	18,454,319	1.0	0.5	8.7	16.9	1.8	6.8	
1961	19,861,644	1.1	0.5	10.4	18.8	1.5	8.6	
1962	20,158,743	1.0	0.5	10.7	18.8	1.0	9.2	

*NR = not recorded

In Problem 6, the number of animals sent to slaughter varies for different years. This fluctuation may reflect higher or lower market prices and the withholding of animals by farmers, or the marketing of younger animals than usual. Thus, apparent changes may be reflected in the frequencies of diseases with known age associations.

Trends such as those shown in Table 6-1 may be difficult to interpret because they represent a huge area, in this case, the United States. A high prevalence in one or a few states may mask a general declining trend. This possibility can be evaluated by studying the spatial distribution of the disease (see Chapter 7).

True secular trends may have many different explanations. Environmental determinants may be active, such as in instances of pollution; or gradual, in systems of animal husbandry that result, for example, in increased crowding of larger numbers of animals or in modification of feeds. A slowly spreading or intensifying infectious agent also may cause trends, possibly in interaction with changed environment or changed characteristics of the host. In addition, host factors may be quite important determinants of secular time trends. The generation time of most farm animals is quite short; and planned breeding and selection for high production traits may result in

stock that, at the same time, carry lethal genes or have increased susceptibility to infectious or noninfectious diseases.

The approach in attempts to explain trends is basically the same as that used in other investigations of diseases in populations (see Chapters 3, 4, and 5); and success depends on the reliability of the available data. The type of information shown in Table 6-1 (based on postmortem examinations in slaughterhouses) probably is diagnostically variable. The purpose of veterinary food protection activities up to now has been almost exclusively to determine whether an animal is fit for human consumption; there have been no requirements for a precise diagnosis. This situation could be improved through attempts to obtain uniform and more precise diagnoses by using objective diagnostic methods (i.e., laboratory tests) whenever possible. The future use of slaughterhouses as a key link in veterinary epidemiological intelligence (see Chapter 14) will require greater diagnostic objectivity.

Data for ascertaining trends are available, too, from sources such as animal hospital records, but these sources have seldom been used. Special animal hospital studies, such as the California Animal Tumor

Registry, offer such possibilities. Within a hospital, the diagnosis is more precise than that derived from existing slaughterhouse data. Even so, some classic difficulties persist in trend evaluation. For example, the California Animal Tumor Registry is based on cooperation with more than 60 veterinary practitioners, who submit samples of tissues suspected of being neoplastic. These submissions depend on the interest and diagnostic acumen of these practitioners and on the owners' uses of veterinary services, which, in turn, may reflect such things as household economics. Trends in these characteristics are likely to occur, but be difficult to measure, and may confuse results.

Secular trends may be revealed by use of the time series methods discussed later, but some examples of seasonal time relationships are illustrated in western equine encephalomyelitis (WE), an infection already considered in Chapter 4.

TIME RELATIONSHIPS IN WESTERN EQUINE ENCEPHALOMYELITIS

The generation of epidemics of symptomatic WE in horses and people in the summertime in various parts of the United States and Canada is dependent upon a time sequence of environmental events. Initially there is a so-called spring amplification period for this virus.

In the western part of North America, this spring cycle of transmission begins when some infective *Culex tarsalis* mosquitoes start their active feeding upon wild birds. These birds then become viremic and, in turn, are fed upon by more mosquitoes, which remain infective for life. The resultant spring build-up of infection in *C. tarsalis* and in nestling sparrows is shown in Figure 6–4. It can be seen that these rates closely parallel one another. Nestling birds are preferred by *C. tarsalis*, possibly because they are quiescent and relatively exposed. This preference is

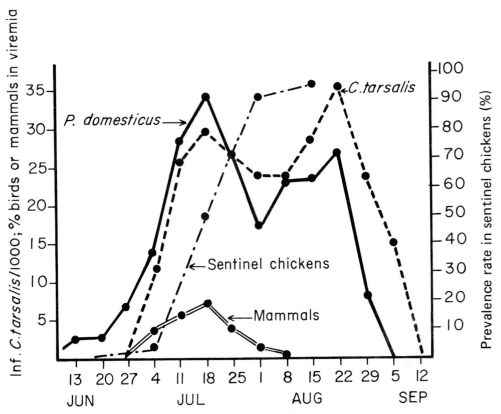

Fig. 6–4.   Western equine encephalitis (WE) virus infection rates in *Culex tarsalis*, nestling sparrows (*Passer domesticus*), and small wild mammals; and WE antibody rates in sentinel chickens, Hale County, Texas, 1965. *C. tarsalis* infection rates are numbers positive per 1000 mosquitoes. Bird and mammal infection rates are the percent in viremia. Sentinel chicken antibody rates are percent with hemagglutination-inhibition (HAI) antibodies. All infection rates are plotted as moving averages (redrawn after Hess, A.D., and Hayes, R.O. 1967. Seasonal dynamics of western encephalitis virus. Am. J. Med. Sci. 253:333).

shown in Figure 6–4 by the time lag for infection in sentinel chicken flocks.

Climatic factors, such as temperature and rainfall, determine the time that spring amplification commences and the level it reaches. Sentinel data provide a useful means for comparing these periods and the rates of spring virus amplification for different years and in different places. Such comparisons (Fig. 6–5) show, for example, that the date at which virus amplification can begin correlates with spring temperatures, which, among other things, partially determine the time when populations of nestling birds will be available in any locale. Spring mosquito population build-up, in turn, is dependent in part upon the rainfall pattern that has preceded it. Figure 6–4 also shows the time relations between this build-up in populations of infective mosquitoes and viremic wild birds on the one hand and the onset of WE infections in rodents.

From these data and their lag relationship to the rate of sentinel chicken infections, it would appear that mammalian infections clearly represent a "spill-over" of virus from a large and highly infected mosquito population that must then resort to feeding upon other than its preferred hosts. Again, in Figure 6–6, this rate of acquisition of infection in small

mammals is shown to precede the parallel epidemic curve of human cases during the summer months. The epidemic curve of horse infections generally precedes that of man by about a week or two. These latter cases of disease in horses and then man occur *only* if a "threshold level" of viral amplification in wild birds and mosquitoes has been reached in the spring, with the result that infective mosquitoes are feeding on purely secondary hosts. Confirmatory data on the time sequence of blood meal preferences by *C. tarsalis* are shown in Figure 6–6.

This time sequence of events prior to horse and human infections with WE virus in the western United States is in contrast with the situation in the eastern part of the country, where the principal spring and summer vector of the virus is *Culiseta melanura*. In the East, cases of WE in horses and man virtually never occur because this mosquito rarely if ever feeds upon mammals.

TIME SERIES METHODS

A time series is merely a distribution of data, say, of illnesses or deaths, according to time of occurrence. Times series analyses are concerned with the detection, description, and measurement of patterns or periodicities from such data. It has already been

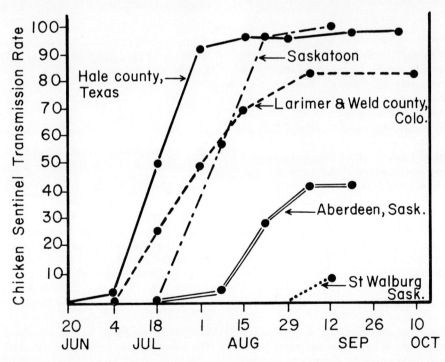

Fig. 6–5. Seasonal patterns of WE antibody (HAI) development in sentinel chicken flocks at five different latitudes from Texas high plains area to west central Saskatchewan during epidemic year, 1965. Transmission rates are percent chickens with HAI antibodies (redrawn after Hess, A.D., and Hayes, R.O. 1967. Seasonal dynamics of western encaphalitis virus. Am. J. Med. Sci. 253:333 using some data from Burton and McLintock).

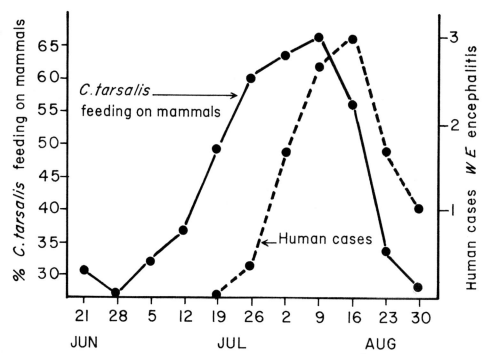

Fig. 6–6. Relationship between increased feeding of *Culex tarsalis* on mammalian hosts and weekly human WE encephalitis case rates during summer of 1964 in eastern Colorado. Data plotted as moving averages (redrawn after Hess, A.D., and Hayes, R.O. 1967. Seasonal dynamics of western encephalitis virus. Am. J. Med. Sci. 253:333).

noted that these patterns are (1) long-term rises or declines called secular trends; (2) cyclical patterns, that is, more or less regular rises and declines with periods of years; and (3) seasonal changes with periods of one year or less. The remaining variations in data with time represent unpredictable, accidental, random, or other short-term and nonperiodic fluctuations in data. Data expressed as a time series may represent the sum of any or all of these components superimposed on one another. Time series analysis helps to isolate each component.

Demonstration of secular trends

Among the ways to identify a long-term trend from a time series are (1) the freehand method, which requires no explanation; (2) the least squares or regression method, which was considered briefly in Chapter 5; and (3) the moving average method. A moving average is a series of data averages centered at each successive measurement point on the time scale. For example, a large pig farm has a 120-month accumulation of monthly neonatal mortality rates (Table 6–2), and one wants to determine whether there is a secular trend in mortality. Twelve-month moving averages calculated from these 120 months' data tend to eliminate or smooth out irregular variations or those with periods of 12 months or less (including possible seasonal variations and the month-to-month fluctuations in deaths representing specific

outbreaks, for example). The result is an approximate trend line. The simple calculations required to obtain moving averages are

$$\overline{Y}_1 = \frac{15.6+15.6+15.8+ \ldots +21.0+16.5}{12}$$

$$= \frac{269.7}{12} = 22.5, \text{ the 12-month moving aver-}$$

age centered between June 15 and July 15, 1966. The next 12-month moving average then is

$$\overline{Y}_2 = \frac{15.6+15.8+19.8+ \ldots +16.5+14.6}{12} = 22.4,$$

which is centered between July 15 and August 15, 1966. The moving average centered on July 15, 1966, then is the mean of $\overline{Y}_1$ and $\overline{Y}_2$ or 22.45%. A disadvantage of this method is the loss of some data at the beginning and at the end of the series, in this example, the first and last six months of observation.

The regression equation for this trend (obtained by the method of least squares, shown in Table 6–3) is $Y = 27.1 + 0.856x$, and is plotted in Figure 6–7. The equation can be used to calculate the monthly mortality rate trend increments as $\frac{0.856\%}{12} =$ 0.071%. By eliminating this monthly increment from each of the observed monthly mortality rates shown for 1966 (e.g., for February, 15.6% - 0.071% = 15.529% (rounded off as 15.5%); for March, 15.8%-2 (0.071%) = 15.7%, etc.), one can see in Table 6–4

Table 6–2.   Neonatal Pig Mortality Rates per 100 Live Births on ARC Pig Farm, 1966-75 (Numeric Data Adapted from Alder, H.L., and Roessler, E.B. 1972. *Introduction to Probability and Statistics*, 5th ed. W.H. Freeman and Co., San Francisco)

Year	Jan.	Feb.	Mar.	Apr.	May	June	July	Aug.	Sept.	Oct.	Nov.	Dec.
1966	15.6	15.6	15.8	19.8	20.5	23.7	26.0	31.7	38.0	25.5	21.0	16.5
1967	14.6	15.7	15.9	20.2	22.7	23.2	28.3	26.0	34.5	34.0	19.5	15.1
1968	13.4	14.3	15.4	17.0	20.3	27.5	36.8	41.3	43.0	36.1	29.4	23.1
1969	16.0	16.2	17.2	17.1	21.0	24.4	37.4	39.4	47.6	33.9	33.2	23.6
1970	15.3	16.1	16.7	18.5	20.9	26.9	35.6	40.4	47.4	35.0	30.9	24.3
1971	16.5	17.8	18.4	18.5	20.7	28.5	35.9	38.5	46.0	34.9	31.5	23.6
1972	17.4	17.9	17.9	18.8	21.1	26.3	36.4	41.7	50.1	33.6	34.1	22.4
1973	17.6	17.4	17.2	18.8	24.0	29.0	38.8	42.2	46.8	35.7	34.3	24.8
1974	18.8	19.0	20.1	20.0	23.6	31.3	41.8	43.2	45.3	38.7	33.9	24.9
1975	19.6	18.7	18.3	20.5	23.9	30.6	38.8	43.6	48.4	43.6	37.3	25.0

what these monthly rates would have been without the effect of the secular trend. These values then represent any cumulated cyclical, seasonal, and unpredictable variations for 1966.

Description of seasonal changes

Similarly, calculation of three-month moving averages from monthly death data helps smooth short-term data fluctuations, such as those that reflect specific outbreaks or accidents of management. The resulting time series emphasizes any seasonal changes in occurrence of deaths. Seasonal data are plotted as moving averages in Figures 6–4 and 6–6.

Using the data on neonatal pig mortality in Table 6–2 and the 12-month moving averages calculated from these data (as illustrated previously), one can calculate so-called *specific seasonals*, that is, an index or ratio in which the *observed* monthly value is

divided by the 12-month moving average value centered on the middle of that month, e.g., for July, 1966, $\frac{26.0}{22.45}$ = 1.16. These specific seasonals for 1967-1974 are shown in Table 6–5. For August, 1972, the neonatal pig mortality rate was 48% above the average for the year centered on that month. Averaging (by the mean or median) these values for each month for all of the years covered by the data (i.e., 1967-1974) gives so-called *typical seasonals*, which are indices of the amount of variation attributable to seasonal influences, in this case, of neonatal pig mortality rates on the farm (Table 6–5).

Specific seasonal and typical seasonal ratios may also be calculated by the ratio-to-trend method. In Table 6–6, this method is used to examine observed monthly incidence rates of respiratory symptoms in

Table 6–3.   Calculation of Trend Line for Neonatal Pig Mortality Data of Table 6–2 by Method of Least Squares (Numerical Data Adapted from Alder and Roessler, 1972)

Year	Y'	x	x²	xY'
1966	22.5	-4.5	20.25	-101.25
1967	22.5	-3.5	12.25	-78.75
1968	26.5	-2.5	6.25	-66.25
1969	27.2	-1.5	2.25	-40.80
1970	27.3	-0.5	0.25	-13.65
1971	27.6	0.5	0.25	13.80
1972	28.1	1.5	2.25	42.15
1973	28.9	2.5	6.25	72.25
1974	30.0	3.5	12.25	105.00
1975	30.7	4.5	20.25	138.15
Totals	271.3	0	82.50	70.65

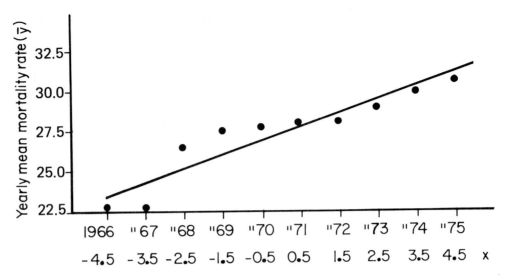

Fig. 6-7. Trend line for neonatal pig mortality rates obtained by method of least squares showing also mean observed rates for each year (adapted from Alder and Roessler, 1972).

calves and trend rates calculated from 10 years' hypothetical data by the method of least squares. The typical seasonals subtracted from the specific seasonals leave the combined cyclical and unpredictable variations shown in column 6 of Table 6-6. Long-term cyclical changes often require more complex time series methods for their isolation and measurement.

In a final example of time clustering of disease, clustering occurred throughout a large area and ultimately was shown to represent multiple common source outbreaks. This example illustrates a concentrated effort at disease investigation, with many pathological, microbiological, and other conventional inputs. However, systematic epidemiological studies were conspicuously lacking from these efforts until an investigator working on a completely different disease problem made an important chance observation in the field and followed it up with a series of prospective trials.

TEMPORAL PATTERN OF BOVINE HYPERKERATOSIS

The unusual temporal pattern of bovine hyperkeratosis in the United States is reflected in Table 6-1. Sporadic cases of this new disease syndrome of

Table 6-4.   Elimination of Trend for Pig Mortality Rates of Table 6-2 (Year 1966) (Numerical Data Modified from Alder and Roessler, 1972)

Month	Y observed rates (%)	Rates after elimination of the trend (%)
Jan.	15.6	15.6
Feb.	15.6	15.5
Mar.	15.8	15.7
Apr.	19.8	19.6
May	20.5	20.2
June	23.7	23.3
July	26.0	25.6
Aug.	31.7	31.2
Sept.	38.0	37.4
Oct.	25.5	24.9
Nov.	21.0	20.3
Dec.	16.5	15.7

Table 6-5.   Specific Seasonals, 1967-1974, for Neonatal Pig Mortality Data of Table 6-2 (Numerical Data Adapted from Alder and Roessler, 1972)

Year	Jan.	Feb.	Mar.	Apr.	May	June	July	Aug.	Sept.	Oct.	Nov.	Dec.
1967	0.64	0.70	0.72	0.90	1.00	1.03	1.26	1.16	1.55	1.54	0.89	0.69
1968	0.60	0.61	0.63	0.68	0.80	1.05	1.38	1.54	1.60	1.35	1.09	0.86
1969	0.60	0.61	0.64	0.63	0.78	0.90	1.38	1.45	1.75	1.25	1.22	0.86
1970	0.56	0.59	0.61	0.67	0.76	0.99	1.30	1.47	1.71	1.26	1.12	0.88
1971	0.59	0.64	0.67	0.67	0.75	1.03	1.30	1.39	1.67	1.26	1.14	0.86
1972	0.63	0.65	0.64	0.67	0.75	0.93	1.29	1.48	1.78	1.20	1.21	0.79
1973	0.62	0.61	0.60	0.66	0.84	1.01	1.34	1.45	1.60	1.21	1.16	0.84
1974	0.63	0.63	0.67	0.67	0.79	1.04	1.39	1.44	1.51	1.29	1.13	0.83
Median	0.61	0.62	0.64	0.67	0.785	1.02	1.32	1.45	1.635	1.26	1.135	0.85
Typical seasonals	0.61	0.62	0.64	0.67	0.785	1.02	1.32	1.45	1.635	1.26	1.135	0.85

Table 6-6.   Computation of Seasonal and Cyclical Variation, Ratio to Trend Method, for Incidence of Respiratory Symptoms in Calves, 1955-65 (Numerical Data Adapted from Arkin, H., and Colton, R.R. 1970. *Statistical Methods*, 5th ed., Barnes and Noble, New York)

Year and month	Incidence rate (%) (A)	Trend (T)	Specific seasonal index (A/T)	Typical seasonal index	Cyclical and residual
1964					
Jan.	62.00	56.79	1.09	1.02*	0.07
Feb.	62.50	56.68	1.10	0.98	0.12
Mar.	60.60	56.56	1.07	0.98	0.09
Apr.	58.00	56.45	1.03	0.93	0.10
May	57.80	56.33	1.03	0.90	0.13
June	58.50	56.22	1.04	0.92	0.12
July	56.40	56.10	1.01	0.89	0.12
Aug.	61.60	55.99	1.10	0.95	0.15
Sept.	65.40	55.87	1.17	1.08	0.09
Oct.	67.40	55.76	1.21	1.14	0.07
Nov.	67.70	55.64	1.22	1.14	0.08
Dec.	67.20	55.53	1.21	1.11	0.10
1965					
Jan.	62.60	55.41	1.13	1.02*	0.11
Feb.	61.30	55.30	1.11	0.98	0.13
Mar.	61.60	55.18	1.12	0.98	0.14
Apr.	57.70	55.07	1.05	0.93	0.12
May	57.20	54.95	1.04	0.90	0.14
June	57.30	54.84	1.05	0.92	0.13
July	54.60	54.72	1.00	0.89	0.11
Aug.	61.70	54.61	1.13	0.95	0.18
Sept.	65.90	54.49	1.21	1.08	0.13
Oct.	67.90	54.38	1.25	1.14	0.11
Nov.	68.20	54.26	1.26	1.14	0.12
Dec.	67.00	54.15	1.24	1.11	0.13

*For example, the average of all January specific seasonals for 1955-65.

cattle were first reported in Germany in 1923. The same disease appeared in the United States in 1942 with diagnosis of an affected herd in Michigan. By 1946, this condition, by then called either X-disease or bovine hyperkeratosis, had been reported from 10 U.S. states and, by 1948, from 27 states. However, most outbreaks occurred in the eastern, central, and southern states. The disease was later diagnosed in a number of other countries including Belgium, Morocco, New Zealand, Australia, Great Britain, and Israel. By 1950, hyperkeratosis had reached serious epidemic proportions in the United States. Difficulties in determining the cause of this disease, despite considerable effort, reflected the lack of a systematic epidemiological effort and undue emphasis upon conventional, piecemeal approaches to "detecting the agent." For this reason, the history of bovine hyperkeratosis is worth recounting.

The reported signs of X-disease were swollen, red blotches on the oral mucosa; lacrimation and salivation; anorexia; hyperkeratosis without itching; reduced milk flow with lowering of fat content; depression; abortion; and pyometra. Papillary growths sometimes occurred in the mouth, and there was an increased tendency for warts to grow. Reduced resistance to infections was evident.

It was noted that X-disease affected mainly younger animals (but no animal under three months), with case fatality rates of 30 to 73%. Reported case fatality rates in older animals were 4 to 37%.

The primary lesions found were cystic dilation of the renal tubules; metaplasia of the epididymis, seminal vesicles, Fortner's duct, and salivary ducts; mucoid papillary proliferation in the large bile ducts and gall bladder; liver fibrosis; cystic dilation of the glands of the stomach and intestinal glands; fibrosis and duct proliferation in the pancreas; and hyperkeratosis, particularly in neck, shoulder, and inguinal regions.

X-disease quickly became a serious economic problem; and a meeting was held in July, 1948, in Washington, D.C., for the purpose of recommending ways to find the causes of the disease and to control it. At that time, a number of institutions became involved in cooperative studies; and, over the following years, a series of investigations were made concerning the etiology of X-disease. Many attempts to transmit the disease from animal to animal were unsuccessful although it was reported once that wart-like lesions occurred in calves after intravenous injection of material from a sick animal. In spite of *many* efforts, no microbial agent that would induce the disease could be isolated.

Sixty different poisonous plants were tested in a survey in 1948, but none produced X-disease. Besides, most of the cases of hyperkeratosis occurred during the wintertime in states where the ground was covered with snow.

The resemblance of bovine hyperkeratosis to scurvy led to studies of the plasma levels of ascorbic acid. Vitamin A levels were subnormal while other vitamins were present at normal levels. Treatment with vitamin A, but not carotene, alleviated symptoms in affected animals, and it was suggested that abnormal vitamin A metabolism was the immediate cause of the disease.

Attempts were also made to reproduce X-disease with arsenic; but, although prolonged feeding produced skin lesions, no other diagnostic signs appeared in three months. Changes in soil management, such as increased use of lime and fertilizers, were considered as causal factors; but examination of tissue samples from affected animals for 50 different elements did not reveal anything abnormal.

It is of special interest now that DDT was also considered; but this compound could not be found in the tissues of affected animals, and feeding DDT did not reproduce the disease. Along with these studies, feed trials were carried out in attempts to locate a source of the agent. They, too, were all negative.

In 1947, a piece of epidemiological information was gathered that might have led to an earlier explanation of the X-disease's etiology than actually was the case. At that time, five affected herds were found within a 15-mile radius of Burlington, Vermont. These herds had in common the fact that they were all fed bread crumbs produced by a bread-slicing machine in a Burlington bakery. In a feeding trial with the same type of bread crumbs, hyperkeratosis was reproduced in calves. A manuscript reporting these findings was sent to a journal for publication, but was rejected, presumably because *some* cattle with hyperkeratosis had not been fed bread crumbs! This situation is a good example of lack of understanding of epidemiological studies and failure to undertake further investigations (successive approximations) of the bread, the machine, the slicing operation, or other factors that should have led to incrimination of the slicing machine lubricant.

Some of these bread crumbs were used again for feeding trials in 1951 and, again, reproduced hyperkeratosis in calves. The results of these 1951 trials were that not all bread crumbs (i.e., from different bakeries) produced the disease. In addition, the disease was never produced by any of the ingredients that are used to make bread. There was no further follow-up. In the meantime, pelleted feeds of various types had also been incriminated, but there was also no follow-up of these discoveries with controlled trials until 1951, when the events recounted next had already occurred.

Another significant epidemiological observation about the cause of hyperkeratosis occurred in

Virginia in 1951. "By chance," a veterinarian working on an unrelated problem observed that calves in herds suffering from hyperkeratosis were licking lubricating oil from the transmission and differential housing of machinery kept in the barnyard. A sample of this lubricant was secured and produced hyperkeratosis when fed to calves. It was shown subsequently, in a series of prospective trials, that the active agent was chlorinated naphthalene (actually a series of highly chlorinated naphthalenes), a fairly recent additive to some lubricants. This same type of lubricant was used for feed pelleters and for bread-slicing equipment. The oil companies discontinued the use of these additives, and the prevalence of hyperkeratosis decreased dramatically in a short time (Table 6–1). Other sporadic cases, a recent one reported from Michigan in 1972, can be traced to wood preservatives containing chlorinated naphthalenes.

The interesting aspect of hyperkeratosis is that it was a "new" disease, which would probably have continued to show an increasing secular incidence trend had the agent not been discovered. Another interesting aspect is the approach taken to unravel the etiology of the disease. The emphasis was on detecting agents; and, although interesting epidemiological observations were made, there were few attempts to follow these up; and no one involved seems to have been interested in systematic studies of temporal and spatial clustering of cases or studies involving properly selected comparison herds free of the disease. The final detection of the agent—after much circumstantial evidence—was based on induction from a chance observation—which, by itself, is not a mean feat. Methods for cluster analysis, which would have been useful in the preceding studies, are discussed in the next chapter.

SOME TIME CONSIDERATIONS IN APPROACHING PROBLEMS AND INTERPRETING DATA

Time concepts can be an important consideration in selecting the appropriate epidemiological approach to a problem.

The alternatives of a cross-sectional, or point of time, approach and a longitudinal, or period of time, approach constantly present themselves to the epidemiologist. To recapitulate, there are the alternative measurement possibilities of prevalence or incidence and the alternative study approaches of the (cross-sectional) survey or the longitudinal study (either retrospective or prospective). There are also the two approaches for calculating age specific rates (from all age groups of an existing population—in which case there is no certainty that prior life periods for different age groups are epidemiologically comparable—and from the successive age interval experiences of a selected population cohort), and the related alternatives of the current life table or the follow-up (cohort) life table. Short time interval versus long-term considerations are also evident in the two epidemiological diagnostic alternatives of intensive follow-up and surveillance.

These alternatives may pose problems to the epidemiologist. He must evaluate the time *he will need* for the approach, and possibly also the cost of the approach, the different presumptions that must be investigated or considered in undertaking the approach, the appropriateness of the approach to a particular form of analysis considered or type result desired, and the availability or suitability of the data. Most of these questions are discussed or illustrated as the particular subjects are discussed in this book.

Chapter 7

SPATIAL DISTRIBUTIONS OF DISEASES AND OF POPULATIONS AT RISK

THE distributions of disease events in space usually are as interesting to epidemiologists as the distributions of these events in time. For this reason, most descriptive studies attempt to define the geographic limits of the disease events of concern, as well as particular patterns of spatial distribution within those limits. Such attempts often are inseparable from similar efforts to determine the limits and spatial distribution of populations at risk. Since the two are related, both are the subjects of this chapter.

GEOGRAPHY OF DISEASES

There are various explanations for the geographic limits of particular diseases.[1] Among the more obvious are the global distribution or habitat range of the susceptible species themselves, particularly of those that may play a reservoir role in infections. Thus, canine distemper seems to be generally distributed throughout most parts of the world where there are dogs. The science concerned with the distributions of animal species is zoogeography, which is considered briefly in this chapter with respect to the enumeration and spatial patterns of populations.

However, many diseases are more restricted geographically than their susceptible reservoir species. The disease may not occur in some areas because a particular portion of a general species population is not susceptible, or because the disease agent may be excluded or may never have been introduced. Chemical toxicoses, for example, are limited geographically by the distribution of the toxic agent itself. Similarly, certain infections are restricted in their geographic distributions because free-living stages of the agent may not be able to survive in particular areas within the ranges of its potential hosts. Thus, some gastrointestinal nematodiases are absent from populations of susceptible ruminant animals in arid areas. For some other diseases, the population density of hosts is too low to maintain an infectious cycle, or the migratory or other movement pattern of the population at potential risk may be such that a cycle cannot be completed. Similarly, a vector-borne infection may be limited solely by the territory habitable by the vector, or more restrictedly by the habits of the vector, including its biting habits. For example, a potential mosquito vector may be a forest canopy dweller and, therefore, not bite any susceptible host species whose biotope is on the forest floor.

Natural geographic barriers such as oceans, mountains, or deserts may aid in the exclusion of diseases. For example, the virus of rinderpest has always been absent from North America, despite the presence of large susceptible populations. However, some other infectious agents, such as the virus of foot-and-mouth disease, have managed to jump these formidable ocean barriers to secure toeholds on the North American continent from time to time.

A disease may be limited geographically for 'a variety of reasons. All of them relate to forces that can act upon the susceptible host (or vector) populations or upon the agents. Any of a variety of determinants of the disease may be among the particular factors responsible in any instance. Especially prominent are the kinds of environmental determinants that are discussed in the following chapter.

Recognition of particular spatial distributions of diseases sometimes considerably precedes their explanation. Thus, equine infectious anemia was associated with a swamp ecosystem long before its agent or vector had been identified or its epidemiology well understood. For some comparatively well-known diseases, an explanation for a particular geographic distribution is still not apparent. Coccidioidomycosis is one such infection; it affects many different animal species, and its fungal agent has a free-living cycle. For relatively unknown reasons, coccidioidomycosis seems to be limited geographically to arid areas of the United States, Mexico, and South America.

Spatial patterns of diseases

It is also of epidemiological interest to determine the spatial *patterns* of disease distributions within these general limits. Whether a specific pattern represents differences in frequency of disease events, for example, among the pens of a feedlot, toward one end or another of a row of stanchions in a cow barn, between different barns or pastures, from farm to farm, or in the different districts of a city or parts of a country, non-random patterns of disease distribution (Fig. 7–1) have explanations that are always of epidemiological interest. In some circumstances, their epidemiological value is increased by repeated observations of spatial distribution in a determined time frame, as, for example, on successive days, weeks, or months (Fig. 7–2). As with geographic limits, it is important to search for associations between the spatial distribution pattern of a disease and possible disease determinants.

CLUSTERING. Of special interest in the case of both infectious and noninfectious diseases is a clustering of disease events. Geographic clustering may represent a true nonrandom pattern of disease frequency per unit of population or merely reflect the different population densities of geographic subareas. It is important to distinguish between these types. Isodemic mapping, a cartographic method to express the spatial distributions of disease events in epidemiologically meaningful ways, and cluster analysis are both discussed later in this chapter.

SPATIAL PATTERNS OF POPULATIONS

Animal populations, like disease events, may be distributed in space in different ways. Individual pens or stanchions may prescribe a more or less uniform distribution following some regular pattern. Otherwise, animals may tend to be distributed at random, or in some more contagious pattern among gregarious species or because of environmental and other constraints (see Fig. 7–1).

One can determine how much the spatial distribution of a population of normal or diseased animals departs from randomness. The method of nearest neighbor, discussed later in this chapter, may be of value for this purpose if the population density (m) has been determined already by some other method and if the samples are large. Under such conditions,

$$m\bar{x}_r^2 \begin{Bmatrix} < \\ = \\ > \end{Bmatrix} 0.25 \longleftrightarrow \begin{Bmatrix} \text{cluster distribution} \\ \text{random distribution} \\ \text{uniform distribution} \end{Bmatrix}$$

where $\bar{x}_r$ is the mean distance to the nearest neighbor.

In the case of clustering, the value of $m\bar{x}_r^2$ is less than 0.25; and, for more uniform distributions than random, it will be more than 0.25, for example, 1.154 for a uniform pattern of hexagonal spacing.

Whether infectious disease distributions merely follow those of the host population is partially dependent upon the ease of introduction and spread of the infectious agent. This choice may reflect, in part, the nature of the population. Therefore, one must distinguish between contiguous and separated populations and between open and closed populations; and one must also consider the question of population density.

Contiguous and separated populations

The ease of movement and spread of infections is particularly dependent upon the degree of contact or interaction between population units of the susceptible species. Island populations of animals and people are discrete, and more or less lack contact with the general species population. In contrast, most ethnically or politically different human populations occupying large land areas tend to overlap and therefore are essentially in continuous contact. Rare exceptions for man include the still highly isolated

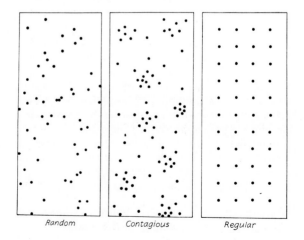

Random *Contagious* *Regular*

Fig. 7–1. Patterns of spatial distribution of diseased or well animals (after Southwood, T.R.E. 1968. *Ecological Methods*. Methuen and Co., Ltd., London).

Fig. 7-2. Series of spot maps representing new cases of equine encephalitis in a river valley on three successive weeks.

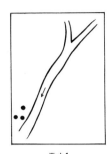 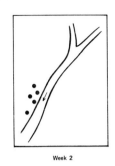 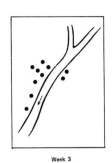

Week 1   Week 2   Week 3

human populations of adjacent coastal areas on the large island of New Guinea.

Separated populations are much more common among both wild animals and livestock than among man and his pets. Wild ruminant herds, certain wild carnivore packs, and various colonial species may exist as discrete populations within the same general land area, with infrequent contact. Also, wild animals of some species may spend much of their lives by themselves, as breeding pairs, or in small families with relatively few outside contact possibilities. Information on relations between populations often is of epidemiological importance and may or may not be obvious for different wild animal populations.

Livestock populations are usually more or less discrete because their owners segregate them into geographically distinct farm or other production units. Where these units are contiguous, opportunities for disease spread may exist; but, in general, the discreteness of livestock populations tends to thwart disease movement. It should be pointed out, however, that contiguous and separated are relative terms. For example, in the Asian Newcastle disease epidemic in southern California in 1972-74, the pattern of movement of feed, eggs, and vaccination crews, essentially removed any separateness among bird populations.

Open and closed populations

Open and closed imply something rather different from the preceding descriptions. Open populations include even those essentially discrete groups in which *individuals* go in and out as part of a more or less regular movement. In contrast, those populations with little or no migration in or out are called closed. For example, dairy farms that raise all of their replacements are essentially closed, while those that continually buy replacements are less so and correspond more to the relatively closed human populations of prisons, boarding schools, and military posts. Dog populations of cities are relatively more closed than are urban human populations insofar as frequent short-term movements in and out are concerned.

Many livestock populations are managed according to the "all in, all out" principle and are essentially closed herds. However, in other instances, premises may never be completely depopulated; and established infections have the opportunity to persist indefinitely. Such has been the case, for example, with pseudorabies in swine in some garbage-feeding ranches in California. Animal purchases and sales increase the chances for introduction of infections into and spread of infections from a population. The more closed a population, the greater the prospects for disease control and the more readily accurate and usable population data can be obtained. On the other hand, the more closed the population, the more likely that it resembles an island, in which case its data may not be as readily generalizable to other "islands."

Population numbers and density

The density of animal populations per unit area may influence the probability of animal contacts and therefore the frequency of transmission of infections (e.g., the secondary attack rate) and the level of herd immunity realized. These considerations relate partially to physical proximity and partially to more complicated relationships such as social distance (discussed in Chapter 9) and increased stress.

The following pages describe some of the variety of methods to enumerate animal populations and to determine population density.

Estimations of population size

Animal population data are expressed either as counts or as population per unit area of space, that is, population density. Among more commonly used measurements of population size are (1) a periodic census or total count of all individuals, (2) an initial census kept up to date through registration of movements in and out (such as births, deaths, immigration, emigration), (3) sampling techniques, such as capture-release-recapture and nearest neighbor, and (4) indirect methods. Where direct censusing is impossible, several different types of sampling estimates may be compared. When these results are not in reasonable agreement, the explanation may be found, for example, in the nonrandomness of the population's distribution.

CENSUSING. For relatively sedentary human or domestic animal populations, total counts of individuals may be undertaken. However, such efforts usually are laborious and expensive and, for that reason, are seldom undertaken solely for epidemiological purposes. Where census data are collected for other purposes (see, for example, the Canadian livestock survey in Chapter 14), the epidemiologist should know about such efforts and make use of them. On occasion, he even may be able to insert his own questions into census questionnaires. Some wild animal populations, particularly large grassland game, may be censused more or less completely by direct aerial counts or aerial photography. Drive censuses also may be undertaken for some species.

POPULATION SAMPLING METHODS.   Usually, sampling procedures are applied to population counting. A variety of population sampling methods have been advocated, but only a few of the more widely applied methods are mentioned in this chapter.

Extrapolation of representative counts. These methods usually involve the random selection of representative subareas for censusing and the extrapolation of these data to the overall study area. For example, the rat population of New York City was estimated by dividing the city into tracts, selecting a random sample of tracts, enumerating the buildings and lots in the selected tracts, selecting a random sample of buildings and lots in each, counting the rats in these selected buildings and lots, and extrapolating these data to the entire city. In 1949, the New York City rat population was estimated by this multistage sampling method, and found to be 250,000 or one rat per 36 people.[2] Table 7–1 shows a comparison of population data on game species; data were obtained from a ground sampling method of selected tracts and direct aerial census in the Mara region of Kenya.

Capture-release-recapture method. This frequently used approach for estimating an animal population (N) is based upon the capture, marking, and release of a sample of animals (M). After an appropriate time interval, a second sample (n) of animals from the same population is captured; and the number of previously marked (i.e., recaptured) individuals (m) in this second sample is noted. It is then possible to calculate an estimate of N from the formula

$$\frac{N}{M} = \frac{n}{m} \text{ or } N = \frac{Mn}{m}.$$

Use of this method, sometimes called a Lincoln Index, or of its innumerable modifications,[3] is based upon the following assumptions:

(1) The marks are not lost, and the capture and marking process does not affect the animal's behavior or survival.

(2) The marked and released animals become completely mixed in the population.

(3) The population of marked and unmarked animals is resampled randomly.

(4) The sampling periods are discrete and comparatively small.

(5) The population studied is closed, or the emigration and immigration can be determined.

(6) No births or deaths have occurred in the time interval between samples, or these events are corrected for.

Nearest neighbor method. This method is a fairly rough order-of-magnitude procedure applicable when estimating relatively sedentary populations, for example, when determining the density per unit area of burrows of burrowing animals, or populations of nestling birds, snails, or ticks. Its ease recommends it for such purposes. A point in the habitat area is selected at random; and the area around it is searched in tight but concentrically expanding circles until an animal (e.g., nest, burrow) is found. The search procedure is then continued until the nearest neighbor is located. The distance between the two sites (r)

Table 7–1.   Enumeration of Plains Game in East African Grassland Area (from Stewart, D.R.M., and Talbot, L.M. 1961. Kenya Game Commission Report).

	Aerial counts Mara, Kenya	Sample estimate Mara, Kenya
Wildebeest *(Gorgon taurinus)*	17,817	15,000
Zebra *(Equus burchelli bohmi)*	20,867	12,000
Topi *(Damaliscus korrigum)*	4111	4000
Buffalo *(Syncerus caffer)*	5934	4000
Elephant *(Loxodonta africanus)*	455	500
Kongoni *(Alcelaphus buselaphus cokii)*	721	1000
Eland *(Taurotragus oryx pattersonianus)*	750	500
Rhinoceros *(Diceros bicornis)*	54	100

is measured. This same overall procedure is repeated several times from different randomly selected points, and the mean distance ($\bar{x}_r$) between nearest neighbors determined.

The mean population density (m) is then calculated as follows:

$$m = \frac{1}{4\bar{x}_r^2}$$

If, for example, several measurements of nearest neighbor for clutches of eggs of ground-nesting birds were 25, 28, 23, 29, 39, and 32 meters, the $\bar{x}_r$ would be 29.3 meters, and m would be 29 egg clutches per 100,000 square meters.

Removal trapping. This technique is based upon the fact that a known number of animals (Y_i) removed from an unknown population (P) on successive trapping occasions (i) reduces that population and therefore the sizes of subsequent catches. Again, certain assumptions must be fulfilled for this method to be valid. Assuming successive animal catches, at equal time intervals, of 65, 43, 34, 18, and 12 animals, population (P) may be estimated by Zippin's procedure,[4] as follows:

$$R = \frac{\sum_{i=1}^{k} (i-1)\, Y_i}{T}$$

where R is a computed ratio, T is total catch, k is the total number of successive trappings, i is the particular trapping, and Y_i is the catch of the ith trapping.

In the example,

$$R = \frac{(1-1)65+(2-1)43+(3-1)34+(4-1)18+(5-1)12}{172}$$
$$R = 1.238$$

If p is the probability of capture on a single occasion and P the estimate of total population,

$$P = \frac{T}{(1-q^k)}$$

From Zippin's graphs (Fig. 7–3) and a k of 5 and R of 1.238, $(1-q^k)$ is read as 0.85.

Therefore,

$$P = \frac{172}{0.85} = 202 \text{ animals.}$$

RELATIVE POPULATION INDICES. Trapping data and even simpler means may be used sometimes to obtain *relative* population indices. Where an independent estimate of population is also available, regression of a relative index on this estimated population

may be undertaken. In this way or through use of various formulas, population estimates may be obtained directly from the index values. One commonly used population index technique is the line transect.

Line transects. By this method, an observer merely walks through a habitat at a constant speed and counts the number of animals he sees in a given unit of time. The total is a population index (Z). Given certain assumptions,[4] the population density (D) may then be estimated as follows:

$$D = \frac{Z}{2RV}$$

where R is the radial distance within which the animal must approach the observer to be observed and V is the average velocity, in the same units, of the observed animal relative to the observer ($V^2 = \bar{\mu}^2 + \bar{\omega}^2$; $\bar{\mu}$ = average velocity of the observer and $\bar{\omega}$ = average velocity of the animal). The greatest difficulty in using this method is estimating the average velocity of the animal.

RELATIONSHIPS OF TEMPORAL AND SPATIAL VARIABLES

Time relationships in disease were considered in Chapter 6. Many types of spatial observations on diseases are made sequentially in a time frame. Reference to these subjects in relation to disease transmission mechanisms appears in Chapters 3 and 4.

Movement and spread of diseases

Just as there are natural geographic *barriers* to the continuity of populations and the spread of diseases, other geographic features such as rivers, valleys, and plains may provide natural *channels* for disease spread over a period of time.[5] Often, detailed historic information is lacking for specific diseases or particular areas.

On the other hand, the progressive movement of some diseases has been well documented. For example, that of bovine pleuropneumonia through Australia is shown in Figure 7–4. Similarly, the spread of rabies through certain wild animal populations has been followed closely in recent years, as, for example, in the southward extension of the infection in vampire bats in southern South America and in its westward progress in foxes in Europe. Also, the movement of Venezuelan equine encephalomyelitis had been followed northward through Central America before it finally reached the United States in 1971. Many explanations exist for the spread of diseases, but only a few are to be considered in this chapter.

MAN AS A FACTOR. Frequently, man is responsible directly or indirectly for the spread of animal, as well as human, diseases. Pastoral migration routes

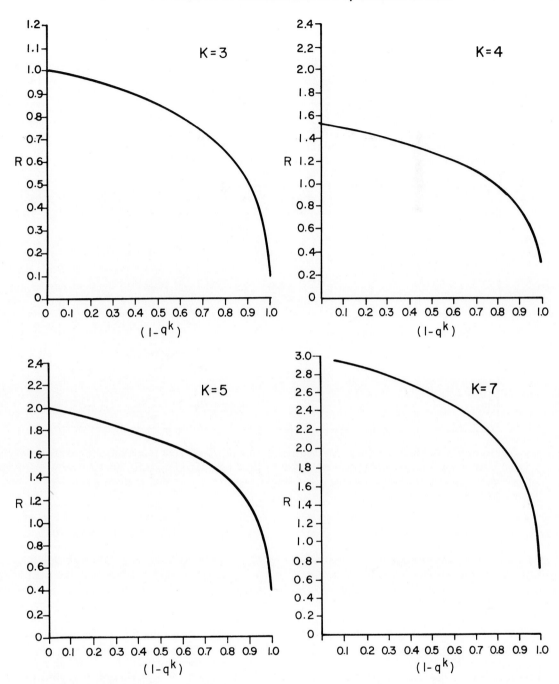

Fig. 7–3. Graphs for estimation of $(1-q^k)$ from ratio R in removal trapping method of wildlife population estimation (redrawn from Southwood, T.R.E. 1968. *Ecological Methods*. Methuen and Co., Ltd., London; after Zippin).

have been involved prominently in the spread of some animal diseases, as for example, African horse sickness through the Middle East beginning in 1959, in the course of which over 170,000 equine animals died. Another instance is the pandemic spread of rinderpest southward in Africa at the end of the last century (see Chapter 4). This occurrence, which

involved both wild and domestic animals, has been extensively documented.[6]

Trade in animals and animal products are other important means for disease spread. African swine fever, which first appeared in Kenya in 1910 in newly introduced domestic swine, remained confined to the African continent until 1957. It then leaped the

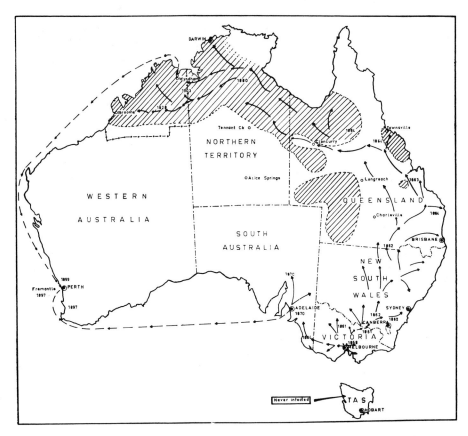

Fig. 7–4.   Spread of bovine pleuropneumonia in Australia. Cross-hatched area represents approximate extent of the infection in remote thinly populated areas in 1953 (after Seddon, H.R. 1953. *Diseases of Domestic Animals in Australia*. Part 5, Volume II. Commonwealth of Australia, Department of Health, Service Pub. No. 10).

ocean barrier to Europe through trade between Portugal and its African colonies. By 1958, over 16,000 Portugese farms were infected; and the virus spread thence into other European countries and, eventually, across the Atlantic ocean to Cuba. Asian Newcastle disease probably entered California in 1971 in wild birds imported for the pet trade.

Man may also be involved in disease spread by other mechanisms. For example, smuggling of animals is known to have played a part in the spread of foot-and-mouth disease, African swine fever, and other diseases. Fowl plague was once introduced into the poultry population of the United States by a careless laboratory worker, and foot-and-mouth disease virus into Canada by an agricultural laborer. Contaminated anaplasmosis vaccine was thought responsible for much of the spread of lumpy skin disease in Africa following its 15-year localization in the Rhodesias.

In 1952, vesicular exanthema of swine, after confinement to the pig-importing state of California for 20 years, was introduced into a livestock center in the American Midwest via dining-car garbage from a transcontinental train. Within a few weeks, transport

of infected animals by road and rail had spread the infection into 42 states! *Rhipicephalus evertsi*, an important two-host tick vector of bovine piroplasmosis and theileriasis, passed through U.S. quarantine on infected zebras in 1960, and transiently established itself in a Florida wild animal park before it was detected and stamped out by vigorous measures.

In yet another instance, the responsibility of man for focally disseminating an avian influenza virus among turkey ranches in Minnesota and adjacent states was demonstrated when the widely scattered occurrence of a new strain of turkey virus was shown clearly to be associated with the movements of a single artificial insemination team. (The semen used on each ranch was obtained on that ranch so semen was not a vehicle.) Veterinarians may be responsible for disease spread in similar ways.

MOVEMENT OF WILD ANIMALS. As in the avian influenza instance, the local distribution of diseases may be difficult to understand without knowledge of their possibilities for spread. Natural migrations of wild animals may be responsible, particularly for infections to which birds are susceptible. Thus, in another example involving influenza, a completely new virus appeared in Oregon chickens a few years ago. It was apparently introduced by wild birds. Supportive evidence for this hypothesis was provided when that virus was found to have the H antigen of classic chicken influenza (fowl plague) virus but the N antigen of another previously known tern influenza virus. Genetic recombinations of influenza viruses are known to occur readily (see Chapter 10).

WIND-BORNE DISEASE. Many infectious agents are transmitted from animal to animal over relatively short distances by the air-borne route (see Chapter 3). Winds may also be responsible for spread of infections over greater distances. Agents may be dispersed by wind directly, or wind may transport the flying vectors of infections. Wind direction and wind speed may be of particular epidemiological importance in connection with this mode of spread of infections. Useful ways to express wind direction and speed data by vector-diagram are shown in Figure 7–5. These particular climatic factors are also epidemiologically important because the combined effects of wind speed, moisture, and temperature accentuate the untoward effects, on organisms, of temperature alone (see Chapter 8). Furthermore, some viruses can survive only long enough for wind-borne transmission if humidity levels are fairly high and if they are protected against sunlight.

Some of the physical characteristics of droplet nuclei from saliva of infected animals were given in Table 3–1. Generally, such particles are a few microns in size and may be transported relatively long distances (50 km, or more) by the air-borne route. Studies, first on wind dispersal of plant rust spores and subsequently of radioactive fallout, have shown that knowledge of surface and upper wind data as well as climatic factors (such as rainfall or snow) that affect particle deposition may allow predictions of the risks of downwind infections and disease spread. Particularly detailed studies have been made of the possibilities of this mechanism with respect to the spread of foot-and-mouth disease in Great Britain.

Wind-borne foot-and-mouth disease virus. Detailed studies of the spread of wind-borne viral infections have used data from several British foot-and-mouth disease epidemics.[7] The initial studies were suggested by the observation that, during the 1967 epidemic, the initial disease spread was entirely downwind. The weather then was wet with continuous southwesterly winds. With a sudden change in wind direction, the direction of disease spread immediately changed.

In all, five British foot-and-mouth disease epidemics have been studied in considerable detail with respect to their spatial pattern of spread with time. In each case, during the initial two weeks of each epidemic,

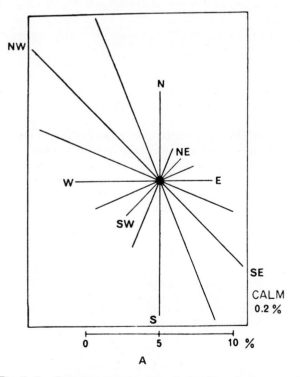

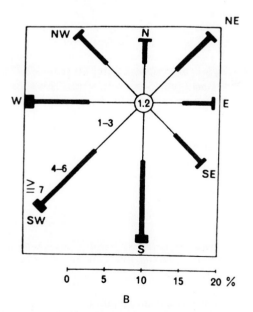

Fig. 7–5. Recommended ways of plotting wind roses: *A*, frequency of wind direction for the year, Hurbanova, Czechoslovakia (1946-1955); *B*, frequency of wind directions for groups of wind speeds (1-3, 4-6, $\geq$ 7, Beaufort) for one year, Torslanda, Sweden (1937-1946) (from Munn, R.E. 1968. *Biometeorological Methods*. Academic Press, New York).

beginning with identification of a single source of virus (i.e., the primary and initial secondary cases on the index farm), disease spread occurred almost entirely in the direction of surface to 1,000-foot winds blowing during periods of precipitation (Fig. 7–6). Rain is important to such dispersal because radioactive fallout studies have shown that the radioactivity of rain is about a million times greater per unit volume than that of the air itself.

The pattern of horizontal particle spread downwind is also a function of the prevailing temperature profile. Vertical spread of viruses (dispersal of virus into high wind zones) is decreased when meteorological conditions are stable, that is, in anticyclonic conditions, particularly in winter, or at night when the wind is not strong. Moreover, decreases in spread, with decreases in incidence of foot-and-mouth disease, were found to be associated with cessation of rainfall, particularly with a series of dry nights.

Predictive value of these associations was demonstrated by British workers in a simulated exercise using epidemiological data from an additional epidemic. Comparable data from radioactive fallout studies also indicate that, on rainy days, cattle downwind from a source will ingest from contaminated herbage 350 times as much radioactivity as they will inhale; but that, on dry days, this ratio is reduced to 70 times as much by ingestion. These findings have interesting implications for the epidemiology of diseases that may be spread by the digestive as well as by the respiratory route.

In the case of foot-and-mouth disease, virus survival also is favored by high humidity and the absence of ultraviolet radiation. These factors also could help explain the observed effects upon its spread on dry nights. Furthermore, the protective effect of high humidity, especially when accompanied by winds, aids in survival of virus spread by other means, e.g., through normal contacts between farms. This variable makes it difficult sometimes to prove wind spread.

One investigator[8] of the spread of foot-and-mouth disease virus during the early days of the 1967-68 British outbreak hypothesized that the mechanism

for an unusual spatial clustering of secondary and tertiary outbreaks, regularly at 18 to 20 km. downwind (Fig. 7–7) and temporally within one incubation period of the initial Bryn farm outbreak, was a meteorological phenomenon known as *lee waves* (Fig. 7–8). The probability of this observed clustering of subsequent outbreaks as a chance phenomenon was shown to be 0.001.

With such an unusual wind pattern, virus material (droplet nuclei) can be borne aloft in discrete air parcels and deposited intact at intervals downwind in volumetric concentrations similar to those borne aloft at the source. In other words, lee waves are known to permit air-borne dissemination of particulate matter in concentrated bundles without the expected uniformity of dispersion and marked dilution from more ordinary wind-borne spread. Although the detailed meteorological data for testing this hypothesis were lacking in the preceding study, the ground conformation data strongly suggested the possibility of lee wave occurrence. However, in such instances agent spread by other means is also likely to result in clustering.

USE OF CARTOGRAPHIC METHODS IN EPIDEMIOLOGY

Maps have obvious value in epidemiology, for they make graphic the spatial limits and distributions of disease events. Several atlases of diseases as well as individual large-scale maps show the broad geographic limits of particular diseases.[9] Smaller-scale maps offer greater detail and, with it, additional possibilities for epidemiological use. Colors, or cross-hatching and other patterns, enable several facets of a disease to be shown on the same map. For example, different levels of prevalence or incidence of a particular disease may be so indicated, or the distributions of different virus strains or vector species or host breeds shown. The possibilities of these types of maps are virtually endless. Figure 7–9 is a monochrome simplification of a detailed full-color map showing known occurrences in Soviet Transbaykalya of various zoonotic

Fig. 7–6. Secondary outbreaks of foot-and-mouth disease in the 1967 English epidemic as related to wind direction and rainfall: (O) primary outbreaks; (●) secondary outbreaks (from Smith[7]).

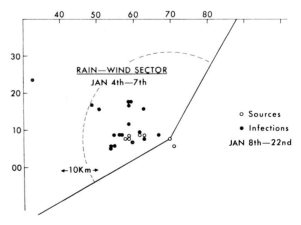

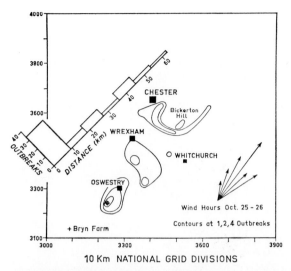

Fig. 7–7. 1967-8 English foot-and-mouth disease data; outbreaks downwind for days 1-10 following initial outbreak on Bryn farm (from Tinline[8]).

infections (rabies, tularemia, tick-borne encephalitis, and alveolar hydatid disease) in mammals according to biome (or transitional area) and known distributions of particular rodent species. The problem with using single maps to display multiple data is, as is the case with other graphs, clutter and "busyness." This problem can sometimes be remedied by use of transparent overlays (see the following discussion).

A *series* of maps is an excellent way to show changes in disease patterns or to portray progress in control programs, as in the malaria eradication maps for Trinidad shown in Figures 7–10 to 7–12. Other less familiar cartographic techniques also recommend themselves for more specialized epidemiological uses.

Spot maps

A *spot map* is one in which such things as individual cases of a disease are plotted to suggest a particular spatial distribution, such as clustering. A time-interval series of such spot maps may allow one to visualize the genesis of an epidemic and its directional movement (see Fig. 7–2). The transparent overlay technique is useful for this latter purpose.

Grid maps

Grid maps have similar value. The Inter-African Bureau for Animal Health, for example, uses one-degree grid maps of Africa to indicate the reported presence of selected diseases during particular time periods (Fig. 7–13). Grids also are used for computer-generated maps.

Isodemic mapping

A cartographic device to examine geographic clustering of cases in terms of population density, or true clustering, is *isodemic* mapping, or construction of *population-by-area cartograms*. By this device, geographic areas (physical or political) are distorted according to their respective population densities (Fig. 7–14 and 7–15). The recommended steps in constructing an isodemic map[10] are:

(1) Select an appropriate scale.

(2) Initiate construction of the cartogram around several prominent geographic features (or political divisions) to assure that the resulting map retains somewhat the shape of the physical map of the same area.

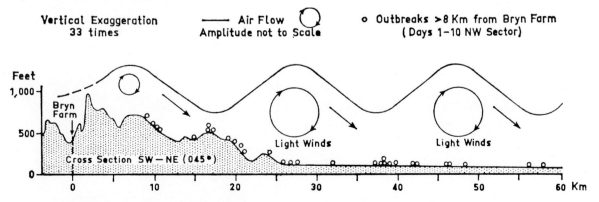

Fig. 7–8. Profile through Bryn farm illustrating lee-wave hypothesis of virus spread in foot-and-mouth disease, England, 1967-68 (from Tinline[8]).

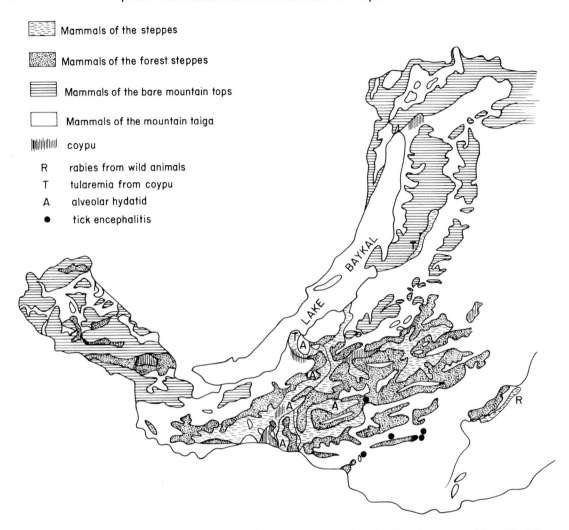

Mammals of the steppes

Mammals of the forest steppes

Mammals of the bare mountain tops

Mammals of the mountain taiga

coypu

R   rabies from wild animals
T   tularemia from coypu
A   alveolar hydatid
●   tick encephalitis

Fig. 7–9.   Map showing distribution patterns for several zoonotic infections by biome (simplified from a color plate in the Soviet *Atlas of Transbaykalya*,1967).

Fig. 7–10.   Map showing malaria eradication in Trinidad, 1945, as evidenced by changes in spleen rate (redrawn from Fonaroff, L.S. 1968. West Indian Med. J. 17:14).

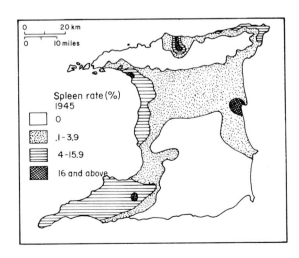

Spleen rate (%)
1945

0

.1–3.9

4–15.9

16 and above

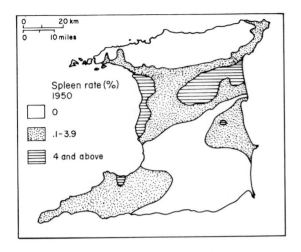

Fig. 7–11. Malaria eradication in Trinidad, 1950. See legend for Figure 7–10.

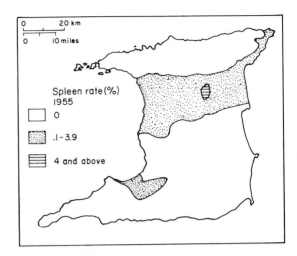

Fig. 7–12. Malaria eradication in Trinidad, 1955. See legend for Figure 7–10.

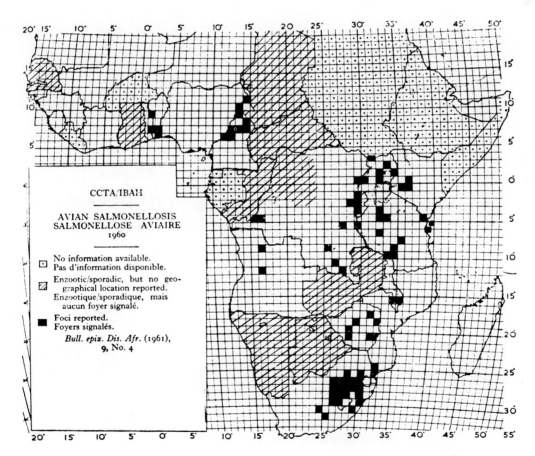

Fig. 7–13. Surveillance program map of reported outbreaks of avian salmonellosis in Africa south of Sahara during 1-year period, 1960, as plotted by one-degree coordinates (source: Inter-African Bureau for Animal Health).

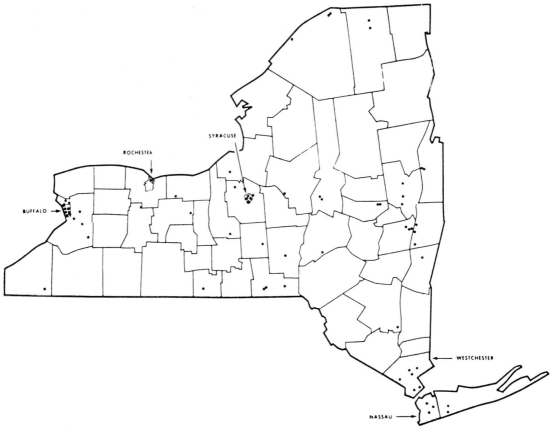

Fig. 7–14. Conventional map of New York. Each dot represents a case of Wilm's tumor in man, 1958 to 1962. Possible clustering of cases is suggested (source: Levison, M.E. and Haddon, W. 1965. Public Health Reports 80:55).

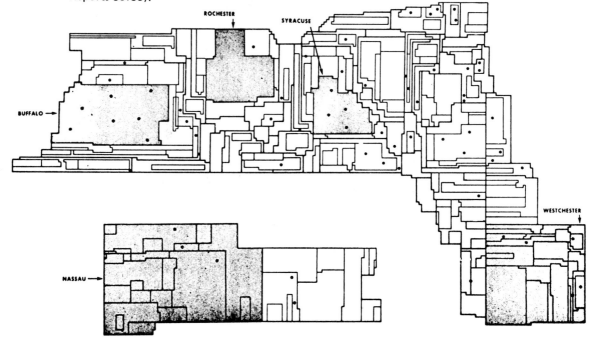

Fig. 7–15. Same cases of Wilm's tumor in man (Fig. 7–14) plotted on population-by-area cartogram of New York (source: Levison, M.E. and Haddon, W. 1965. Public Health Reports 80:55).

(3) Give constant positions to important geographic areas (e.g., cities for man) of high population concentration. The positions and size of 2 and 3 then provide the framework of the cartogram and positions of the other geographic units.

(4) Avoid unnecessary complications of attempting to retain geographic shapes of other areas plotted. Instead, formalize them into rectangular masses so that the demographic weighting of areas is visually apparent. In this situation, loss of true geographic positions and relationships is preferred to highly "gerrymandered" areas difficult to weigh visually.

(5) Distinct population aggregations within the same political area may be displayed best as noncontiguous groupings.

In the absence of known isodemic maps for animal diseases, the example of this technique shown in Figures 7–14 and 7–15 is of the human population of New York with respect to an apparent clustering of cases of a rare tumor. Similar maps distorted for factors other than populations also enable visual control of other variables when plotting a distribution of cases.

Transparent overlay maps

A helpful technique for epidemiological purposes is the use of *transparent overlay maps*. With them, cases, a great number of useful environmental, host, and agent variables, or other epidemiological information can be plotted on a series of transparent maps of the identical geographic area and scale. Superimposed on each other in different combinations and displayed with an overhead projector or a radiograph reader, transparent overlays permit a quick examination of (1) time sequences of cases or other distributions and (2) apparent associations between diseases and other variables. They also offer many other possibilities. A convenient format is to use cardboard frames for overhead projector transparencies, with maps prepared on clear plastic sheets. (Transparent adhesive plastic sheets in various colors are also available.)

Isopleth maps

Epidemiology has made relatively less use of isopleth maps, which enable one to plot the distribution of continuous variables such as climate, and the levels of prevalence or incidence of a disease (Fig. 7–16).

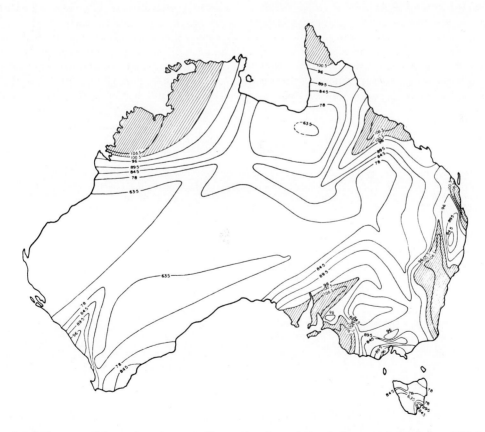

Fig. 7–16. Isopleth map of human male mortality ratios (actual deaths/expected deaths) x 100 for cerebrovascular lesions, Australia (from Schwabe, C.W. 1969. *Veterinary Medicine and Human Health*, Williams & Wilkins Co., Baltimore; after Learmonth and Nichols, 1965).

Isopleths of these latter for morbidity have been referred to as *isomorbs*, and death rate plots are called *isomorts*.

Computer-generated maps[11]

This technique, as most employed, is essentially the programming of a computer to position a given symbol by its x and y coordinates on a grid. In the simple example given in Figure 7–17, the selected grid pattern is longitude and latitude; and the computer plots political boundaries and locations of congenital anomalies in swine. More complicated epidemiological data, requiring greater computer memory capacity, can be plotted as isopleths (Fig. 7–18) or as choropleths (i.e., region or area plot), based geographically on political units (Fig. 7–19). Less frequently used are computer-mapped data displayed by plotting machines and on cathode ray tubes. In the latter case, there can be direct interaction with the computer; and permanent records of maps can be produced by photography.

CLUSTER ANALYSIS

In its broadest sense, cluster analysis refers to procedures by which individuals are formed into "natural" groups. Often the number of groups is not specified in advance, but a system of groups is sought such that the individuals within groups resemble each other much more closely than do individuals among groups. One of the approaches used for such cluster formation problems is numerical taxonomy.[12] In this section, however, emphasis is not on forming clusters, but on detecting whether clusters of cases of diseases may have occurred.

Aggregation of cases of disease in time, space, or in time and space is of epidemiological interest because such clustering may help in identifying a common environmental factor or source of exposure, thereby facilitating disease control or prevention. This interest has existed to some extent for centuries. In a global sense, clusters of cases of disease in time correspond to disease pandemics. In the same sense, finding clusters in space may be analogous to identifying areas in which the disease exists at high endemic levels. If one can identify areas of time-space association with disease incidence, then, essentially, he can define an epidemic of the disease.

Disease clusters in time

In studying whether a disease shows clusters in time, a simple technique is to divide the time scale into (say k) equal intervals, express the incidence of disease in the population as a proportion, and test for the significance of differences among these proportions by the usual chi-square test for $2 \times k$ contingency tables.

If the disease under investigation exhibits some known periodicity, such as seasonal incidence, and interest is in whether there may be additional clusters, time series methods can be used to calculate "expected" frequencies for each period, and then the chi-square test can be performed in the usual way.

On the other hand, if incidence of the disease is very low and if the population at risk remains

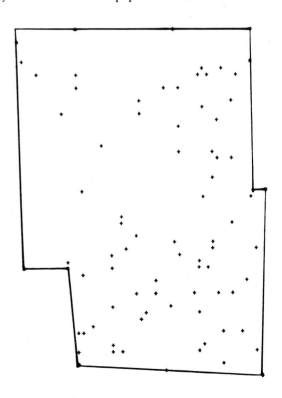

Fig. 7–17. Computer-generated map of Nodaway County, Missouri, showing locations of farms from which congenital malformations in swine were reported during given time period (from Wright, H.T., Marienfeld, C.J., and Silberg, S.L. 1969. "Place" in environmental epidemiology; a rectangular coordinate method. Public Health Rep. 83:427).

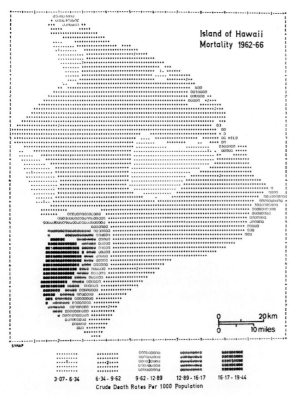

Fig. 7–18. Computer-generated isopleth map of human crude death rates on island of Hawaii using 20 data points corresponding to death rates for census tracts. Isomorts were computed mathematically from the data points using the Synagraphic Mapping Program (SYMAP), Version 5, of the Laboratory for Computer Graphics and Spatial Analysis, Harvard University, Cambridge. (Note: Preferably the class intervals on this figure and Fig. 17–19 should have been exclusive.) (From Armstrong, R.W. 1972. Computers and mapping in medical geography, *In* McGlashan, N.D.[11]).

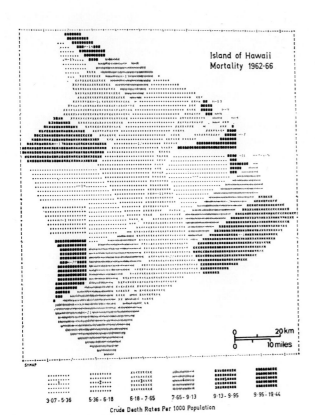

Fig. 7–19. Computer-generated choropleth map of human crude death rates on island of Hawaii using same mortality rates as in Figure 7–18 but plotted by line-printer as choropleth map with census tracts as units. This computer graphic was constructed using the Synagraphic Mapping Program (SYMAP), Version 5 of the Laboratory for Computer Graphics and Spatial Analysis, Harvard University, Cambridge (from Armstrong, R.W. 1972. Computers and mapping in medical geography, *In* McGlashan, N.D.[11]).

relatively constant over the k time periods, under the null hypothesis that there is no clustering, the number of new cases appearing in each of the different intervals would probably follow the Poisson distribution. In this circumstance, a reasonable analytic strategy would be to fit a Poisson distribution and then test for goodness-of-fit by the chi-square test.[13]

Disease clusters in space

The methods used for detecting clusters in time are readily adapted for studying clustering in space. In general, the population under study can be divided into groups such as administrative areas, geographic regions, and climatic areas, depending upon what factors are being considered relative to the disease under investigation. Since the usual subdivisions of the population in space would not produce equally sized subpopulations, the Poisson distribution would not be applicable. However, the usual contingency table methods can be applied in testing for possible associations between disease incidence and spatial factors.

Disease clustering in time and space

In studying possible infectious or environmental determinants for rare diseases such as leukemias, some cancers, or certain congenital malformations, clusterings in time *and* space are usually of more interest than either clusters in space or in time. Various statistical procedures for analyzing such "micro-epidemics," particularly leukemia, have been reported;[14] but all have been subject to methodologic or analytic problems. In particular, the numbers of cases occurring in a given period of time have generally been small, and the analyses were done *after* some initial observations that an "unusual" incidence had occurred. Furthermore, case identification has been generally more complete in an area of suspected clustering than in other areas. For these reasons, it has been difficult to derive meaningful inferences from most reported studies on clustering of diseases. A final difficulty lies in the fact that "epidemics" of nonoccurrence seem to have been ignored com-

pletely, and data from such times and places could provide useful clues on the etiology of various diseases.

Clustering of diseases in time and space may occur as "familial" aggregation (including dam-sire-offspring groups in animals), nonfamilial clusters, or a spurious phenomenon arising from faulty case ascertainment procedures. Although familial aggregation of disease would usually arise from infections transmitted among family members, particularly those housed together, or may be due to genetic causes, the commonly shared social and environmental conditions within herds or common housing facilities may contribute to the incidence of the disease in related groups of animals. Apparent familial aggregation may also be a partial result of the fact that human siblings and animal siblings from species giving multiple births tend to be fairly similar in age.

As mentioned earlier, several methods have been used for studying possible time-space associations in cases of diseases. For example. Knox (1964b)[14] studied childhood leukemia in Northeast England, and found 96 cases occurring in the 10-year period from 1951 to 1960. It was pointed out that, if the disease were caused in part by an infectious agent or resulted from some common environmental factors, then cases occurring close together in space should also be clustered in time. Knox arranged the 96 cases by adjacency in time and space by constructing all possible pairs ($\frac{96 \times 95}{2} = 4560$ pairs). By selecting 1 km as the criterion for the space adjacency and 60 days as the limiting time criterion, five pairs of cases were adjacent in time and space (Table 7-2). Although the data arrayed thus appear as a 2×2 table, the chi-square test for association could not be used because the independence assumption was violated severely.[15]

If the time and place in which cases occur are not related, one can calculate an expected frequency of pairs on the basis of proportionality to the marginal totals. For example, the number of pairs of cases adjacent in time and space would be $(25 \times 152) \div 4560 = 0.83$. Using a Poisson approximation, with the mean equal to the expected frequency

Table 7-2.   Distribution of Pairs of 96 Cases of Leukemia in Children Under Six Years of Age, by Adjacency in Time and Space (Knox, 1964b[15])

Time apart (days)	Distances apart (km.)		Total
	0-1	>1	
0-59	5	147	152
60-3651	20	4388	4408
Total	25	4535	4560

(0.83 in the example), the probability of observing five or more pairs of cases that are adjacent in time and space is calculated as follows:

$$P(5 \text{ or more}) = 1 - P(0, 1, 2, 3, \text{ or } 4)$$

$$= 1 - \sum_{i=0}^{4} \frac{\mu^i e^{-\mu}}{i!}$$

Replacing μ by its estimate $\bar{x} = 0.83$ produces

$$P(5 \text{ or more}) = 1 - \sum_{i=0}^{4} \frac{(0.83)^i e^{-0.83}}{i!}$$

$$= 1 - e^{-0.83} \sum_{i=0}^{4} \frac{(0.83)^i}{i!}$$

$$= 1 - 0.9983 = 0.0017.$$

This approximate test reflects a highly significant excess of cases that are adjacent in time and space. One additional technique, which has been applied fairly widely, is a regression approach proposed by Mantel.[14] In his report, several other methods were summarized and criticized.

Closely associated with spatial distributions of diseases are various environmental variables (see Chapter 8).

Chapter 8

ENVIRONMENTAL DETERMINANTS OF DISEASES

$\mathbf{M}$EDICAL ecology was introduced in Chapter 4 as an historic approach to epidemiology. It is the study of the relationships between a population of animals (or interacting populations of animals) and their *environment* insofar as the effect upon these target populations is disease. From an ecological standpoint, living and nonliving *agents* of disease are environmental factors, *immediate* environmental factors. However, because of the almost total preoccupation of 19th and 20th century medicine with a search for such specific immediate determinants of disease, most epidemiologists have tended quite rightly to regard specific agents of disease as environmental variables of such importance that they must be considered separately from other more remote variables of environment *per se*. That approach is followed in this chapter and in Chapter 10.

Thus, those determinants of disease event frequency that are not functions of an agent or of some characteristic of the host population are considered environmental. Consequently, environment includes a number of possible physical and biological variables that may partially determine given disease patterns and frequencies. Since the time of Hippocrates' *Airs, Waters and Places*,[1] medicine has paid some attention to disease in relationship to such more remotely operating environmental determinants. The importance of wind, humidity, and ultraviolet radiation were mentioned in the last chapter's discussion of foot-and-mouth disease in the United Kingdom.

PHYSICAL ENVIRONMENT

Of major concern are the effects of physical features of the micro- and macrohabitats of the population at risk upon the frequency and pattern of disease events. Some of the principal variables involved are topography, climate, shelter, and soils. A number of general disease relationships of topography are discussed in Chapter 7.

Climate

Climate is determined by a variety of variables acting in combination. These climatic factors are among the more important physical determinants of disease patterns. The study of climate and weather in relationship to disease is an area of interest to biometeorologists as well as to epidemiologists and thus recommends itself to collaborative efforts.[2]

Climatic factors not only affect a host population directly, but also act upon vector populations, as well as upon free-living stages of infectious agents. Factors of particular epidemiological importance include temperature, barometric pressure, radiation, oxygen concentration, precipitation, humidity, wind speed, and wind direction. The general aspects of climate of greatest interest to the epidemiologist are ground-level climate and other so-called microclimates. It is important, therefore, to differentiate between macro- and micrometeorology.

MACROMETEOROLOGY. Ordinary weather data recorded routinely by government agencies describe macroclimates; these data are based upon use of collecting points and procedures that tend to dampen out small-scale microclimatic differences and permit the plotting of meaningful isopleths for large geographic areas. For example, macrometeorological data on surface weather usually are obtained from standardized instruments housed in so-called Stevenson screens and located in the open at a fixed height over short grass. These general types of weather data for a geographic area are not necessarily representative of the climatic values of a grass sward in a particular pasture, a poultry house, a shaded barnyard, or a city street. They are, however, the types of weather data most generally available.

MICROMETEOROLOGY. Weather values obtained by placement of sensing apparatuses in the specific *biotopes* for which the data may be required, for example, on the soil surface for some nematode larva, within a "climatological sheath" such as a calf barn, or at the interface of two ecosystems, are micrometeorological. To understand the differences between the macroclimate of an area and specific microclimates, consider that the near-ground temperatures at sunrise in New Jersey correspond to those of the 6-foot macroclimate of southern Canada or northern Maine. Therefore, inappropriate sampling procedures for weather data could result in misleading conclusions.

CLIMATIC TYPES. A number of different classifications have been proposed for climatic types. One that has epidemiological value is given in Table 8–1, with type-climatograms in Figure 8–1.

DISEASE AND CLIMATE. Severe weather may directly cause illness or death of animals. Extremes of heat and cold, for example, may act as immediate physical *agents* of disease.[3] Newborn animals are particularly susceptible to climatic extremes, particularly of temperature. For one thing, they dehydrate very rapidly. All animals are born wet, and have a high ratio of surface area to body mass; some species also have little initial control over their body temperature. While newborn lambs begin to show func-

tional thermoregulatory control within several hours, piglets are not able to regulate their body temperature effectively before about six days. One result is that piglets born and maintained on cold damp floors readily develop a specific metabolic disorder called "nutmeg liver."[4]

More commonly, stress induced by climatic factors may interact with endocrine function, state of nutrition, genetic predisposition, or the innate or acquired resistance to infections of animals; and may thus provoke activity on the part of latent or opportunistic pathogens. In these ways, climatic stress may determine or influence the occurrence, the frequency of occurrence, or the severity of various diseases. Examples of such apparent relationships in pendulous crop in turkeys and in pregnancy toxemia in ewes are considered in this chapter, while more complicated relationships of climatic stress to calf mortality are discussed in Chapter 13.

Climatic stress and pendulous crop. This epidemically occurring disease of turkeys is characterized by marked distention of the crop with food stasis and

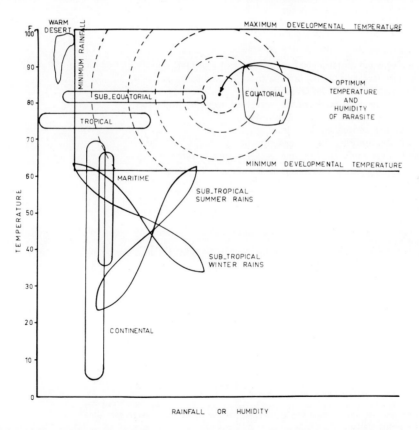

Fig. 8–1. Theoretical climatograms for different world climates. The climatic conditions for each month are plotted and lines drawn to connect them. Developmental conditions for the free-living stages of a hypothetical parasite are superimposed, thus making a bioclimatogram indicating transmission periods for the parasite (from Cameron, T.W.M. 1958. *Parasites and Parasitism*. John Wiley & Sons, Inc., New York).

Table 8–1. Koeppen's Climatic Classes and Main Climatic Types* (Adapted from Levine[9] After Crutchfield, H.J. 1960. *General Climatology*. Prentice-Hall. Englewood Cliffs.)

| | Major category (class) | | Seasonal distribution of precipitation | | |
| | | | Full year wet | Winter dry | Summer dry |
Symbol	Description	Subclass			
A	Tropical rainy climates; hot all seasons	—	—	—	—
B	Dry climates	S	—	—	—
C	Warm (mesothermal), temperate, rainy climates; mild winters	—	f	w	s
D	Cold (microthermal), humid forest climates; severe winters	—	f	w	s
E	Polar climates	T	—	—	—
		F	—	—	—
Af	Hot; rainy in all seasons				
Am	Hot; seasonally excessive rainfall				
Aw	Hot; winter dry				
BSh	Semi-arid (steppe); hot				
BSk	Semi-arid; cool or cold				
BWh	Desert; hot				
BWk	Desert; cool or cold				
Cfa	Mild winter; moist all seasons; hot summer				
Cfb	Mild winter; moist all seasons; warm summer				
Cfc	Mild winter; moist all seasons; short, cool summer				
Cwa	Mild, dry winter; hot summer				
Cwb	Mild, dry winter; short, warm summer				
Csa	Mild winter; dry, hot summer				
Csb	Mild winter; short, warm, dry summer				
Dfa	Severe winter; moist all seasons; long, hot summer				
Dfb	Severe winter; moist all seasons; short, warm summer				
Dfc	Severe winter; moist all seasons; short, cool summer				
Dfd	Severe, extremely cold winter; moist all seasons; short summer				
Dwa	Severe, dry winter; long, hot summer				
Dwb	Severe, dry winter; cool summer				
Dwc	Severe, dry winter; short, cool summer				
Dwd	Severe, extremely cold winter; moist, short summer				
ET	Polar climate; very short summer				
EF	Perpetual ice and snow				

*Definitions of symbols

A = Tropical; mean temperature of coldest month above 18°C. (64.4°F.)
B = Dry; no temperature limitation
C = Mesothermal (middle or intermediate temperature); mean temperature of coldest month between 18 and –3°C. (64.4 and 26.6°F.)
D = Microthermal (small or little heat); mean temperature of coldest month less than –3°C. (26.6°F.); mean temperature of warmest month above 10°C. (50°F.)
E = Arctic; mean temperature of warmest month below 10°C. (50°F.); EF = mean temperature of warmest month below 0°C. (32°F.)
S = Steppe
W = Desert (from German Wüste)
T = Tundra
F = Eternal frost

a = Mean temperature of warmest month above 22°C. (71.6°F.)
b = Mean temperature of warmest month under 22°C.; at least 4 months above 10°C. (50°F.)
c = Only one to four months above 10°C.; coldest month above –38°C. (–36.4°F.)
d = Temperature of coldest month less than –38°C.
f = Moist (from German feucht); driest month with a mean precipitation of at least 60 mm. (2.4 in.)
g = Ganges type of temperature trend; maximum before summer rainy season
h = Hot; annual temperature above 18°C. (64.4°F.)
i = Isothermal; difference between warmest and coldest months less than 5°C. (14°F.)
k = Cold winter; annual temperature less than 18°C.; warmest month above 18°C.
l = Mild; all months 10 to 22°C.
m = Monsoon regime of precipitation; short dry season compensated for by heavy rains during rest of year
n = Frequent fog
p = Infrequent fog, but high humidity, low rainfall, and relatively cool; summer months 24 to 28°C. (74.2 to 82.4°F.)
s = Summer dry period; driest month with a mean precipitation of less than 40 mm. (1.6 in.) and less than 1/3 that of the wettest month of the winter half of the year
u = Coolest month after summer solstice
v = Warmest month in autumn
w = Winter dry period; driest month with a mean precipitation of less than 60 mm. (2.4 in.)
x = Maximum rainfall in spring or early summer; dry in late summer

fermentation, mucosal ulcers, secondary infections, and unthriftiness, with death in about 50% of affected birds. Pendulous crop was first described in the Central Valley of California in the 1930s. The disease was observed to occur only in the extremely hot, dry summers characteristic of that area, and only in turkeys of the Bronze breed. Interestingly, similar populations of Bronze turkeys raised 60 miles away on the milder California coast were unaffected, as were Bourbon Red populations kept in the Central Valley.

Pendulous crop is now recognized to be a disease with genetic as well as climatic determinants (Fig. 8-2). A hot, dry *environment* causes turkeys to consume excessive amounts of water, which must be regarded as the actual *agent* of this disease. In birds of the Bronze breed with a genetic *host* predisposition to the condition, this abnormal water consumption causes a usually irreversible stretching of the crop, with occurrence of the sequelae mentioned.

Climatic stress, nutrition, and pregnancy toxemia. Another illustration of the indirect effects of climatic stress (and possibly other climatic factors) upon the incidence of disease is provided by the case of pregnancy toxemia in ewes in Wales.[5] Observations on 20,000 Welsh ewes showed that this disease usually occurred in ewes carrying twin lambs, and almost always in chronically malnourished ewes or in well-nourished ewes that were unable to graze during winter period of severe climate.

An index of the incidence of this disease was developed by combining the amount of excess rain (i.e., above a 16-inch threshold value for the November to March period) and the accumulated tempera-

ture deficit below 43°F. Applying this approach to the data from the 20,000 ewe population, a formula was derived for predicting expected numbers of cases of pregnancy toxemia. Use of this predictor during a three-year period resulted in expected (and observed) numbers of cases of pregnancy toxemia of 70(63), 431(401), and 757(770). The regression line for the observed numbers for 1955-1965 is shown in Figure 8-3.

MEASUREMENT OF CLIMATIC IMPACT. High and low ambient temperatures are the most obvious causes of climatic stress. However, the effects of both are influenced by other climatic factors such as humidity and wind speed. Biometeorologists have proposed several indices for determining the cumulative effects of such climatic variables, although most existing indices have been calculated for man rather than for other animal species. Several of these types of combined measures are mentioned in the following paragraphs.[6]

Wind chill. The *wind-chill index* is an attempt to integrate effects of temperature and wind speed since, at temperatures below freezing, strong winds magnify convective heat losses from the body. One expression of this is

$$Q_H = (10\sqrt{\mu} + 10.45 - \mu)(33 - T_a)$$

where Q_H is the wind-chill index, μ is the mean wind speed in meters/second, and T_a is the air-temperature in degrees Celsius. Nomograms have been prepared on so-called *wind-chill temperature*, which expresses the comparative human response to wind plus temperature in terms of temperature only. For example, a

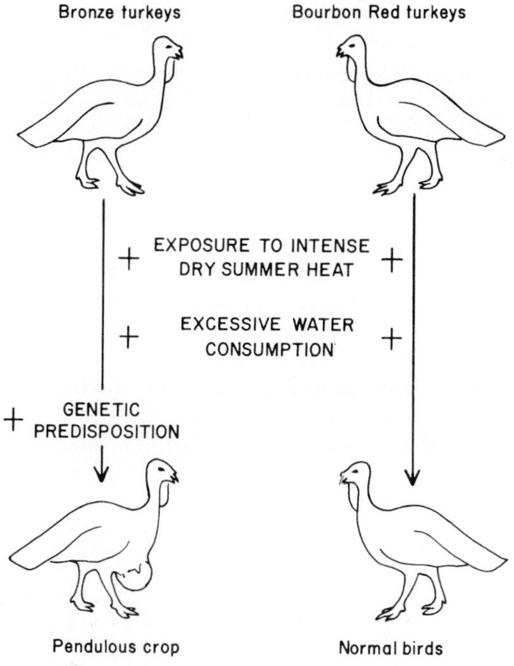

Fig. 8-2. Interaction of climate (environment), genetic predisposition (host), and excessive water consumption (agent) in etiology of pendulous crop of turkey.

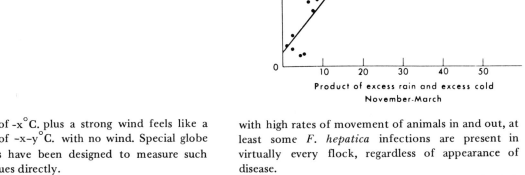

Fig. 8–3. Incidence of pregnancy toxemia in population of Welsh ewes plotted against combined rainfall-temperature index, 1955-65 (from Smith, L.P. 1970. Weather and animal diseases. World Meteorological Organization. Technical Note No. 113).

temperature of -x°C. plus a strong wind feels like a temperature of -x–y°C. with no wind. Special globe thermometers have been designed to measure such combined values directly.

Combined temperature-humidity. From the standpoint of comfort or body response to climate, humidity affects apparent temperature just as wind speed does. Wet-bulb thermometers are used in attempts to measure the combined effect of these factors.

Effective temperature. This index is an attempt to combine the three effects of temperature, humidity, and wind speed in terms of an apparent or *effective temperature*. A nomogram designed for this purpose for response of human beings is shown in Figure 8–4. Other combined measures based upon effective temperature for man are *annual cumulative stress* and *temperateness index* (Figs. 8–5 and 8–6).

CLIMATE AND THE TIMING OF DISEASE EVENTS. Climate is also of epidemiologic importance as a determinant of temporal patterns of disease occurrence and transmission. One example of this, smog disease, was considered in Chapter 2. Other comparatively well-studied examples are some of the arthropod-borne viral infections and fascioliasis.

Climate and fascioliasis. In England, a parasitologist and biometeorologist have collaborated on studies designed to forecast epidemic periods of transmission of *Fasciola hepatica* and the optimal times for implementation of preventive measures.[7] Because sheep flocks in England are open populations

with high rates of movement of animals in and out, at least some *F. hepatica* infections are present in virtually every flock, regardless of appearance of disease.

The vector snail for this fluke in England is *Lymnaea trunculata*, which lives on water-saturated pastures. Such soil moisture conditions are more likely to be found in poorly drained areas of clay soil over impervious rock than in well-drained soils, such as sandy soils, areas of sloping land, or places where the top soil overlies porous rock. Under conditions of high topsoil moisture and a near ground-level air temperature above 10°C, snail eggs hatch, and snails develop and complete their life cycle. If the favorable moisture and temperature conditions persist, the *Lymnaea* population becomes numerous and extends its habitat. At the same time, individual snails reach a larger size. The biotopic conditions of soil moisture-temperature required for the snail are necessary, too, for the eggs of *F. hepatica* to develop and hatch. With prolongation of the optimal temperature-moisture levels, infestations of pasture grass with the metacercariae of the fluke build up rapidly.

Studies of past data on the yearly incidence of clinical fascioliasis in sheep in endemic areas of Wales, plus data on mean air temperatures, rainfall, and rain-days, and calculated potential evapotranspiration were used to derive a combined moisture-temperature parameter that would correlate closely with disease frequency. This index proved valuable in prediction of a higher than average incidence of clinical fasci-

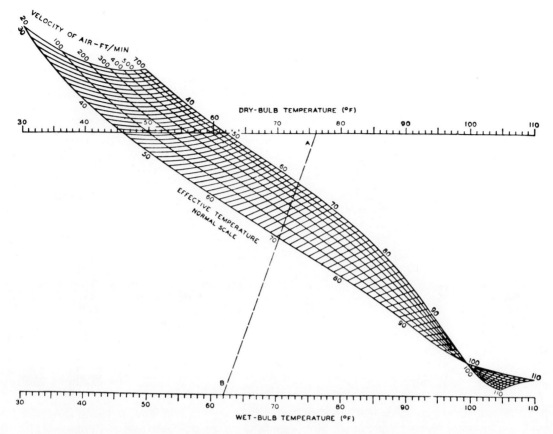

Fig. 8–4. Nomograms for determining effective temperature (E.T.) for sedentary persons, normally clothed, from measurements of dry-bulb and wet-bulb temperatures and air speed. To use the chart, draw a line A-B through measured dry- and wet-bulb temperature; read effective temperature or velocity of desired intersections with line A-B. For example, given 76°F D.B. and 62°F W.B., read 69 E.T. at 100 fpm velocity or 340 fpm required for 66 E.T (from Munn, R.E. 1970. *Biometeorological Methods.* Academic Press, New York).

oliasis in southwest England and Wales in 1968 and the occurrence of the disease that year on farms in nonendemic areas of East Anglia.

Since indices such as these have local predictive value, they are useful in the practice of preventive veterinary medicine. Some effects of wind speed and wind direction upon *spread* of infections are discussed in Chapter 7. In Chapter 13, there is an example of the use of statistical techniques such as multiple regression for investigation of effects of multiple climatic variables upon disease frequency.

FURTHER EPIDEMIOLOGICAL TECHNIQUES WITH RESPECT TO CLIMATE. Sources of technical methods to measure ground-level climate are listed in the chapter notes.[2] For the United States, recorded weather data are available for many stations from the National Climatic Center of the U.S. Department of Commerce, as well as from state governments, airlines, and other sources. Some of these records are stored on computer tapes. Specific types of information available include daily maximum, minimum, and average temperatures; weather types; precipitation by type and water equivalence; wind direction; maximum and average wind speed; hours of sunshine; and sky cover.

Bioclimatograms. A particularly useful visual device for epidemiological studies of climate as a disease determinant is the bioclimatogram. This graph is merely a representation of the sum of two selected climatic variables (e.g., temperature and precipitation) for a geographic locale, usually by month, and for a one-year period. Superimposed on this climate graph are relevant biological data, such as minimum or maximum survival or development temperatures and rainfall for the free-living stage of a pathogen, or of a vector species. Type bioclimatograms are shown in Figure 8–1. The examples in Figure 8–10 indicate possible transmission periods for *Haemonchus, Ostertagia,* and *Trichostrongylus* in several areas of the United States.

Use of degree days. This measure is the *accumulated departure* of mean temperatures on successive days from a reference level, as for example, days over 70°F. in the example on WE encephalomyelitis in

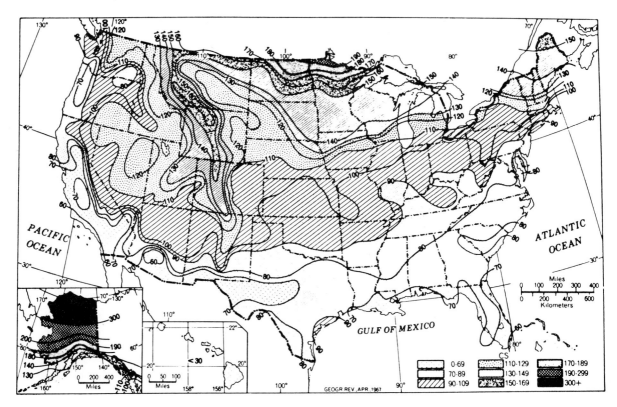

Fig. 8–5. Annual cumulative stress (combined measure of temperature, humidity, and wind speed) for United States (from Munn[2]; reproduced, with permission, from the Geographical Review, vol. 57, 1967, copyrighted by the American Geographical Society).

Chapter 6. This measure of "exposure" is analogous to total dosage of some chemical pollutant for which daily concentration values and a threshold value are available.

Shelter

Shelter is a physical variable closely related to climate. The basic function of shelter is to shield or buffer animals against the effects of sun, wind, precipitation, and other climatic variables, thereby providing what meteorologists call a climatological sheath. Such shelters are either natural or man-made; and, depending upon the system of husbandry, animals may be confined to them or have resort to them free choice.

More elaborate shelters may provide not only facilities for at least partial *control* of temperature, air circulation, humidity, light, and other environmental variables, but also sanitary amenities such as solid, dry, and readily cleanable surfaces; facilities for provision of clean water and feed; facilities for the removal of wastes; plus other special comfort and safety features such as bedding and constraints.

Thus, the design features of animal shelters may alter disease risks and frequencies of disease events. Because of a shelter's relation to health and the fact that physical facilities are usually expensive parts of

the fixed costs of animal production, those involved in their design or modification should consider all these possible influences. In addition to climatic shielding and control, other important variables with respect to shelter relate to the population density of animals. As indicated previously, crowding is a stressing factor; and it also relates directly to ease of disease transmission, as well as to the general level of environmental sanitation.

The variety in possible combinations of features of housing facilities for animals is such that categorization and comparison of effects of individual housing variables in epidemiological analyses may be difficult; and the positive or negative effect of one design feature may tend to obscure or cancel others. Little use has yet been made of prospective epidemiological trials in the rational design of animal housing, although special buildings and chambers designed for a multiplicity of climate controls are available increasingly for biological research in general. The *biotron* of the University of Wisconsin, for example, contains 48 climate control laboratories of a variety of kinds, some of them specially adapted for large animal studies.

Beyond such research facilities, which could be used for prospective epidemiological studies, environmentally controlled housing is becoming increasingly

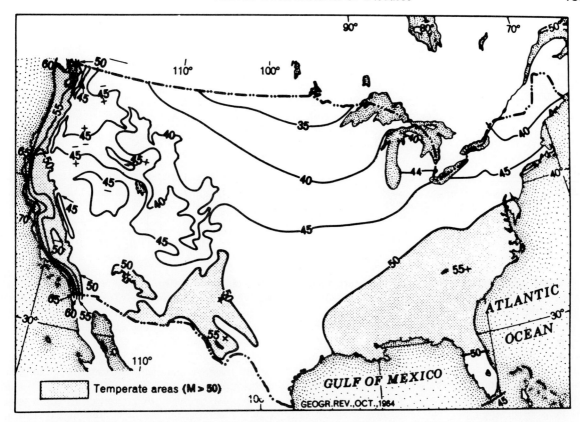

Fig. 8–6. Temperateness index (combined measure of temperature, humidity, and wind speed) for the United States (from Munn[2]; reproduced, with permission, from the Geographical Review, vol. 54, 1964, copyrighted by the American Geographical Society).

commonplace for certain branches of animal agriculture in some countries. The broadest application of this approach has been in the poultry industry where light, temperature, humidity, and air circulation are commonly regulated. To date, however, little has been done to relate such possibilities for environmental regulation to studies of disease frequency or to design of rational programs for disease control.

To indicate one important epidemiological relationship of climate control in animal housing, it has been determined that the air throughput of most modern intensive poultry houses is in the range of 1 to 2 million cubic feet per hour. Due to the "filter and trap" effect of the building, such conditions may expose housed animals to greater inhalation risk from air-borne infectious agents than is experienced by unhoused birds. Also, if such buildings house infected birds, the air effluent may be particularly rich in air-borne agents.

Soil

Although soil types may be of significance in several ways, epidemiologists have paid relatively little direct attention to this variable. Soils in part reflect long-term climatic patterns and partially determine the nature of plant communities and conse-

quently the animal species present in a given ecosystem. The distribution of soil types may explain the distribution of the natural foci of particular infections.

Soil types may also affect available moisture levels in a particular microclimate. This factor, plus the porosity and chemical composition of the soil, may influence such things as the ability of free-living stages of pathogenic agents, such as hookworm larvae, to develop or to survive on the soil surface, and affect the likelihood that such agents as bacterial spores and helminth ova will remain viable and available to animals, since these spores and ova remain on the soil surface for varying periods of time. For example, certain hard ticks (Fig. 8–7), as well as the orbatid mite vectors of the cattle tapeworm *Moniezia expansa*, survive best in moderately moist soils but die off in soils that are either too wet or too dry. Bedrock composed of limestone and dolomite appears to be a geographic marker for the distribution of *Leptospira pomona* infection.[8] Again, helminthiases associated with die-offs of snowshoe hares in the Soviet Union are localized in areas of hard soils, close groundwaters, and ample precipitation (Fig. 8–8). On well-drained soils, the mortality rates are lower.

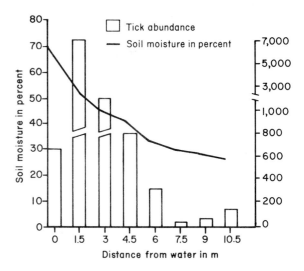

Fig. 8–7. Spatial distribution of sexually mature hard ticks in relation to water content of soil in floodplain (redrawn from Naumov, N.P. 1972. *The Ecology of Animals*. University of Illinois Press, Urbana; after Moskacheva, 1960).

Methods for combined soil-climate measurements relative to surface or subsurface conditions include (1) determination of evapotranspiration (actual or potential), a combined estimate of direct evaporation losses plus soil moisture losses from transpiration through plants, and (2) various direct measurements of soil moisture. Evapotranspiration thus represents the return of water from the soil to the atmosphere and is, therefore, the reverse of precipitation. The relationship between the two determines whether a climate is dry or moist. For example, the average annual precipitation for Urbana, Illinois, is 91.3 cm.; and the average annual potential evapotranspiration,

70.8 cm., for a net soil moisture balance of 20.5 cm. per year. An example of attention to combined effects of climate and soils upon disease transmission is given in the following study of gastrointestinal nematodes of ruminants.[9]

TRANSMISSION OF GASTROINTESTINAL NEMATODES. Mixed parasitisms, particularly in ruminants, represent a type of epidemiologically complex multivariate problem that requires attention worldwide. Much research has been done on experimental infections with single parasite species (pure infection groups) under one set of environmental conditions. This situation, however, bears little resemblance to

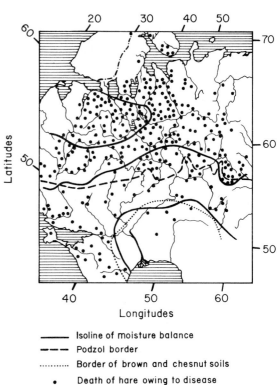

Fig. 8–8. Distribution of epidemic hare die-offs from helminthic infections in western USSR from 1884 through 1941. Epidemics are most frequent in areas of hard soils, close groundwaters, and ample precipitation. The hares are distributed throughout the entire area (redrawn from Naumov, N.P. 1972. *The Ecology of Animals*. University of Illinois Press, Urbana).

these disease complexes as seen in nature. Levine developed an approach to this problem in a preliminary methodological study. First, he compared the nematode species population profiles of sheep and cattle raised in Urbana, Illinois; Beltsville, Maryland; Experiment, Georgia; and central and northeast Texas (Fig. 8–9). It is clear that different species predominate in mixed gastrointestinal parasitisms in different geographic areas.

Next, he related the climates of the same areas (more or less) to optimal transmission conditions of certain parasite species in terms of climatic type (see Table 8–1), bioclimatograms (Fig. 8–10), potential evapotranspiration-precipitation patterns (Fig. 8–11); and potential transmission periods (Fig. 8–12). Only through such detailed epidemiological groundwork does one *begin* to identify the important local determinants of mixed gastrointestinal parasitic diseases and acquire the knowledge necessary to predict

their consequences and begin to combat them. Multivariate statistical tools such as multiple regression and discriminant analysis lend themselves admirably to this type of complex epidemiological task, provided the prerequisite data are quantifiable.

In addition to the types of soil and climate factors considered in the preceding study, particular organic constituents of soils may provide an optimal medium for growth of saprophytic pathogens, such as the fungal agents of cryptococcosis and histoplasmosis. Soils may also contain specific chemical agents of disease, available to animals either directly from the soil or indirectly through water or plants. Some of these agents occur in toxic amounts naturally, as does selenium; or may result from industrial or other contamination, as with fluorides and lead. In an interesting situation in California, rupture of the aorta in swine occurs endemically in an area of high zinc content of soil. Excess zinc competes with the

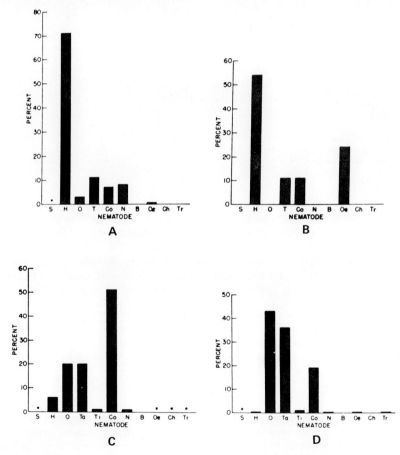

Fig. 8–9.   Nematode species profiles of sheep and cattle from different regions in United States. S = *Strongyloides papillosus*; H = *Haemonchus*; T = *Trichostrongylus*; Ta = *Trichostrongylus axei*; Ti = *Trichostrongylus colubriformis* and other intestinal *Trichostrongylus* species; Co = *Cooperia*; N = *Nematodirus*; B = *Bunostomum*; Oe = *Oesophagostomum*; Ch = *Chabertia*; Tr = *Trichuris*. *A*, Beltsville, Maryland (data from Kates, 1950); *B*, Urbana, Illinois (data from Levine and Clark, 1961); *C*, Experiment, Georgia (data from Ciordia et al., 1962); *D*, Central and northeast Texas (data from Bell et al., 1959) (from Levine, N.D.[9], which should be read for more complete data).

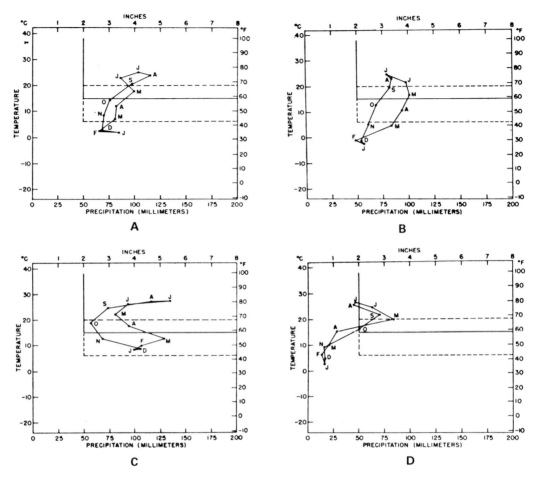

Fig. 8–10. Bioclimatographs for different regions of United States in relation to epidemiology of ruminant gastrointestinal nematodes. Optimum conditions for pasture transmission of *Haemonchus*: 5 cm or more total monthly precipitation and 15 to 37°C mean monthly mean temperature. Optimum conditions for pasture transmission of *Trichostrongylus* and *Ostertagia*: 5 cm or more total monthly precipitation and 6 to 20°C mean monthly mean temperature. *A*, Beltsville, Maryland, 1921-1950, Cfa climate; *B*, Urbana, Illinois, 1903-1954, Cfa climate; *C*, Columbus, Georgia, 1921-1950, Cfa climate; *D*, Lubbock, Texas, 1921-1950, Bsk climate. See Table 8–1 for climate types (from Levine, N.D.[9]).

nutrition of copper causing a copper deficiency and reduced linkage of collagen in connective tissue. Conversely, specific soil deficiencies, particularly deficiencies of phosphate and cobalt, are associated with a number of animal diseases.

BIOLOGICAL ENVIRONMENT

Epidemiologists consider that biological environmental determinants of disease include the influences of all biological factors (other than specific biological agents of disease) on the particular population of the animal species at risk. Such factors include the plant communities that characterize the ecosystem under study; the associated populations of other vertebrate and invertebrate species, particularly those that may serve as reservoirs of infection or as vectors; and man. Chapter 4 has developed the first two of these groups of possible biological determinants of disease pat-

terns. This discussion is limited, therefore, to consideration of man as an epidemiological variable in animal diseases.

Man as a biological determinant of animal diseases

People may influence the frequency of animal diseases in a great variety of ways. Transients and visitors, including salesmen, deliverymen, service personnel, and veterinarians or other consultants, all may be specifically involved in the introduction of diseases to new premises. Several examples have been given elsewhere in this book.

Probably far more important as human epidemiological variables, however, are management personnel and their practices. Despite this fact, there has been a tendency among veterinarians to dismiss so-called management factors in disease as outside their area of interest or influence. This "dismissal"

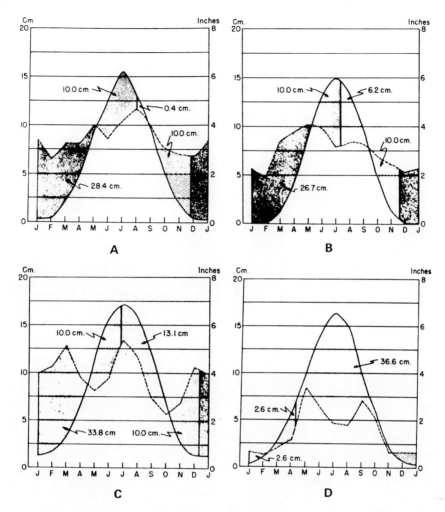

Fig. 8–11. Potential evapotranspiration and precipitation for different regions of United States. *A*, Beltsville, Maryland, 1921-1950, Cfa climate; *B*, Urbana, Illinois, 1903-1954, Cfa climate; *C*, Columbus, Georgia, 1921-1950, Cfa climate; *D*, Lubbock, Texas, 1921-1950, Bsk climate. See Table 8-1 for climate types (from Levine, N.D.[9]).

becomes an untenable position for a veterinarian as attention in the economically developed countries is focused more and more upon prevention of endemic, insidious, and epidemiologically complex animal diseases that take a marked but inadequately measured toll in the cost of production of animal protein and other valuable animal products. The general subject of changing patterns of disease problems in such countries is detailed in Chapter 17. Specific management factors as disease determinants must be sorted out, examined, and, if need be, corrected as part of future applications of epidemiology in veterinary practice. The following type of disease problem is one in which such factors are prominent.

HYPOTHETICAL SITUATION ON A DAIRY FARM. The owner of a large dairy farm has called in a veterinarian to face a problem of high neonatal losses. He examines some of the sick calves and discovers that

they suffer from diarrhea. The herd manager assures him that every calf receives colostrum promptly and has its navel disinfected. The veterinarian performs necropsies on a few moribund and dead animals and sends appropriate tissues to a state laboratory. While waiting for the laboratory report, he probably prescribes an antibiotic regimen, and possibly other supportive therapy. He may attempt to learn how soon after birth the deaths of calves have occurred; but quite often the calf records will not be adequate for this purpose, and he must rely on the manager's opinion. More often than not, no one knows the frequency and pattern of death losses now or before the veterinarian was called in.

From the laboratory, he may find that all the calves examined have harbored a single specific pathogen; or, more often, a series of autopsy specimen reports may indicate presence of a spectrum of coliforms,

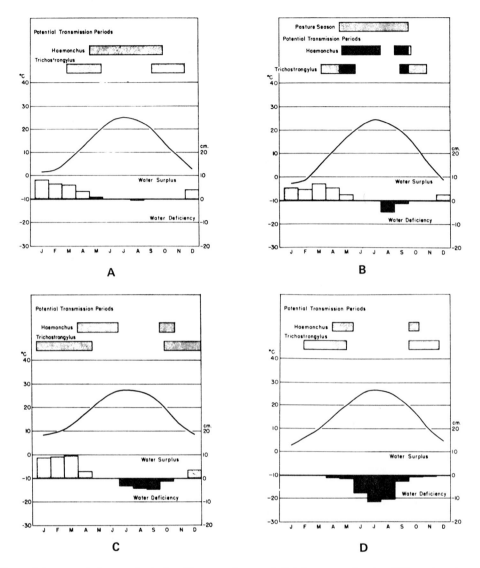

Fig. 8–12. Potential transmission periods for *Haemonchus* and *Trichostrongylus* in different regions of United States. *Haemonchus*: 15-37°C (55-99°F) mean monthly temperature and not more than 2.0 cm (0.8 inches) monthly water deficiency. *A*, Beltsville, Maryland, 1921-1950, Cfa climate; *B*, Urbana, Illinois, 1903-1954, Cfa climate; *C*, Columbus, Georgia, 1921-1950, Cfa climate; *D*, Lubbock, Texas, 1921-1950, Bsk climate. See Table 8–1 for climate types (from Levine, N.D.[9]).

salmonellae, and, if looked for, a virus or two. If the problem continues and a program of therapy is ineffective, the veterinarian, in desperation, may make an autogenous vaccine from one of the isolates and give it a try. Either enough calf losses continue to make the herd manager think that the problem is still bad, or the situation may improve temporarily.

In the meantime, the farmer's neighbor (or an equipment salesman) may suggest a new $35,000 calf-rearing barn in place of the portable pen system then in use. This suggestion entails a large enough commitment to enthuse even an absentee owner; but, when the barn is built and the losses still continue, more or less, the veterinarian, who has visited frequently enough by then to have observed a

number of generally slipshod husbandry practices, concludes that management factors are to blame for these calf deaths. He leaves the scene more or less comfortable in the knowledge that he has done all he could professionally—if obviously not enough. It is doubtful that he will be called there again. Lumped into his ubiquitous catch-all of management factors are a number of specific or general determinants of epidemiologically complex, multicausal disease problems such as neonatal mortality. A possible epidemiological approach to problems of this type is suggested in Chapter 13.

MANAGER FACTORS. Certain management practices, such as those with respect to housing and those that relate to efforts to control the physical environment, have already been considered in this chapter. Many of the others pertain to specific aspects of husbandry, such as systems of record keeping; feeding and breeding regimens; transportation, restraint, and other animal handling procedures; measures followed immediately before, at, and following the birth of offspring; systems for care of neonatal animals; and product harvest procedures such as those for milk, eggs, and wool. Some management variables pertain to environmental hygiene, animal hygiene, and rou-

tine medical and surgical procedures. Still others, however, are more specifically manager factors than management factors; and reflect, in part, the attitudes and sense of responsibility on the part of managers, herdsmen, and other animal handlers. Such things include not only intent, but also thoroughness, consistency, and other nebulous components of "tender loving care."[10] Little serious attention has been paid to the influence of such factors upon the frequency of disease and death.

Chapter 9

HOST DETERMINANTS OF DISEASES

THE occurrence of some diseases is strongly associated with a particular host variable such as sex, or a disease may occur only in animals of certain age groups. For some situations like these, an explanation may be readily apparent, and it may or may not have any practical consequences from an etiologic or preventive medical standpoint. For other diseases, particularly those of essentially unknown etiology, associations between a specific host variable and a disease may be hypothesized from descriptive studies and subsequently established on a statistical basis. Rarely, however, does such a single discovery result in a substantial causal hypothesis about the disease. Instead, a variety of alternative and equally attractive explanations may suggest themselves.

Still, this association may have been a useful finding. If associations of this disease with *different* independent host variables can be demonstrated from studies of other populations of animals, one explanation may be common to *each* of these instances. Causal hypotheses derived by this process of agreement, mentioned in Chapter 1, are usually productive from an etiological standpoint; and they may identify a more direct determinant, which can then be manipulated in ways that many host variables *per se* cannot.

It is intuitively easy to accept the idea that metabolic diseases and the well-characterized hereditary diseases have strong host factor determinants. However, infectious diseases may also have host determinants that manifest themselves within a species either directly or indirectly. The fact that susceptibility and resistance to infectious diseases are variables capable of genetic transmission was first clearly demonstrated by experimental epidemiological studies with colonies of mice.[1] The generality of these observations has been substantiated since in studies of other animal species, including man. For example, of 24 human diseases studied using identical twins, five of the 12 that showed evidence of an hereditary factor were infectious diseases.[2]

ACTION OF HOST DETERMINANTS

Host determinants may act not only by influencing whether an agent of disease will come into contact with a host or will be taken into the host's body, but also, in the case of infections, by affecting such things as the outcome of the infection for the host (e.g., disease or no overt disease) and for the agent (e.g., its multiplication, development, and/or shedding). The point to note is that the types of events that an agent triggers in a host, including manifest lesions and clinical signs, are *mainly under host control*.

In other words, not only is the severity of the signs generally determined by the host, but so are such outcomes as death or recovery, including the possibility of clinical recovery with persistence of the agent (i.e., a carrier state). Usually, death of a host is a detrimental outcome for a living agent of disease as well as for the host; and long-term evolutionary changes tend to make host species and agent species more compatible and their relationship more commensal than parasitic (see Fig. 2–4).

Similarly, except for some metazoan parasites, egress of a living agent from the host seldom reflects activity on the part of the agent; but it may be a direct result of some host activity such as coughing, defecating, or urinating. Less often, the agent may be shed more passively such as in secretions from surface lesions. In congenitally acquired infections, shedding of a living agent also may occur *in utero*, with its passage to the eggs or offspring of the host. Other living agents are not shed by the host at all, while still others require the active aid of vectors.

Some host determinants of disease may act through a variety of defense mechanisms available to the host animal. For example, hair and skin form barriers to some types of agents and are less penetrable generally than are the conjunctivae or the mucosae of the respiratory or intestinal tracts. Thus, skin thickness, hair density, and mucosal integrity are all possible host variables of epidemiological importance. In the event that an agent does successfully enter a host's tissues, the physiological defense systems of the latter may respond. Thus, different mechanisms exist to eliminate or neutralize toxic agents, while such things as inflammatory processes, phagocytes, antibodies, and interferon may act directly on living agents. The degree to which the host possesses or can mobilize such defenses depends in part upon its physical and chemical constitution, including its general immune competence; and these characteristics, in turn, are functions of both the animal's genetic make-up and such environmental influences as diet, climatic or other stress, exercise, fatigue, and existing or previous disease conditions. A few examples will show some of the many ways that different host determinants may interact with agent and environmental determinants and together produce a diseased individual or a population with a given frequency of disease.

Shipping fever, a disease complex primarily of young cattle, occurs when they are exposed to strenuous transportation or other stress and various infective agents, some of them purely opportunistic pathogens. These relationships in shipping fever are only partially understood. Conversely, rats that have been kept under crowded or other stressful conditions develop *less* severe disease when infected with *Trichinella spiralis*. In this instance, the hypertrophy of the adrenal glands- induced by stress reduces the host's cellular response, which in turn increases its susceptibility to the parasitic infection but, paradoxically, also reduces the severity of the disease.

Nutritional status (e.g., a state of protein deficiency) is another host variable that, under experimental conditions, has been shown to affect host response to infectious agents.[3] Physical body build also may be a disease determinant, as evidenced in the German shepherd dog's increased susceptibility to hip dysplasia. Similarly, body build may play a role in the susceptibility of hosts to infectious diseases, since certain insect vectors (e.g., some mosquitoes) respond to the body size of a potential host, just as they may respond to its coat color.

The preceding examples, some of which are discussed in more detail later, suffice to illustrate possibilities for interactions of host determinants of disease with factors of agent and environment. They should suggest, too, that in few real-life situations can host factors in disease be considered in isolation, because they themselves may be partially functions of an animal's environment. It should also be borne in mind that one type of host factor, for example physiological state, may be confounded with others, such as sex, age, or another specific genetic characteristic. The following discussion of different classes of host determinants of disease is based upon their categorization, as shown in Table 9–1.

INTRINSIC HOST DETERMINANTS

Host variables that may determine in part the pattern of occurrence or frequency of a disease are either extrinsic or intrinsic. Many of the latter are, in turn, genetically determined.

Species

Animal species differ in their clinical response to the same disease agent (or closely related agents) and also in their resistance to the same infectious agent. For many agents, there is a broad range of more or less susceptible host species in which the agents may or may not produce a disease. Overt disease is for this reason—and also for other reasons—not a reliable indicator of the extent of a disease agent's activity. For many, perhaps all, infections, the true host range in nature is unknown.

Some examples of multihost infections are discussed in Chapter 4. Psittacosis is another interesting example. The agent of that infection was originally believed to be limited to the parakeet, with man serving only occasionally as a blind or dead-end host from which the agent was not transmitted. Only many years later was it learned that the agent of psittacosis infects a number of other birds and mammals in nature; that is, it is a multihost agent that is associated with disease in some species of hosts but not others. The explanation for this phenomenon of different species manifestations (of *relative* specificity of infections) is not known for psittacosis or for other infections, but it can be surmised that infection without disease in many cases results from an evolutionary development resulting in a "climax state" in the host-parasite relationship. The phenomenon of relative specificity of infections is of particular epidemiological significance in that it may from time to time manifest itself in the occurrence of so-called "new" infectious diseases. As pointed out already, bluetongue first appeared in South Africa as a new disease only after Merino sheep were introduced into that country. Subsequently, it was found

Table 9–1.   Some Host Determinants of Disease

Intrinsic					Extrinsic	
Genetic						
Species, breed, physical type	Hereditary defects, resistance	Sex	Age	Physiological state	Animal use	Level of husbandry

that local wild ungulates were already infected but showed no clinical disease. Similarly, African swine fever showed up in Kenya, Uganda, and in other African countries only after these areas imported European breeds of swine. In this case, bushpigs were the reservoir host; they were infected without clinical signs and were able to transmit the agent to domestic swine.

Vesicular stomatitis virus is another agent that can infect a number of host species with different outcomes. Raccoons are susceptible, but their infection is inapparent and no virus is shed. Deer, on the other hand, develop lesions and may serve as amplifier hosts. Cattle, swine, and horses develop an acute disease. The maintenance or reservoir host for vesicular stomatitis virus has not yet been identified; but it is known that invertebrate animals can also become infected, and the virus is morphologically similar to some viruses that infect plants. Recent studies on marine mammals indicate that they may be maintenance hosts for a clinically similar viral infection, vesicular exanthema of swine—a disease formerly believed to have been eradicated globally.

As stated in Chapter 4, it is probable that most vertebrate animal species are susceptible to infection with a much wider range of agents than has been demonstrated. Yet we still tend to regard man and the guinea pig as two unusually susceptible species. This assumption is probably not at all accurate. In nature, the guinea pig inhabits a particular grasslands ecosystem in which it is exposed to a fairly narrow range of infectious agents. However, extensive laboratory use shows that the guinea pig has a great susceptibility range to infections. Many infectious agents have been demonstrated in man largely because he intrudes into a wide range of ecosystems, and thus has almost infinite opportunities for exposure; besides, his illnesses are subject to far closer scrutiny than are those of any other species. It should not be surprising to find any animal species susceptible to a particular infection, given favorable circumstances, as for example in the case of trematode parasitism of fish, discussed in Chapter 4.

Many infectious agents associated with vertebrate diseases also infect invertebrates, generally without serious consequences. There are some exceptions however, one being the agent of plague, which could be regarded as a disease of fleas for which vertebrates, such as ground squirrels, serve as inapparently infected maintenance hosts. These examples show that many infectious agents have wide host ranges and that the outcome of infection may vary greatly among host species.

There are also agents in nature that apparently infect only one or a few species; that is, some or most potential host species seem to possess absolute resistance. However, as research evidence accumulates, such agents continually decline in numbers. The

recently discovered susceptibility of armadillos to the leprosy bacillus is a case in point.

Breeds

Differential response to agents of disease is found not only among species but also among breeds or races within a given species. Many of these interbreed differences relate to diseases that are not known to be infectious, such as the higher prevalence of carcinoma of the eye in the Hereford breed compared to other cattle breeds and, among dogs, the predisposition to ruptured intervertebral disks in the dachshund and hip dysplasia in the German shepherd. The reasons for some of these breed associations are known or can be surmised. The predisposition to eye cancer in Hereford cattle is probably related to lack of protective pigment in the eyelids; and bodily structure can explain the predispositions seen in dachshunds and German shepherds. Since physical type is an intrinsic variable closely related to breed, differences within species of animals are often immense. Nowhere are they as great as those in the species *Canis familiaris*, whose breeds vary in size from the Chihuahua to the Irish wolfhound. This particular differential suggests that large dog breeds are especially suitable for studies on cancer.

In other cases of breed associations, no explanation is apparent. For example, pendulous crop in turkeys is breed-associated, as explained in Chapter 8; but the exact reason is unknown. Examples of interbreed differences in resistance to infections are also known, as for example, resistance to bovine trypanosomiasis. Other examples are given in the following section on hereditary defects and disease resistance. The special host-related phenomenon of herd immunity is discussed separately.

HEREDITARY DEFECTS AND DISEASE RESISTANCE

Hereditary genetic host characteristics are inseparable from characteristics such as species, breed, and sex since those also are genetically determined. Even animal use, an extrinsic host factor, is to a large extent genetically determined. The intent here is to discuss a genetic approach to epidemiological problems and to give examples of diseases in which genetic explanations of patterns of disease occurrence have been offered.[4]

Morphological and biochemical defects that are present at birth, though congenital, need not be hereditary. There are many examples of agents (e.g., x-rays, chemicals, microorganisms, dietary deficiencies) which, when acting on the pregnant dam, may induce nonhereditary congenital changes in the fetus. Such agents are called *teratogens*. A single teratogen may produce a variety of defects, and the same type of defect can be induced by widely different teratogens. The sensitivity of the fetus to such teratogens varies considerably at different stages of pregnancy. It is generally greatest when a particular organ is in the stage of most rapid differentiation, that is, early in pregnancy. Such congenital abnormalities may not show up until later in life as is the case with functional sterility.

Ultimately, the decision about whether a defect is hereditary is based on studies involving cross-breeding of suspect "carrier" animals of the responsible gene or genes. Such studies are not often performed unless a congenital malformation occurs with high frequency. For example, cyclopian malformation in lambs occurred for many years before decisive epidemiological studies were undertaken.

Cyclopian malformation in lambs

Though cyclopian malformation in lambs was recognized for some time, it was not considered economically important until 1959 when an increased incidence of this abnormality was reported from western Idaho. Its yearly incidence among the newborn of different bands of affected sheep varied from less than 1% to more than 8%. Ranchers called the affected lambs "monkey faced." A shortening of the upper jaw was a consistent finding; and hydrocephalus, harelip, cleft palate, and displacement of the nose commonly occurred. Other features of the abnormality were fusion of the cerebral hemispheres, absence of the olfactory bulbs, and occasional absence of the pituitary gland. When the eyes were displaced centrally, usually only one optic nerve was present. In extreme cases, there was only a single median eye. There was extensive edema and accumulation of fluid in the thoracic and abdominal cavities. Affected lambs often were born after gestation periods that were prolonged by six to nine weeks, and they were much heavier than normal lambs. The geographic distribution of the disease was limited to sheep ranges in southwestern Idaho, and the incidence seemed to depend on using forested areas for grazing during the breeding season.

Prior to 1956, most medical observers assumed that cyclopian malformation was hereditary. Most sheep farmers, however, did not believe the anomaly was hereditary. Because of this controversy and because the validity of a genetic hypothesis had not been tested, breeding experiments were eventually initiated. Forty-eight "carrier" ewes (i.e., ewes that had earlier given birth to malformed lambs) were kept with 12 rams (all sons of "carrier" ewes) in a geographic area not normally associated with the occurrence of cyclopian malformation. All 88 of these lambs were born after a gestation period of usual length, and all were normal. Two abortions had been associated with pneumonia, and there was one other. These three fetuses were normal.

Under the assumption that a single locus, autosomal recessive gene was responsible for these congenital cyclopian defects, the outcomes shown in Figure 9–1 would have been expected. Assuming further that half of the 12 rams used were AA and half Aa, one can calculate that the observed outcome of this breeding experiment would occur by chance less than once in 1000 times. The hereditary (i.e., host factor) hypothesis was therefore rejected.

The following alternative hypotheses were considered for possible determinants: (1) altitude anoxia, (2) a poisonous plant, (3) excess or deficiency of a nutrient, (4) a toxic mineral element, or (5) combinations of (1) to (4). Ultimately, a series of epidemiological experiments proved that the agent of cyclopian malformation in lambs actually was a specific *agent*, the poisonous plant, *Veratrum californicum*, which grows only at high altitudes and in certain places, both factors of environment.

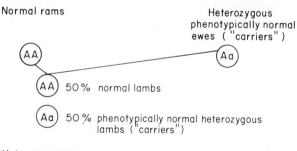

Normal rams — Heterozygous phenotypically normal ewes ("carriers")

AA × Aa

AA — 50% normal lambs

Aa — 50% phenotypically normal heterozygous lambs ("carriers")

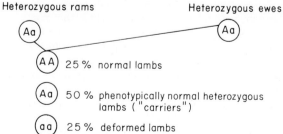

Heterozygous rams — Heterozygous ewes

Aa × Aa

AA — 25% normal lambs

Aa — 50% phenotypically normal heterozygous lambs ("carriers")

aa — 25% deformed lambs

Fig. 9–1. Expected outcomes of breeding experiments to study congenital cyclopian malformation in lambs.[5] The hypothesis is that malformation results from a single recessive autosomal gene.

Epidemiological considerations in genetic theory

Other disease conditions, including some malformations, *are* hereditary, however; to understand their basis, one must consider some of the operative mechanisms.

MENDELIAN INHERITANCE. Characteristics transmitted according to Mendel's laws are transmitted in their entirety or in no way at all; and they remain undiluted by transmission over many generations. Inheritance of the characteristic depends on which alternative gene at a particular locus is transmitted from parent to offspring. The principle is that alleles segregate. Alleles are genes that occupy the same locus on homologous chromosomes. The inheritance of a gene on one chromosome is stochastically independent of the inheritance of a gene on another; but this rule is not true for genes that occupy different loci on the same chromosome. Such genes are linked and tend to be transmitted together. Several examples of randomly segregating "unilocal" genetic defects are given below; but, first, it is important to consider alternative genetic possibilities.

GALTONIAN INHERITANCE. Although this type of inheritance is probably not qualitatively different from simple mendelian inheritance, different methods have to be applied in the analysis of so-called galtonian inheritance. While the outcomes of mendelian inheritance are distinct classes (e.g., tall or short pea plants, absence or presence of certain anatomical defects), galtonian inheritance results in progeny that exhibit a more continuous spectrum of a characteristic, such as a range of body weights or degrees of resistance to disease. A galtonian character can be imagined to be dependent on many loci that contribute more or less equally to the control of the character. Such a system is called "multilocal."

A number of laws in population genetics are of importance for epidemiological studies. However, the assumptions behind many of these laws are not fulfilled for populations of domesticated animals because such populations are extensively manipulated to obtain and maintain desired genetic characteristics (e.g., high productivity) in the breeding stock. On the other hand, genetic experiments—though often expensive—can be performed with domestic animals to reveal the nature of genetic defects. The still-increasing use of artificial insemination in livestock breeding has made it possible to propagate desired characteristics, such as egg and milk production, and has also increased the risk of spreading genes that are responsible for anatomical or functional defects that lower disease resistance. To what extent this risk of defects is or has been occurring is not known, but some of the following examples illustrate the potential. The first examples are mendelian while the latter ones, dealing with atrophic rhinitis, leucosis, nutritional diseases, and mastitis, are all of a galtonian nature.

Recessive defects in livestock

At least 90 lethal or semilethal hereditary anomalies are known in livestock.[4] There are probably many more, but the genetics of most livestock anomalies is poorly documented. Most of the known genetic defects in livestock are due to recessive genes. One well-known defect is beef-cattle dwarfism, which is due to a single autosomal gene. This defect has been observed in many breeds and was for a while widespread in Hereford cattle in the United States. The homozygote is a "snorter" dwarf that exhibits symptoms characteristic of achondroplasia (short legs, short body, short broad head, distended abdomen, and labored breathing); growth is slow, bloat common, and early mortality high.

Figure 9–2 shows the number of dwarfs, carriers, and "free" calves expected when at least one parent has the gene. This figure illustrates the mode of inheritance and also suggests ways of controlling this defect. The heterozygote, the carrier, is phenotypically undetectable (in spite of many attempts) and can be identified only by breeding. The most efficient detection approach would be to breed a suspected carrier (heterozygote) with a dwarf, since 50% dwarfs would be expected in the progeny (Fig. 9–2,C). However, dwarfs are expensive and difficult to maintain; and an alternative test, namely mating a sire with his daughters or with his full or half sisters, is used in practice. The number of sire-daughter matings required to test that there is less than a 5% probability that the sire is a carrier is 23. If this trait were sex-limited, 46 matings would be required! These facts explain why congenital malformations in livestock have been investigated only to a limited degree. Methods other than experimental mating are available for such tests (as mentioned later), provided that sufficient record data are available.

Dominant defects

Dominant defects are rare in domesticated animals. In the case of dominance, the heterozygotes exhibit the defect and therefore tend to be eliminated by selection. Sometimes the anomaly is lethal when homozygous, resulting in death of the affected animal *in utero.*

Sex-limited and sex-linked anomalies

Both cryptorchism and scrotal hernia are sex-limited anomalies, but evidence of the mode of inheritance is lacking. Sex-linked traits represent a different concept—the responsible genes are located in the X or Y chromosomes that determine sex. Not many examples are known for animals; but in dogs—as well as in man—hemophilia is one disease determined by a recessive sex-linked gene located in the X-chromosome. The heterozygous female is normal, but half of her male offspring exhibit this trait.

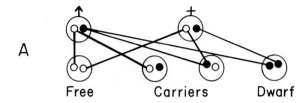

A

Free   Carriers   Dwarf

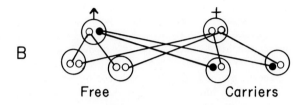

B

Free   Carriers

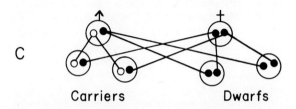

C

Carriers   Dwarfs

Fig. 9–2. Expected offspring from mating of bulls and cows with genes for dwarfism. *A*, both parents as carriers; *B*, one carrier parent; *C*, one carrier and one dwarf parent.

Defects with hereditary disposition but mode of inheritance unknown

Harelip, cleft palate, atresia ani, and amputated or deformed legs are examples of hereditary defects of unknown inheritance. Some of these defects may not be hereditary but may be caused by physical or chemical insult *in utero*. Unless these defects are proven nongenetic, animals that have them should never be used for breeding even if the defect can easily be corrected by surgery.

Disease resistance

Some variations in resistance to development of overt diseases are genetically determined. The mechanism of inheritance has in no case been explained, but the degree of inheritance has in some cases been measured.

NUTRITIONAL DISEASES. Nutritional diseases are particularly well known in domesticated animals, since the minimal requirement of almost all essential nutrients had been established for these species sometime before it was established for man. It is recognized that, within species, different groups of animals vary considerably in their response to nutritional deficiencies. For example, the White Leghorn is known to be more resistant to deficiencies of thiamine, vitamin D, and manganese than are several other breeds of chickens.

INFECTIOUS DISEASES. Inheritance of resistance to infectious agents has been well documented for mice, as mentioned earlier; and it has been convin-

cingly shown that genetically controlled resistance also occurs in chickens. For example, by selection, there was established a line of White Leghorns that had a markedly increased resistance to *Salmonella pullorum*. In this instance, it was found that increased resistance derived from the ability of newly hatched birds to increase their body temperature to 41 to 43°C. in a short time.

The heritability (i.e., the proportion of the total variance of the phenotype transmissible from parent to offspring) for resistance to leucosis in chickens has been estimated to be 0.08 to 0.15; and 20 years of selection has established lines of Leghorns that have a high resistance to this disease.[6] These lines also were bred for high egg production and low overall mortality. Although there is much to recommend them, similar experiments have not been carried out to any great extent with larger farm animals because the cost in animal maintenance, animal testing, and time is high. However, limited results indicate that heritability of resistance to mastitis in cattle can be as high as 0.2 to 0.4, and heritability of resistance to atrophic rhinitis in swine has been reported to be 0.3. The complexity of an infectious disease in which genetic determinants have a strong influence is particularly well illustrated by Aleutian disease in mink.

Aleutian disease in mink.[7] Beginning about 1945, mink farmers in the western United States began to report unusually high mortality among their stock. Preliminary investigations revealed that these excessive deaths were due to a characteristic syndrome that had not been previously described in mink. Its first clinical signs were loss of weight (in spite of normal food intake) and increased thirst. A few animals developed nervous symptoms, such as abnormal behavior, bizarre postures, and paralysis; and there was occasional bleeding from the mouth and nose. Almost all animals showing signs died, most of them within one month after the onset of disease. Few affected mink survived beyond two months.

Prominent postmortem findings were an enlarged spleen and lymph nodes. Often, the liver was also enlarged and, in acute cases, the kidneys. Pale foci were observed on the surfaces of the kidneys and the liver. Microscopically, mononuclear cells, apparently mature plasma cells, were found in the kidneys, liver, and lymph nodes. In addition, many animals showed universal vascular changes consisting of deposits of eosinophilic material in and around the walls of the small arteries. Necrotic foci were sometimes seen in the walls of the arteries; this situation was accompanied by infiltration with leucocytes, histiocytes, and fibroblasts. In the kidneys, acidophilic deposits were found in the mesangium of the glomeruli, some glomeruli being completely destroyed and replaced with connective tissue. In some cases, ulcers occurred in the gastric and oral mucosae. Bacterial examinations yielded inconsistent results.

The incidence of this disease was found to vary considerably among farms. No characteristic geographic distribution pattern was observed; and, after a few years, the disease was reported in other areas of the United States and in Canada, Japan, Germany, and the Scandinavian countries. The incidence seemed to be age-associated since mortality was highest among older animals. However, autopsy surveys revealed that the prevalence of lesions also was high among kits; so it was concluded that there was no true age association, but that the disease had a long subclinical stage.

Sex association was found in breeding animals, with highest mortality in males. It was believed that this factor was due to stress although special tests for sex-linked hereditary defects apparently were not made. No association was found between feed and the disease.

Mortality followed a seasonal pattern. Among breeding females, losses were highest in May during whelping and nursing; and a smaller increase occurred in November when the weather conditions worsened. The highest mortality among kits occurred in early November.

A strong breed association was also observed. Initial reports stated that the disease occurred only in blue types of mink. These mink have a light, gun-steel blue color, which became much in demand beginning around 1940. The gene responsible for this color is recessive and is called the Aleutian gene because the color resembles that of the Aleutian fox. Mink homozygous for the Aleutian gene, aa, possess the blue color while heterozygous, Aa, mink and mink without the Aleutian gene, AA, do not. Through extensive inbreeding and crossbreeding of Aleutian mutants, the blue mink became widely distributed inside and outside the United States.

Because this disease syndrome is rather complex, efforts were directed toward a simple method to identify the disease. When it was found that the syndrome was invariably accompanied by a markedly increased concentration of gammaglobulin in the blood serum, a simple—though not specific—iodine agglutination test was developed for application in the field.

It was a common belief that this disease was inherited, so breeding experiments were carried out to verify this belief. The experiments used the iodine agglutination test as a diagnostic tool. One such trial gave the results shown in Table 9–2. Segregation seemed to exist, but the data were not easily interpreted. Examination of the experimental procedures revealed that the data were not strictly comparable, in that the proportions of barren females were 32% and 20% for the first two groups of animals and 0% for the last group. The number of stillbirths and neonatal death rates, as well as litter sizes, also differed among these groups.

Other studies revealed that lesions in other breeds of mink were almost as prevalent, but less extensive than in blue mink. Finally, it was shown that this disease is transmissible and that a specific slow virus is involved. Aleutian disease is now known to affect most breeds of mink, but its highest mortality occurs in blue mink. The reason seems to be that blue mink are inferior with respect to antibody response, a

Table 9–2.   Results of Breeding Experiment to Study Possible Genetic Basis for Aleutian Disease of Mink[7]

Group	Females Iodine* test	Females Aleutian gene test	Males Iodine test	Males Aleutian gene test	Ratio of iodine positive: negative among offspring
1	+	aa	+	aa	1:1
2	–	aa	–	aa	1:1
3	–	Aa	–	Aa	1:2

*Iodine agglutination test for immunoglobulin level

characteristic associated with abnormal granulation in all leucocytes. There seems to be a genetic linkage between these defects and the single-locus Aleutian characteristic.

Similar syndromes also have been found in Hereford cattle, Karakul sheep, and man (so-called Chidiak-Higashi syndrome). In man the syndrome is characterized by nystagmus, partial albinism, photophobia, and abnormal granulation in all leucocytes. Human patients with this syndrome are highly susceptible to infections and seldom live beyond seven years of age. This condition has been shown to be associated with a single-locus recessive gene in man as well as in Hereford cattle.

Application of hereditary resistance in disease control

The case for using genetic manipulations for getting rid of morphological or functional hereditary defects is strong. However, with respect to resistance to infectious diseases in livestock, genetic possibilities have been little explored. The past emphasis in veterinary medicine has been almost exclusively on treating the hosts (including vaccination) or more directly eliminating the agent, rather than boosting the hereditary resistance of the host. The former approach is probably sound when dealing with rather specific and well-defined agents such as *Mycobacterium tuberculosis* and *Brucella abortus*. However, when agents are ubiquitous, as in mastitis, or ill-defined and difficult to trace, as in a number of other infectious disease complexes, genetic measures might well be the most economical. Through good record-keeping, enough information can be collected about a relatively common disease to permit breeding for resistance without resorting to costly experiments. The principles involved (selection, crossbreeding) are the same as those in breeding for improved economic performance in livestock; and they have been applied, as mentioned previously, for breeding disease resistance into certain lines of poultry.

Epidemiological aspects of population genetics

One of the main purposes of epidemiological studies in population genetics is to obtain information about pathogenesis. The most solid inferences can be made with data from populations over which the epidemiologist has control, but these data are often not available. In the absence of such data, the most fortuitous situation occurs when a genetic trait is unilocal and the phenotype is clearly separable, e.g., in the homozygous beef cattle dwarf. Even then, however, unilocal traits may not operate in the simple, classic way. For instance, epistasis or incomplete penetrance may occur. With the latter, an identifiable manifestation of the disease may be available for study. For example, blood cholesterol levels and blood pressure have been used in this

manner in epidemiological evaluations of the genetics of coronary disease in man; and, in the example of Aleutian disease in mink, gammaglobulin levels were used similarly. In human studies in epidemiology, extensive use also has been made of associations with "marker genes" in exploring coronary disease, hypertension, and other diseases; but experience has shown that association is difficult to demonstrate. More successes have been achieved in epidemiological studies of chromosome anomalies.

If attempts to demonstrate classical mendelian inheritance fail, one must have recourse to nonsegregational methods that are more inductive in character. Nonsegregational methods include comparison of breeds (e.g., prevalence of carcinoma of the eye of Hereford and other cattle breeds), study of isolated populations, and twin studies. Care has to be exercised in such studies to exclude the effects of confounding variables such as place, time, and husbandry conditions.

Another factor to note is that a multilocal genetic mechanism may have a dichotomous expression. For example, in disease resistance, there may be a threshold level beyond which the probability of infection is greatly increased. This case may be mistaken for an autosomal dominant disorder at one locus. However, a true dominant tends to persist intact over an indefinite number of generations while a multilocal characteristic dissipates.

Sex

Some diseases are definitely sex-associated. For example, parturient paresis, mastitis, and other diseases related to specific female structures or functions occur only in females, and *vice versa* for males. Other conditions may be associated with desexing; for example, an increased incidence of urinary calculi has been reported in castrated male cats although other investigations have been unable to demonstrate such an association. Apparent sex-associated disease conditions frequently relate to other factors such as age or use of an animal; so care must be exercised in interpretation. It is, for example, frequently observed that neonatal mortality is higher for male dairy calves, but it is also known that female dairy calves generally receive better care.

Another possible pitfall in studying sex association is that there is an unequal sex distribution in most animal populations. The numbers of males and females at risk therefore can differ considerably, and this difference must be taken into account.

Age

Age is another host variable that must always be considered in epidemiological studies, not only because age association may assist in understanding the pathogenesis of the disease in question, but association with age in a disease is often so strong that it results in various indirect effects.

Numerous factors may influence age associations. Some are simple, while others are poorly understood. For example, certain infectious diseases, such as canine distemper and infectious bronchitis in chickens, have a much higher incidence in younger than in older animals, the reason being that older animals often possess protective antibodies from an infection acquired when young. This age distribution explains acquired herd immunity, as discussed later, and is absent for such diseases only in "virgin" populations, that is, populations that have not been exposed to the particular infectious agent for at least a generation. In human populations, a similar situation is seen in some so-called childhood diseases such as measles.

Although many infectious diseases have a high incidence among the young, the disease is often milder in younger than in older individuals. This characteristic is especially true if the young acquire their infections when maternal antibodies still have a protective effect. Advantage is sometimes taken of this situation in veterinary medicine by deliberately exposing young animals so that they will acquire a mild disease and remain resistant for the rest of their life. With protozoal infections, in which the organism persists in the host, this resistance is called *premunition*—a measure used in several countries against piroplasmosis in cattle.

A poorly understood but disease-related function of age is the influence, apart from antibody levels and other extraneous factors, of the ageing process upon the frequency of so-called degenerative diseases (e.g., cancer, hypertension, and coronary disease). Human studies in epidemiology in recent years have concentrated upon such phenomena. It is known in veterinary medicine that certain lines of animals age faster than others and that physiologic age is determined by genetic constitution and by environment, especially during early development. It might be argued that diseases associated with the ageing process are of little importance with respect to food animals since most of them have a truncated life span; they die young in the slaughterhouse. However, age-associated disease phenomena may occur also in young animals, particularly those exposed to disease agents early in life or even *in utero*. Second, dairy cows and other producing animals generally go out of production *because* of disease conditions (e.g., infertility, mastitis), but it is not known whether these diseases are truly associated with ageing processes. Research resulting in the prolongation of the productive life of animals would no doubt be of economic importance. A valuable research situation for such studies in cattle exists in India where cattle frequently are maintained in "old cattle homes" until they die natural deaths.[8]

Diseases of infancy and degenerative diseases have unimodal age distribution curves, the first curve peaking at a young age, the latter at old age. Sometimes bimodal age distribution curves are seen for diseases. The general explanation is that one is dealing with clinically or pathologically similar diseases that are not identical in young and old animals, or that two different sets of determinants are active, one in the young age group, another in the older. An example of such a bimodal distribution occurs with cat leukemia.

STUDY OF AGE ASSOCIATIONS. There are several general techniques used in studying age association. The first is to calculate age specific morbidity or mortality rates in order to gain information about a possible age association and also to compare rates for populations with different age distributions. Second, a standard population often is used as a basis for adjustment of rates between populations of different age composition. This latter permits overall morbidity and mortality rates to be expressed by just one number. This single expression may make comparisons between several populations easier, but it may also make interpretation difficult. Methods used for rate adjustment were illustrated in Chapter 5.

Where samples of populations are being compared for an association between occurrence of a disease and an hypothesized determinant, and the disease is also age-associated, another approach is to match cases and "controls" by age. From the following data, it can be seen how age may readily be confounded with other variables resulting in difficulties in interpretation of data.

AGE DISTRIBUTION OF AN INFECTIOUS DISEASE. An epidemic of an infectious disease affected cattle in a number of dairy herds. Each herd contained Holstein and Guernsey cattle, and these two breeds were considered at equal risk of exposure to infection. However, the attack rate for Guernseys was 49.1% and for Holsteins 45.2%; and their case fatality rates were; respectively, 27.8% and 22.6%.

The detailed distribution of these cases and deaths is shown in Tables 9–3 and 9–4. Note that while the overall attack rate is higher for Guernseys than for Holsteins, the table shows that the recorded attack rates are a little higher *in each age group* for Holsteins than for Guernseys. These tables also reveal that the age distribution is quite different in these two breeds. One could easily draw a fallacious conclusion if this age distribution were not taken into account. Calculations of relative risk in age groups 5.5 to 6.5 years and over 8.5 years reveal no significant differences between breeds. Still, the slightly higher attack rate in each age group of Holsteins is statistically significant if it is tested by a nonparametric test. The sign test is a useful "quick and dirty" nonparametric statistical test. Its use is illustrated with data in Tables 9–4 and 9–5.

One can record a + (plus) for every age group in which the age specific attack rate for Holsteins

Table 9–3.   Sicknesses and Deaths of Cattle by Breed in Epidemic of Infectious Disease of Cattle in American Middle West in 1960.

| | | | | | Age (in years) | | | | | | |
	<0.5	1.5	2.5	3.5	4.5	5.5	6.5	7.5	8.5	>8.5	Total
No. Guernsey cattle at risk	91	107	128	154	139	156	124	127	119	108	1253
No. Guernsey cattle sick	0	15	48	72	73	89	72	76	89	81	615
No. Guernsey cattle dead	0	0	2	4	11	21	28	32	36	37	171
No. Holstein cattle at risk	476	455	580	577	612	502	477	332	197	68	4276
No. Holstein cattle sick	0	89	239	280	328	297	291	206	150	53	1933
No. Holstein cattle dead	0	2	10	17	51	70	116	85	61	24	436

exceeds that for Guernseys, record a – (minus) for the reverse, and ignore age classes in which the rates are the same. Using Table 9–4, one records nine +'s and no –'s; and in Table 9–5 one records five +'s and two –'s. If there are no differences due to breed, then one should expect to observe about equal numbers of + and – signs being recorded.

Using a two-tailed test for the binomial distribution, one can calculate the probability of observing something as strange as, or stranger than, that

observed. In other words, in Table 9–4, one calculates the probability of all +'s *or* all –'s.

$$P(9 \text{ +'s } or \text{ } 9 \text{ –'s}|p=0.5, n=9) = {}_9C_9 p^9 q^0 + {}_9C_0 p^0 q^9$$

$$= 2(1)(1/2)^9 = \frac{2}{512} = \frac{1}{256} = 0.0039.$$

Thus, if there really are no attack rate differences attributable to breed, one would expect all age-

Table 9–4.   Age Adjustment of Morbidity Rates for Infectious Disease by Cattle Breed (see Table 9–3)

Age (in years)	Standard population (Guernsey plus Holstein)	Age-breed specific A.R. %		Difference (+, −)	Expected sick	
		Guernsey	Holstein		Guernsey	Holstein
<.5	567	0	0		0	0
1.5	562	14.0	19.6	+	79	110
2.5	708	37.5	41.2	+	266	292
3.5	731	46.8	48.5	+	342	355
4.5	751	52.5	53.6	+	394	404
5.5	658	57.1	59.2	+	376	390
6.5	601	58.1	61.0	+	349	367
7.5	459	59.8	62.0	+	275	285
8.5	316	74.8	76.1	+	236	241
>8.5	176	75.0	77.9	+	132	137
	5529	49.1	45.2		2449	2581

Age adjusted A.R.:

Guernsey $\dfrac{2449}{5529} \times 100 = 44.3 \ (443/1000)$

Holstein $\dfrac{2581}{5529} \times 100 = 46.7 \ (467/1000)$

Table 9–5.   Age Adjustment of Case Fatality Rates for Infectious Disease by Cattle Breed (see Table 9–3)

Age (in years)	Standard population (Guernsey plus Hostein)	Age-breed specific case fatality rate %		Difference (+, −)	Expected dead	
		Guernsey	Holstein		Guernsey	Holstein
<.5	0	0	0		0	0
1.5	104	0	2.2	+	0	5.0
2.5	287	4.2	4.2		12.1	12.1
3.5	352	5.6	6.1	+	19.7	21.5
4.5	401	15.1	15.5	+	60.6	62.2
5.5	386	23.6	23.6		98.4	91.1
6.5	363	38.9	39.9	+	141.2	144.8
7.5	282	42.1	41.3	−	118.7	116.5
8.5	239	40.4	40.7	+	96.6	97.3
>8.5	134	45.7	45.3	−	61.2	60.7
	2548				608.5	611.2

Age adjusted case
fatality rate: Guernsey $\dfrac{608.5}{2548} \times 100 = 23.9\%$

Holstein $\dfrac{611.2}{2548} \times 100 = 24.0\%$

specific rates for one breed to exceed those for the other breed less than four times in a thousand. This unlikely prospect leads to the conclusion that there is a significant difference in attack rates by breed.

In the same way, in Table 9-5, calculate the probability

$$2 \cdot P(5 \text{ or } 6 \text{ or } 7 \text{ +'s} \mid p = 0.5, n=7) =$$

$$= 2 \left\{ {}_7C_5 p^5 q^2 + {}_7C_6 p^6 q^1 + {}_7C_7 p^7 q^0 \right\}$$

$$= 2 \left\{ \frac{21}{128} + \frac{7}{128} + \frac{1}{128} \right\} = \frac{58}{128} = 0.4531$$

Thus, in seven classes, the probability of observing five or more classes in which one breed's age-specific case fatality rate exceeds that of the other breed is about 45%. From these data, there is little evidence of any difference in case fatality rates between the two breeds.

In using the sign test in this way, some precautions should be observed. First, the number of individuals in each age category should be sufficiently large so the age-specific rates will be meaningful. Also, the number of age classes should be at least eight, and preferably greater than eight (in case of ties). In a very large study, with many age classes, the usual normal approximation to the binomial may be adequate for a preliminary examination.

Many other nonparametric tests may be of value in epidemiological studies. Of these, the Wilcoxon test for paired data may be of some value in comparing rates as has been done in the example with the sign test. The Wilcoxon test has the advantage over the sign test in that the *magnitude* of the difference between pairs is also used in the Wilcoxon test. For a description of that test, the reader is referred to any of several elementary statistical texts.

Physiological state

Categorization of animals by physiological state, for example, virgin or number of pregnancies experienced, dry or fresh, pregnant or open, and stage of estrous cycle, is often possible in veterinary medicine; and husbandry practices frequently attach importance to classifications of these types. Likewise, studies of vector populations may be concerned with whether vectors are gravid, engorged, or depleted. Similar categorizations involve molt, intermolt, hibernation, and estivation. Such physiological states may be associated with particular disease phenomena.

EXTRINSIC HOST DETERMINANTS

"Animal use" and "level of animal husbandry" are veterinary analogs of "occupation" and "socioeconomic status" for man. They are closely related and can be considered together. They also overlap with some of the management factors mentioned in the previous chapter.

Care of animals includes type of feed, handling and disposal of manure, general sanitation and housekeeping, separation of susceptible (often young) animals from possible carriers, avoidance of introducing unknown animals into the herd, or application of quarantine for new animals; and all are recognized by experience as important factors related to disease frequency. For example, in considering the differences between apparently similar farms and herds in the same area and at the same time, it often seems obvious that animal husbandry and management practices are very important determinants of disease. However, few well-controlled studies have been carried out to determine their actual importance under field conditions. The explanation is not difficult to find. Some such animal husbandry factors are difficult to measure; and, unless the disease condition studied is rather common, studies tend to become cumbersome and expensive. Furthermore, the lack of sufficient field data makes rational planning for livestock development difficult—a particularly serious problem in a period of rapid structural changes in agriculture, such as is occurring now (see Chapter 17).

In dealing with effects of husbandry factors, measurements of health of animals may be based not only on usual morbidity and mortality parameters but also on such measures of performance of animals as growth rate, egg production rate, milk production rate, and feed conversion rate. Such data, which already have been mentioned in Chapter 5, can be and often are obtained for animals and are excellent relative indicators of health, particularly when one is concerned with disease in terms of unit cost of production. Until now, veterinarians have been little involved in studies on such extrinsic determinants of disease, and few real epidemiological studies have been carried out. If veterinarians are to continue their valuable service to agriculture in the developed countries, there is little doubt that the emphasis will be more and more on identification of disease determinants related to animal husbandry and on rational preventive measures that take them into consideration. Epidemiological studies are indispensable for such purposes.

A few brief examples can serve to illustrate some of the types of effects of management. Crowding is known to facilitate the spread of infectious agents, but it may also have another indirect effect upon disease frequency. As already mentioned, crowding of rats definitely increases their susceptibility to *Trichinella spiralis* infection. Certain types of housing and husbandry induce tail-biting in swine, and this biting results in disseminated abscesses. Nutritional deficiencies also may affect the resistance of animals to infections. Again, cattle maintained on permanent pasture are more likely to be infected with parasites than those kept under other conditions. Movements

of cattle to mountain foothills in California at a certain time of the year elevates the risk of their acquiring a disease called foothill abortion; and there are strong indications that the pattern of movement of cattle between pastures of different quality in California strongly influences the incidence of pulmonary emphysema. Many of these husbandry measures are indirect causes of exposure to new environmental factors that may relate to disease frequency.

Similarly, present or previous disease history may affect a host's response to disease agents. Infection of man with *Entamoeba histolytica* or turkeys with *Histomonas meleagridis* depends on preexisting enteric bacteria. Hepatic necrosis (black disease) caused by clostridia in lambs is predisposed by infection with *Fasciola hepatica*. Such mixed or synergistic infections probably are more common than is now believed.

Evidence of the relationship between fatigue and resistance to infection is conflicting. Observations suggest that truck transport of pigs can cause a flare-up of intestinal *Salmonella* infections manifesting themselves in increased shedding rates. Another complex disease in cattle, known as shipping fever, has long been associated with the stress of transport.

Shipping fever in cattle

This disease was described first (1917) in Pennsylvania as "stockyard pneumonia" and later was reported in other states and also in Canada, Great Britain (as transit fever), Germany (as infectious bronchopneumonia), and Japan (as bovine influenza). The economic losses from this disease in the United States in 1972 were estimated as $95 million. Shipping fever manifests itself as a respiratory infection with high fever. It occurs in cattle, particularly in young cattle, that have been transported. The attack rate is about 20 to 40% after a 5 to 10 day incubation period, and the case fatality rate is 12 to 25%. At least 10 different bacterial agents and eight different viral agents have been "associated" with this disease.

However, no single agent has reproduced the disease in the absence of transport or similar stressing conditions. More than a dozen husbandry factors other than, or in relation to, transport have been listed as having an influence on the development of shipping fever. These include nutritional state, lack of water, fatigue, crowding, hot weather, cold weather, abuse and rough treatment, dusty or muddy pens, fright and excitement, recent castration, dehorning or branding, and weaning. The currently most attractive hypothesis is that shipping fever is produced by a stress-provoked viral infection, which creates minor lesions favorable to the pathogenesis of opportunistic bacterial pathogens. However, specific stress factors have not been well studied with respect to their relative importance nor, as a result, is there any way to tell which ones should be emphasized most in undertaking rational preventive measures.

INTERPRETATION OF STUDIES OF HOST DETERMINANTS

When explanations are being sought for host associations, careful consideration should be given to the characteristics and composition of the host population. Often only a fraction of the population is at risk; and this fraction may be a special group with respect to age, sex, breed, or other host variables. In addition, the group may not be at risk for any biological reason but only as the result of some extrinsic host factor. An apparent host association may actually result from comparing noncomparable populations, or it may reflect only indirectly another variable that is more directly causal.

The following list may be useful as a check for some of the aforementioned possibilities:[9]

(1) Error of measurement. An example is use of a wrong denominator, such as using the total populations in comparing abortion rates in Jersey and Hereford herds, ignoring the fact that the sex ratios in herds may be quite different for these two breeds.

(2) Difference in more directly associated factors. In the example of disease in a mixed Guernsey and Holstein herd, it was found that different age distributions were much more important than a breed difference.

(3) Differences in environment. Anaplasmosis is more prevalent in Hereford cattle than in Holstein cattle in California, but probably because some Herefords are taken to a different environment (i.e., the mountains) in the summer and therefore are more exposed.

(4) Difference in bodily constitution. This possibility would include intrinsic host determinants such as those mentioned already in cases of hip dysplasia in German shepherds and ruptured intervertebral disks in dachshunds.

A final phenomenon that can be discussed with respect to host factors in the epidemiology of disease is herd immunity.

HERD IMMUNITY

There are several types of immunity in individual animals. Immunity may be innate, for example, the resistance of horses to foot-and-mouth disease virus or the relative resistances of Romney Marsh sheep to gastrointestinal parasites. Innate immunity is probably a complex phenomenon of physiological and genetic origin, but it has not yet been adequately explained. Acquired immunity, on the other hand, results from presence of protective antibodies that are either produced in the individual (active immunity) or transferred from another individual (passive immunity).

Populations also differ in immunity. Resistance in populations is called herd immunity and represents the *proportion* of resistant animals in the population. *Innate* herd immunity reflects a population that is resistant to an infection for some reason other than previous exposure of the present individuals of the herd or their immunization. Several examples of innate herd immunity are known for domestic animals; and, as mentioned earlier, lines of chickens with innate herd resistance to *Salmonella pullorum* have been developed by breeding. An example in wild animals is the increase in resistance to myxomatosis that occurred in European rabbit populations in Australia by a rapid process of selection in the years after introduction of the myxomatosis virus. Examples in man are the higher resistance to syphilis and tuberculosis in Caucasians compared to American Indians and Eskimos. Historic accounts also indicate that, when syphilis first appeared in Europe, it was a much more acute disease than now.

The mechanisms responsible for high levels of *innate* herd immunity are poorly understood. The most convincing body of evidence concerns malignant falciparum malaria in man. While some black African and several other human populations are highly resistant to falciparum malaria, in most other populations its occurrence results in high mortality. Several years ago it was observed that these innately resistant populations carry very high frequencies of one or more of three genetically determined metabolic polymorphisms of red blood cells (sickle cell trait, thalassemia, glucose-6-phosphate dehydrogenase (G-6-PD) deficiency). While these polymorphisms also are seen in other human populations, their frequencies are very low because their homozygous occurrences often are lethal and heterozygosity also confers a disadvantage to the carrier.

The explanation for herd immunity in falciparum malaria is that the altered red blood cells of the heterozygous carrier of each of these polymorphisms are resistant to invasion by or multiplication of *Plasmodium falciparum*; therefore, the trait carriers in these populations survive in malarious zones (survival of the fittest) with a consequent build-up of their frequencies in that population. In other words, falciparum malaria over a period of generations selects for sickle cell, thalassemia, and G-6-PD carriers that are resistant to malaria. If such an unusual selection pressure then is removed from the population, the frequencies of these otherwise undesirable genes would be expected to begin to decline. That this decline takes place can be seen when populations of Black Americans long removed from hyperendemic areas of falciparum malaria are compared with related populations of western Africans.

Acquired herd immunity results from development of protective antibodies in a population after its earlier natural exposure to the agent or to immunization. In the case of populations subjected to mass immunization, the level of herd immunity (proportion of population resistant) is the product of (1) the potential efficacy of the vaccine under controlled conditions, (2) the percentage of animals actually vaccinated (corrected for migrations—in and out—of unvaccinated and vaccinated individuals), (3) percentage of immunologically competent animals among vaccinates, (4) percentage of vaccine doses maintained under optimal conditions, and (5) percentage of vaccine doses administered properly.

To be effective, herd immunity does not require that *every* member of the population be protected. If the proportion of resistant animals is high, there is little risk that an occurrence of the disease will affect all susceptibles should the agent be introduced. The laws of probability for contact are such that only a few sporadic cases usually occur (Fig. 9–3). Thus, the probability of an epidemic depends not only on the proportion of resistant individuals in the herd but

also on the frequency of contacts, which reflects the "social distance" between the individuals.

The dynamics of most contact-transmitted infectious processes are such that, if 70 to 80% of the population can be made resistant, large-scale outbreaks fail to materialize (see Fig. 9–3). This fact explains why good protection is obtained by vaccinating even though less than 100% of susceptibles are vaccinated or by using *en masse* a vaccine that is not efficacious in all individuals.

Changes in level of herd immunity may occur when new susceptible individuals are introduced into a population. Such changes lead gradually to a lowering of herd immunity with resulting epidemics. This explains the two- to three-year cyclic patterns for both epidemic measles in human beings and canine distemper in dogs in cities. After an epidemic, herd immunity protects the population; but, as young are born, the proportion of susceptibles increases, and eventually there are enough for a new epidemic (see

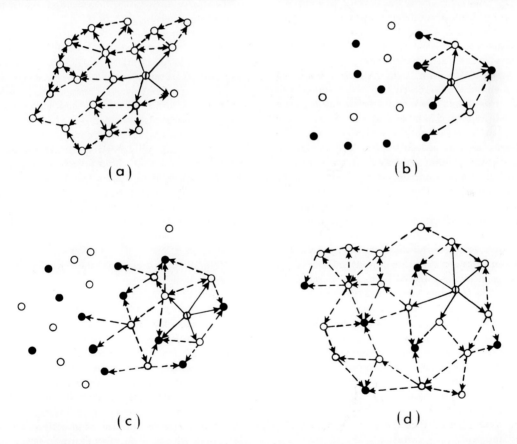

(a)

(b)

(c)

(d)

Fig. 9–3. Hypothetical spread in cattle herd of contact-transmitted infection such as rinderpest upon introduction of one infected animal (primary case). *A,* Nonimmune population (21 of 21 animals affected); *B,* recovered (immune) population after birth of one calf crop (3 of 19 animals affected); *C,* same herd after birth of second calf crop (7 of 27 animals affected): and *D,* same herd after birth of third calf crop (18 of 24 affected—all susceptible animals). Key: ⓘ primary case, ○ susceptible animal, ● immune animal, → and - -→ contacts (from Schwabe, C.W. 1969. *Veterinary Medicine and Human Health,* 2nd ed. The Williams & Wilkins Co., Baltimore).

Fig. 9–3). Panum made his classic observations on acquired herd immunity in human measles in the remote Faroe Islands. There, between 94 and 97% of the population contracted measles when it was reintroduced in the 19th century after an absence of 65 years. There were many deaths among the adult population. If a routine vaccination program is stopped, a population gradually loses its herd immunity. This situation, which is now taking place with respect to human smallpox in the United States, is potentially dangerous unless there remains the capacity to vaccinate enough individuals in a short time to reinstate a high level of herd protection.

Problem 9 relates some of these ideas about the influences of temporal, spatial, environmental, and host variables on disease frequency and patterns of occurrence by approaching an epidemic of disease involving a large number of animals.

Problem 9. A disease in dairy cattle in a township of 78 farms[10]

On May 21, 1960, several dairy farmers in the same township in a middle western state asked their veterinarians to see sick animals in their herds. Complaints in all cases were essentially the same: sudden loss of condition, dehydration, paleness of mucous membranes, increased rate of breathing, and dramatic drop in milk production. Temperatures were between 40 and 41°C. On one of the farms, a cow died after an illness of only several hours. Necropsy showed only an enlarged soft spleen of "blackberry jam" consistency. Other animals died subsequently. Additional necropsy findings were thin and watery blood and taut livers, which were mottled and very dark mahogany in color. A provisional diagnosis of some infectious disease was made, and penicillin therapy was started.

More cows on these farms became ill, and other farms began to report the same illness. Animals began to die on each of the affected farms. Local veterinarians, who were soon at a loss to control the spread of the epidemic, reported the episode to the state veterinarian and requested help in making a diagnosis and in coping with the disease.

You are the epidemiologist sent to investigate. You examine a number of sick animals and confirm the clinical picture. Should you necropsy additional animals? If so, indicate exactly what should be taken for laboratory analysis.

How should each of these types of specimens be prepared and sent? (The distance to the laboratory is 120 kilometers.)

With the information you have thus far, what are your provisional diagnoses?

Indicate fully what further background information you would desire.

While waiting for the laboratory reports, you and several colleagues begin to carry out intensive follow-up investigations on each of the 78 dairy farms in the township (Fig. 9–4). This investigation takes a considerable period of time to complete. You report a summary of your findings as follows:

(1) All animals were in pasture.

(2) The summer was a wet one, and streams and wells were full.

(3) Animals sometimes congregated along fences, and animals from different farms could come into contact in that way.

(4) Dairy husbandry was generally good and barn cleanliness excellent, although there were excessive accumulations of manure in most barnyards because of the unusually wet weather. Flies were common even though farmers were using approved insecticides properly.

(5) None of the farmers raised their replacements entirely; and all bought some replacements this particular year. Some farmers banded together to buy replacement heifers.

(6) Although there was no intermingling of animals between farms, except as noted, there was much traffic between farms in borrowed machinery and equipment. Human traffic between farms was frequent. Veterinarians were constantly at work in the community, and the township had just completed its area testing for brucellosis.

(7) No ticks were found on any of these animals.

This epidemic continued relatively unabated into November, and your field investigations continued. The first killing frost was on October 29.

Laboratory reports received on June 1 had confirmed that the index cases necropsied had died of *Anaplasma marginale* infections. Serological tests for anaplasmosis were carried out on the entire cattle population.

Table 9–6 summarizes the chronology of this epidemic by farm.

Complete this table.

Table 9–7 gives the age distribution of cattle by farm; Tables 9–8 and 9–9 (see also 9–3) summarize the epidemic by breed and age and include the serological data. Using appropriate graphic and cartographic methods, write a full epidemiological description of the chronology of this epidemic. Advance any appropriate hypotheses concerning its spread, mode of transmission of the agent, and possible changes in the frequencies or patterns of infection or severity of infection, with time and from farm to farm.

Interpret your data in terms of your hypotheses. In doing so, carry out all pertinent analyses for which you have data. For example, examine the question of breed susceptibility.

What other types of data, if any, might you want to complete this study?

Summarize your conclusions and suggest possible needs for future surveillance or some directed action.

When you have completed this problem, you may wish to review the discussion accompanying Tables 9–4 and 9–5.

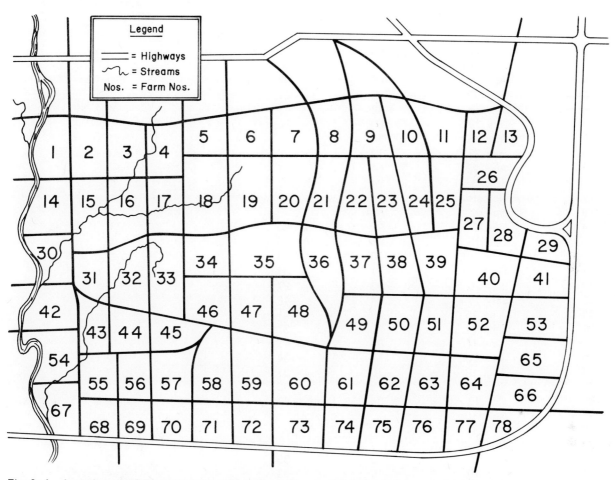

Fig. 9–4. Location of 78 farms in a township affected by a cattle disease (text Problem 9)

Table 9–6.   Chronology of Epidemic of Bovine Anaplasmosis Involving Township of 78 Farms in American Middle West in 1960

Farm no.	Date of first appearance of illness in herd	No. cattle at risk	No. cattle sick	A.R. (%)	No. cattle dead	Case fatality rate (%)
1	Nov. 4	78	34		5	
2	Oct. 12	43	16		2	
3	Sept. 15	71	30		3	
4	Aug. 18	86	32		7	
5	Aug. 17	65	31		3	
6	July 19	82	40		4	
7	July 20	80	36		3	
8	July 25	56	27		2	
9	July 25	79	36		4	
10	Aug. 20	64	31		4	
11	Sept. 16	84	39		3	
12	No cattle					
13	No cattle					
14	Nov. 7	93	40		26	
15	Oct. 16	86	39		2	
16	Sept. 19	70	34		2	
17	Sept. 20	71	34		3	
18	July 20	60	27		2	
19	July 19	94	46		6	
20	June 15	88	41		11	
21	June 11	79	37		10	
22	June 17	89	43		15	
23	July 20	77	34		2	
24	Aug. 18	70	31		2	
25	Sept. 15	75	33		4	
26	Oct. 12	84	41		6	
27	No cattle					
28	No cattle					
29	No cattle					
30	Nov. 5	85	39		3	
31	Oct. 16	79	39		4	
32	Sept. 14	84	48		2	
33	Aug. 15	89	44		4	
34	July 20	86	39		2	
35	June 12	85	41		15	
36	June 22	86	44		13	
37	May 21	82	38		24	
38	May 21	86	39		23	
39	June 10	81	37		18	
40	July 20	99	50		7	
41	Aug. 15	81	34		4	
42	Nov. 2	84	41		5	
43	Oct. 11	79	38		6	
44	Oct. 10	84	37		5	
45	Sept. 11	96	48		8	
46	Aug. 15	88	40		5	
47	July 20	93	41		7	
48	June 18	77	38		17	
49	May 21	75	35		20	
50	May 21	84	38		25	
51	June 9	92	41		23	

(Continued next page)

Table 9-6. (Continued)

Farm no.	Date of first appearance of illness in herd	No. cattle at risk	No. cattle sick	A.R. (%)	No. cattle dead	Case fatality rate (%)
52	June 14	84	37		21	
53	June 18	88	44		30	
54	June 12	82	36		24	
55	July 20	86	39		5	
56	July 24	94	46		6	
57	Aug. 21	95	43		6	
58	Sept. 17	82	36		3	
59	No cattle					
60	Sept. 20	93	43		5	
61	No cattle					
62	Nov. 8	88	40		5	
63	Oct. 11	89	43		26	
64	Sept. 10	87	40		6	
65	Aug. 15	77	35		6	
66	July 20	79	33		5	
67	June 20	91	44		23	
68	June 15	81	41		21	
69	June 13	84	38		19	
70	July 19	81	39		5	
71	July 22	71	27		3	
72	Aug. 19	89	38		6	
73	Aug. 21	77	33		4	
74	No cattle					
75	No cattle					
76	Sept. 20	56	19		2	
77	Sept. 20	76	33		5	
78	No cattle					
Total		5529	2548		607	

Host Determinants of Diseases

Table 9-7.   Age Distribution of Animals in Epidemic of Bovine Anaplasmosis Involving Township of 78 Farms in American Middle West in 1960

Farm No.	Age (in years)										Total
	<0,5	1.5	2.5	3.5	4.5	5.5	6.5	7.5	8.5	>8.5	
1	8	10	8	12	18	8	5	4	5	—	78
2	3	5	4	7	10	8	2	1	3	—	43
3	6	8	8	10	11	8	7	6	5	2	71
4	5	10	11	12	12	14	10	4	4	4	86
5	8	6	10	8	7	5	7	6	5	3	65
6	10	12	12	10	9	9	8	6	3	3	82
7	7	7	10	9	10	12	11	9	5	—	80
8	3	6	5	7	9	12	8	3	2	1	56
9	9	8	8	10	11	10	12	5	4	2	79
10	6	6	7	9	9	8	8	7	3	1	64
11	8	5	13	13	12	11	10	8	3	1	84
12	No cattle										
13	No cattle										
14	4	5	9	9	12	14	11	9	10	10	93
15	9	8	9	13	11	12	10	6	6	2	86
16	7	6	12	9	11	10	7	4	4	—	70
17	8	8	9	10	9	10	8	5	3	1	71
18	4	7	9	12	11	8	6	3	—	—	60
19	12	13	11	10	11	12	9	7	5	4	94
20	11	9	10	12	14	10	8	7	3	4	88
21	9	7	14	10	10	9	10	6	3	1	79
22	5	11	10	12	14	12	10	7	5	3	89
23	7	8	13	11	12	9	9	5	3	—	77
24	8	6	11	10	11	7	7	5	5	—	70
25	10	6	12	11	10	8	7	6	3	2	75
26	9	8	10	12	12	11	9	7	5	1	84
27	No cattle										
28	No cattle										
29	No cattle										
30	6	7	10	11	14	12	10	8	4	3	85
31	7	6	11	10	12	12	8	10	3	—	79
32	4	9	11	11	12	10	9	10	6	2	84
33	8	6	13	12	9	8	10	11	8	4	89
34	7	8	12	10	11	14	10	6	4	4	86
35	9	6	10	12	11	13	9	7	5	3	85
36	10	7	13	13	9	11	10	8	5	—	86
37	9	6	12	12	9	10	10	6	5	3	82
38	6	7	9	12	13	9	11	9	6	4	86
39	9	7	13	9	10	6	9	10	6	2	81
40	5	11	10	12	14	13	12	10	7	5	99
41	7	8	13	11	12	9	10	6	3	2	81
42	10	9	11	14	12	8	9	5	4	2	84
43	9	8	8	10	11	10	12	5	4	2	79
44	8	5	13	13	12	11	10	8	3	1	84
45	14	13	11	12	10	9	9	9	5	4	96
46	11	9	10	12	14	10	8	7	3	4	88
47	10	10	9	11	14	12	9	9	5	4	93
48	7	8	13	11	12	9	9	5	3	—	77
49	10	6	11	10	11	7	7	5	5	3	75
50	7	7	10	9	10	12	11	9	5	4	84
51	12	13	11	10	11	12	9	7	5	2	92
52	10	6	12	11	10	8	8	7	7	5	84

Table 9–7. (Continued)

Farm No.	<0.5	1.5	2.5	3.5	4.5	5.5	6.5	7.5	8.5	>8.5	Total
53	4	9	11	12	10	9	10	11	8	4	88
54	9	6	12	12	9	10	10	6	5	3	82
55	10	9	11	14	12	8	9	7	4	2	86
56	11	9	10	12	14	10	9	8	8	3	94
57	12	13	11	10	11	12	9	7	5	5	95
58	7	8	13	11	12	9	10	6	3	3	82
59	No cattle										
60	11	11	8	12	9	10	9	10	8	5	93
61	No cattle										
62	11	8	11	13	10	9	9	8	7	2	88
63	3	6	7	8	10	9	10	12	12	12	89
64	9	11	12	10	11	9	9	6	5	5	87
65	12	13	11	10	11	8	6	3	3	—	77
66	9	8	8	10	11	10	12	5	4	2	79
67	10	10	9	11	14	9	10	8	7	3	91
68	9	7	14	11	10	9	10	6	3	2	81
69	11	9	10	12	12	9	8	7	3	3	84
70	10	8	12	11	10	8	7	7	3	5	81
71	8	8	9	10	9	10	8	5	3	1	71
72	12	11	12	10	11	8	8	7	5	5	89
73	10	11	9	11	11	7	9	5	4	—	77
74	No cattle										
75	No cattle										
76	7	9	7	7	6	6	5	5	3	1	56
77	11	11	10	8	9	7	6	7	5	2	76
78	No cattle										
Total	567	562	708	731	751	658	601	459	316	176	5529

Table 9–8. Summary of Data by Breed and Age in Epidemic of Bovine Anaplasmosis in American Middle West in 1960 (see Table 9–3)

	<0.5	1.5	2.5	3.5	Age (in years) 4.5	5.5	6.5	7.5	8.5	>8.5	Total
Guernsey cattle A.R. (%)	0	14.0	37.5	46.8	52.5	57.1	58.1	59.8	74.8	75.0	49.1
Holstein cattle A.R. (%)	0	19.6	41.2	48.5	53.6	59.2	61.0	62.0	76.1	77.9	45.2
Guernsey cattle case fatality rate (%)	0	0	4.2	5.6	15.1	23.6	38.9	42.1	40.4	45.7	27.8
Holstein cattle case fatality rate (%)	0	2.2	4.2	6.1	15.5	23.6	39.9	41.3	40.7	45.3	22.6
No. Guernsey cattle survivors	91	107	126	150	128	135	96	95	83	71	1082
No. Guernsey cattle reactors to complement fixation test	8	41	60	77	79	97	81	84	78	71	676
Guernsey cattle complement fixation reactor rate (%)	8.8	38.3	47.6	51.3	61.7	71.9	84.4	88.4	94.0	100	62.5
No. Holstein cattle survivors	476	453	570	560	561	432	361	247	136	44	3840
No. Holstein cattle reactors to complement fixation test	49	191	293	307	358	313	311	220	129	44	2215
Holstein cattle complement fixation reactor rate (%)	10.3	42.2	51.4	54.8	63.8	72.5	86.1	89.1	94.9	100	57.7

Table 9–9. Summary of Morbidity, Mortality, and Test Reaction Data by Age in Epidemic of Bovine Anaplasmosis in American Middle West in 1960

| | Age (in years) | | | | | | | | | | Total |
	<0.5	1.5	2.5	3.5	4.5	5.5	6.5	7.5	8.5	>8.5	
No. cattle at beginning of epidemic	567	562	708	731	751	658	601	459	316	176	5529
No. cattle sick (including those which died)	0	104	287	352	401	386	363	282	239	134	2548
Age specific A.R. (%)	0	18.5	40.5	48.1	53.4	58.7	60.4	61.4	75.6	76.1	48.4
No. cattle dead	0	2	12	21	62	91	144	117	97	61	607
Age specific case fatality rate (%)	0	1.9	4.2	6.0	15.5	23.6	39.7	41.5	40.6	45.5	23.8
Survivor cattle	567	560	696	710	689	567	457	342	219	115	4922
Reactors (among survivors) to complement fixation test	57	232	353	384	437	410	392	304	207	115	2891
Age specific complement fixation reaction rate (%)	10.1	41.4	50.7	54.1	63.4	72.3	85.8	88.9	94.5	100.0	58.6

Chapter 10

SPECIFIC AGENTS AS DETERMINANTS OF DISEASES

INFECTIOUS agents have received much attention as determinants of diseases; and epidemiology is still considered by some people to be synonymous with the study of transmission, survival, and actions of infectious agents. There are several reasons for this attitude, the most important being the series of remarkable discoveries in the microbiological sciences—from their beginnings about 100 years ago up until the present day. The apparent ease with which microbiologists were able to isolate and incriminate a large number of living agents associated with diseases resulted in medicine's preponderant emphasis on *the* agent. Then, Robert Koch formulated his famous postulates, an approach to "proving" such causal associations.

At the same time, the attractive hypothesis of a specific agent for each disease received reinforcement through other important discoveries, by physiologists and biochemists, of distinct chemical agents of disease that fulfilled etiological roles similar to those of the microbes. The interest was on the pathogenesis of disease more than on the *occurrence* of disease or on the causal web that determines the patterns of disease occurrence in populations. In other words, epidemiology was almost totally neglected.

IMMEDIATE AND REMOTE DETERMINANTS

It is interesting that, even during the early period of emphasis upon specific disease agents, John Snow was able to establish the mode of transmission of human cholera and the method for its control by purely epidemiological means some 30 years before Robert Koch identified *Vibrio cholerae* as its agent. Similarly, Daniel E. Salmon succeeded in *eradicating* contagious bovine pleuropneumonia from the United States several years before Edmond Nocard and Emile Roux discovered its mycoplasmal agent! These unconventional achievements were harbingers of others.

First, consider Koch's postulates for establishing the causal relationship of an infectious agent and a disease.

(1) The agent must be shown to be present in every case of the disease through its isolation as a pure culture.

(2) The agent must not be found in cases of other diseases.

(3) The agent must be capable of reproducing the disease in experimental animals.

(4) The agent must be recovered from the host in which the experimental disease was produced.

Although Koch's postulates remain useful guidelines for infectious disease studies, they are increasingly questionable ones. Considering all types of host response to infection, one finds, for example, that infections with saprophytic mycobacteria may mimic the response of the host to *Mycobacterium tuberculosis*. It is a common phenomenon for essentially the same clinical disease to be associated with more than one agent; psittacosis and pasteurellosis in birds, as another example, may result in almost identical clinical manifestations. Postulate one, thus, is etiologically unsatisfactory in that it assumes that each agent causes clinically distinct manifestations. Koch's postulates also disregard mixed infections and such relatively common phenomena as healthy carriers. The third postulate has in some cases been fulfilled only by using unusual methods of transmission, such as intracerebral injection—a process that could not occur in natural disease transmission. In some other instances, the disease has been reproduced only with the aid of a predisposing factor, such as infection with another agent or some other insult to the host.

Clearly, Koch's postulates exclude many commonly occurring situations with respect to infections. Just when some of these facts were becoming evident to microbiologists and epidemiologists, pathologists and clinicians were beginning to find it increasingly necessary to employ such expressions as predisposing causes, secondary causes, contributing causes, and similar hedging terms in referring to the etiologies of many other diseases and to reasons for death. Thus, the dominant hypothesis in medicine for virtually all of its most creative century was the overly simplistic one of *the* specific agent as *the* cause of each and every disease.

Although most students of diseases now see the causes or determinants of diseases in more complex terms—in a more epidemiological perspective—the "one agent-one disease" idea still predominates in the views not only of the public, but also of many medical practitioners. Many veterinarians in particular are further guilty of still *assuming* not only that virtually every newly disclosed disease condition has *an* agent, but also that it is infectious!

In fact, while an agent may be a living parasite, it certainly also may be a toxic substance, a physical force, or any identifiable factor that alone or in combination can cause an impact on a host with an effect or response recognizable as disease. Substances that cause disease when absent, such as vitamins and essential minerals, also are considered agents. To reiterate, the epidemiological conception of disease causality is one of multiple, interacting determinants, prominent among which are a great variety of living and nonliving elements in the host's environment, which are designated as *agents*.

What must be visualized clearly are the distinctions between immediate and remote causes of disease, in other words, direct versus indirect causes. One difficulty in visualizing such sequences of forces or variables and their relationships to one another, and the disease—the web of causation—is to decide how far one wants to or can go in either direction.

For example, clostridia and *Diphyllobothrium* spp. commonly are regarded as agents, or causes, of diseases. In the first case, however, clostridial spores may be present in an animal's tissues when no disease occurs. The probability of presence of the spores in the animal may be related in turn to more or less definite environmental or husbandry variables. Something, like migrating *Fasciola* or a surgeon or an infarct, must create anaerobic conditions for vegetative clostridia to arise in the tissues and multiply. Then, given suitable circumstances, they produce metabolic end products that are toxic to the host. These toxins act by inducing chemical lesions that lead to the physical lesions, signs, and symptoms recognized as the disease. Thus, clostridial agents are not as immediate, or as remote, a cause of some specific diseases as they might be.

Similarly, man or dog acquires *Diphyllobothrium* spp. by eating raw fish, a circumstance that might have identifiable and preventable causes. The worm in turn may or may not deprive its host of a meaningfully large part of its dietary vitamin B_{12}. Whether it does may depend on its location in the host's gut, which may be influenced by other dietary factors. Deficiency of B_{12} affects certain enzyme systems; and specific chemical, then physical, changes occur. Is the cause and/or agent of the most serious form of diphyllobothriasis, vitamin B_{12} (in a negative sense), the cestode, the act of eating raw fish, the circumstances affecting that act (e.g., occupation) or those related to the eater (e.g., age, sex, nationality), or something else? Epidemiologists are interested in *every* stage and link in these webs of causation,

particularly the stage or linkage most amenable to attack.

PROPERTIES OF LIVING AGENTS

Diseases caused by invading living agents are called infectious and, sometimes, communicable or contagious. Distinction between these terms and other remarks about the characteristics of infections are presented in Chapter 2. The properties of living agents, such as their size, structure, metabolism, nutritional requirements, and ability to grow or survive freely in the environment, all vary enormously. While these characteristics are of epidemiological importance, they are dealt with properly in textbooks on microbiology. Other properties of parasites—of living agents—related to their action in the host are described by the following terms.

Infectivity has reference to an agent's ability to lodge itself in a host. *Pathogenicity* refers to an agent's ability to induce disease. *Virulence* is sometimes used synonymously with pathogenicity; but others use it in referring to the property of an agent that determines the severity of a resulting infection as measured by its case fatality rate or the extent of permanent host debilitation.

As mentioned in Chapter 2, *latency* of an infection refers to the ability of an agent to remain quiescent in a host and, therefore, difficult to detect. It is a term that implies, however, a potential for activity. When an agent is readily detectable, that is, being shed by secretions or excretions of the host, or can be recovered or identified from blood or tissues, the infection is said to be *patent*. The *prepatent period* of the agent usually is shorter than the *incubation period* of the disease, which is the time from infection to onset of observable signs and symptoms of illness. Sometimes, however, marked disease may occur before an infection becomes patent, as, for example, in acute hookworm disease in puppies.

The time period during which an infected host can transmit the infection to other susceptible hosts is called the *period of communicability*. During this period direct shedding takes place, or the agent can be transmitted by vectors. The period of communicability may have little relationship to the duration of the disease. Again, the term *carrier* generally is used to designate the individual infected host that can communicate the infection in the absence of manifest disease. The different varieties of carriers are mentioned in Chapter 2. The *antigenicity* or *immunogenicity* of an agent is its ability to induce production of antibodies or immunity in the host.

AGENT INTERACTIONS

As indicated in the brief discussion of Koch's postulates, some diseases occur only as a result of mixed infections. Chapter 9 mentions the interaction of liver flukes and clostridia in black disease, and the interaction of viruses and bacteria in shipping fever. Examples also include those in which an infectious agent depends on the presence of another, harmless microorganism. Thus, *Entamoeba histolytica* in man or the dog apparently requires the presence of intestinal bacteria in order to cause an intestinal amebic infection. These interactions between living organisms also are examples of multiple causality of disease, a concept fundamental to epidemiology (see Chapter 2). However, as stressed earlier, multiple causality also may involve interactions of agents with important host factors. Thus, such ubiquitous nonhost-specific agents as salmonellae, *Coxiella burnetii*, *Coccidioides immitis*, and *Toxoplasma gondii* sometimes produce disease, sometimes do not; and there is the increasingly observed phenomenon that microorganisms not ordinarily considered pathogenic agents sometimes are involved in disease processes as so-called opportunistic pathogens.

AGENT CHANGE

The recognized ability of some living agents of disease to alter their properties by recombination and/or mutation has important epidemiological implications. There is great variation in the genetic stability of different living agents. Influenza virus provides an instructive and well-documented example. The human influenza pandemic that began in 1918 was caused by a strain A virus that later was shown to be closely related to swine influenza virus strain 15. During human epidemics between 1918 and 1957, different virus strains also related to these two were recorded. Then a distinctly different virus, A2, appeared in China in 1957 and caused another human pandemic. So-called Hong Kong virus first appeared in 1968; and a further pandemic occurred. The minor changes in virus, such as those that occurred between 1918 and 1957, were referred to as antigenic *drift*; the major agent changes, such as the ones in 1957 and 1968, as antigenic *shift*. Major agent changes, such as the latter, could result from mutation of virus or virus recombination. In either case, widespread infection and disease could result in spite of the common presence of antibodies (i.e., herd immunity) to earlier virus strains in the populations of potential hosts.

In the instance of influenza in man and most other susceptible animals, antigenic shift and the appearance of previously unknown virus strains result from virus recombination. The resulting viruses are new in the sense that they represent previously unknown hemagglutinating (H) and/or neuraminidase (N) antigens or some new combination of previously known antigens. These changes can arise by hybridization or recombination of two influenza viruses, for example, an H_1N_1 virus and an H_2N_2 virus recombining to yield also H_1N_2 or H_2N_1. There is suggestive evidence, for example, that human Hong Kong virus arose as a recombinant of an avian influenza virus and the previously existing human so-called Asian virus. Evidence for this hypothesis includes a close resemblance in amino acid sequences between the human Hong Kong virus and a known avian virus. Another important change in an agent is represented by the ability of enteric bacteria to transfer to other enteric bacteria certain extrachromosomal genes, plasmids, that result in multiple drug resistance.

INFECTIONS WITHOUT AGENTS AND AGENTS WITHOUT DISEASES

There are diseases of an infectious nature for which no agent has been identified. Human cholera is a classic example of an infectious disease that was well described epidemiologically long before its agent was detected. "Cat-scratch" fever is another such disease that has been well documented epidemiologically, but still has no recognized agent.

On the other hand, a number of virus strains that have been isolated can infect invertebrates as well as vertebrates but have not been shown to produce disease in any species of host. Such viruses have been called "orphan" viruses. Some cytopathogenic orphan viruses, such as ECHO viruses, have been isolated repeatedly in tissue culture from man and other animal species in absence of disease. This repeated isolation without disease also has been the case for certain arboviruses and adenoviruses. Whether such isolates represent opportunistic pathogens that cause disease only under specific circumstances is still, in many instances, unknown.

This latter phenomenon is related to the question of so-called new diseases. New diseases can occur when truly new agents show up in a population's environment; for example, highly chlorinated naphthalenes gave rise to hyperkeratosis in cattle (see Chapter 6), but it seems doubtful that many radically new living agents would suddenly appear. Living agents do change, as explained for influenza virus; but the agent changes generally are minor, and the disease (i.e., its signs, symptoms) usually remains essentially the same despite the antigenic pattern change. Some other diseases appear to be new in the sense that they show up in a new host or in a new area, such as African horse sickness in southwest Asia, African swine fever in Europe, or bluetongue in European-type sheep. In most of those instances, the agent was already present subclinically in its maintenance host or was endemic to another area. Chapter 4 provides examples of new diseases that result from the escape of an agent from its usual ecological niche.

Of similar interest is the question of disappearing diseases. There is no proof that an animal disease agent has ever completely disappeared globally. It was believed for a long time that vesicular exanthema virus had been completely eradicated; but what is apparently this same virus has been isolated recently from marine mammals on the California coast.

Some of the concepts presented in this chapter can be strengthened by considering lessons about infections learned from the unusual circumstance of the release of myxoma virus in Australia as a biological control measure.

Problem 10. Myxomatosis in Australia

Myxoma virus was the second animal virus discovered. It was first reported by Sanarelli in 1898 as the cause of an explosive epidemic in a laboratory colony of European rabbits (*Oryctolagus*) housed in the Institute of Hygiene in Montevideo. Subsequently, it was found to occur endemically in the South American wild rabbit, *Sylvilagus*. In contrast to infections of *Oryctolagus* with "wild" virus, which were 100% fatal, mortality in *Sylvilagus* was almost entirely absent.

How might you explain this difference in case fatality rates in these two genera of rabbits?

In 1950, myxoma virus was deliberately introduced into South Australia as a biological control measure against the European rabbit pest *Oryctolagus*. It was transmitted mechanically by biting insect vectors, particularly by mosquitoes. A typical census of rabbits in one part of the epidemic area of Australia following the 1950-51 release of virus showed 4455 dead rabbits and five live rabbits. In the 1951-52 epidemic, a similar census over a larger part of the epidemic area yielded 2964 dead rabbits and 258 live rabbits. This trend continued into 1952-53 and thereafter. Serological studies indicated that exposure to virus had been 100% in these areas in each of these years, and that the living rabbits observed had recovered from infection.[1]

Use the data from these censuses to calculate the case fatality rates for each year.

Considering the concepts discussed in this chapter, as well as in Chapter 9, what explanations would you offer for this rate trend?

If you were an epidemiologist involved in this biological control program, how might you experimentally test these possible explanations? Be specific about the epidemiological experiments you would devise.

NONLIVING DISEASE AGENTS

Chemical agents are other well-known determinants of diseases in animals. Some of these agents occur naturally, such as poisons produced by plants or animals (e.g., snakes, insects), while others are manmade or are introduced into a population's environment by man. Examples of these latter are mercury compounds used as fungicides in grain. These particular agents have caused a number of outbreaks of poisoning in domestic animals—and, via their meat, in human beings—in the last few years.

Classic examples of the actions of chemical agents are the instances of livestock deaths on two occasions of air pollution in the Smithfield Market, London (see Chapter 2). Many other chemicals in our environment affect animals. Beside the direct harm that they may suffer in that way, animals may serve as monitors of environmental pollution in general and of potential hazards to man. Chapter 14 describes a proposal for the design of such monitoring systems.

Physical agents such as heat and cold, humidity, sunlight, and traumatic abuse are all known to affect animals; and the indirect or interacting effects of such agents may be far more extensive than suspected. Such associations are just beginning to be identified. For example, apparently normal transport conditions may elicit shipping fever in some cattle. Neonatal calf mortality may be strongly associated with the weather conditions on the calf's day of birth. Transport by truck as compared to transport by railroad, and transport on cool, rainy days compared to transport on dry days, both have been shown to relate significantly to the number of food-poisoning *C. perfringens* in the cecal content of beef cattle in Brazil.[2] The effect of physical agents is, in many cases, complex and indirect; for example, they may influence animals' physiology or behavior. For these reasons, they are not easily differentiated from certain host or environmental factors.

Chapter 11

IDENTIFICATION OF DISEASE DETERMINANTS: USE OF CASE-CONTROL STUDIES

THIS chapter and the next are concerned with alternative approaches to the identification and further study of possible determinants of observed frequencies of diseases or other epidemiologically interesting events. The discussion first elaborates on differences between association and cause, a subject introduced in Chapter 2.

SIGNIFICANCE AND CAUSE

A statistically significant association between a variable and a disease may represent any of several biological possibilities, not all of them causal. One possibility is that a direct causal relationship does exist; that is, the presence or level of some factor A relates directly to the presence or level of disease B. An alternative, but still causal relationship, is the indirect one; namely, factor A relates in one of these ways to factor A', which relates directly to disease B. Indirect causal relationships may be even more remote and involve other intermediate factors, e.g., A'' and A'''.

On the other hand, a statistically significant association can occur between a variable A and the presence or frequency of a disease B, and not even indirectly reflect a causal relationship. Instead, the association might occur simply because both the variable A and the disease B are related in some way to a third factor C, which may or may not be causal and which is not being controlled or corrected for in the analysis. For example, in Problem 2 in Chapter 3, decreased hatchability in chicks was caused by an erratically functioning heat source being used to eliminate mycoplasmas from fertile eggs. Other noncausal variables also were statistically associated with that disease because they represented other maneuvers performed (or not performed) on many of the same eggs that had received heat treatment, or on the hens from which these eggs came. Therefore, *to be considered epidemiologically causal, a statistically valid association should make biological sense* and not be explainable by such other relationships.

The preceding distinctions are very important ones because many epidemiological studies yield indirectly causal associations, either because a more directly causal explanation, such as some specific factor or agent, has not been suggested or because this more directly causal factor is difficult to study epidemiologically. Moreover, an indirect determinant of disease sometimes may be manipulated to control a disease more readily than a more direct determinant can. For example, 19th century veterinarians learned that a then well-defined cattle disease, bovine pleuropneumonia, would not occur in healthy cattle unless they came into very close *contact with an existing case* of the disease. That contact was its cause—bovine pleuropneumonia is contagious. Making use of that indirect type of causal information only, Daniel E. Salmon succeeded in eradicating bovine pleuropneumonia from the United States by making it improbable for such an association to take place. It was several years later that Nocard and Roux discovered the directly causal microorganism, the first known mycoplasma, and only comparatively recently have there been alternative means available to combat bovine pleuropneumonia and related diseases via their agents.

Similarly, Theobald Smith's discovery that the hemoprotozoan *Babesia bigemina* was the *direct* cause of Texas fever of cattle in the United States contributed little to eradication of that disease from this country. Eradication could have been accomplished just as readily without such knowledge because there were then no means to affect *Babesia* directly by chemotherapy or to prevent infection with it by immunization. Rather, Frederick Kilborne's and Cooper Curtice's epidemiological discovery of the *indirectly* causal association of the tick *Boophilus annulatus* with Texas fever was the event which permitted that disease to be controlled and eventually eradicated from large cattle populations. Although the act of cigarette smoking *per se* bears a similar indirect relationship to lung cancer in man, this epidemiological discovery offered the first means to combat that important disease, even in the absence of knowledge of any more directly causal factor. Subsequently, that discovery stimulated research on specific carcinogens in cigarette smoke.

These examples show that there are different types of indirect association between factors and diseases. Use of certain vaccines was not part of the web of causation of decreased egg hatchability in Problem 2. However, the tick is a part of the web of causation of Texas fever, and only a slightly more remote cause of that disease than is its protozoal agent. Moreover, it would be almost impossible to show that *Babesia*, independent of ticks, could function as a determinant in the nature of Texas fever.

A statistical test such as χ^2 may reflect merely the probability that an observed association has arisen by chance, but show nothing about its causal or noncausal nature or its medical importance. Applying other statistical tests such as relative risk gives an indication of the magnitude or strength of a demonstrated association, while calculating an attributable risk may show the medical importance of an association, if it is a causal one. Calculation of second stage relative risks is one way to help decide in certain situations whether an observed association is causal. Other kinds of evidence also may help in making logical judgments on this important question. Some of these were mentioned in Chapter 2. Here, careful planning of a study, identifying and minimizing as many likely biases as possible, is of utmost importance (see also Chapter 5).

APPROACHES TO STUDY OF HYPOTHESIZED CAUSES OF DISEASE

To examine a possible association between an hypothesized determinant of a disease and the disease's frequency, one can visualize three situations in which this association might be demonstrated.

In the first situation, there is a population of animals; into one randomly formed subgroup or cohort of these animals, the hypothesized determinant is deliberately *introduced*. Another cohort is kept free of the hypothesized determinant. Both cohorts are followed up until there is a decision on

whether a statistically significant difference exists in the incidence of the disease between the two groups.

In a second situation, in a population of animals it is *observed* that some individuals possess the determinant and some do not, and that these two cohorts subsequently experience a statistically significant difference in incidence of the disease.

Finally, in a third situation, diseased and nondiseased individuals in an animal population are observed, and it is noted that the prevalence of an hypothesized determinant differs significantly between these two groups.

Certainly, these three expressions of an association are not identical. The initial two are population-based situations that are being followed *prospectively*, while in the third the already diseased (and disease-free) animals are first examined and then observed *retrospectively* to learn which in each group possess the hypothesized disease determinant.

The question is whether a *causal* relationship exists between this hypothesized determinant and the disease; but only in the first situation, which is a direct experiment, can one refer confidently, in the results, to a causal association. Frequently, direct experiments such as those of Kilborne on Texas fever may be difficult or impossible to carry out. One then must resort to one or both of the observational alternatives, as did John Snow. The first of these alternatives (the second situation mentioned), together with direct experiments, often are called *cohort studies*, while the latter observational type (the third situation mentioned) is called a *case-control* study (Fig. 11-1). Prospective studies start with groups (cohorts) of animals with and without the factor and follow them along to the event (e.g., sickness or death). Retrospective studies usually begin with a group of preexisting cases, then involve selecting a suitable control group of animals and determining which in each group have the factor.

As illustrated well by Frederick Kilborne's and Cooper Curtice's work on ticks and piroplasmosis, veterinarians long ago had developed the now-familiar prospective approach to epidemiological problems of animal disease. At the level of experi-

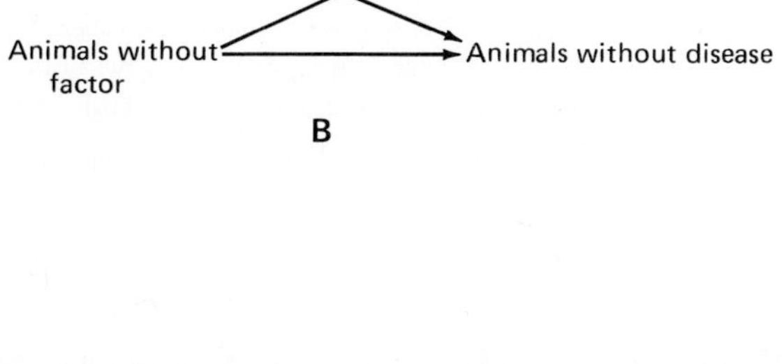

A

B

Fig. 11-1. *A*, Retrospective case-control approach to epidemiological problems. *B*, Prospective cohort approach to epidemiological problems.

mental and "clinical" trials, this prospective strategy also has provided the foundation for comparative medical research. Because a direct experimental approach to medical unknowns is generally impossible to apply to human subjects, the field of experimental medicine has always been largely one of prospective cohort trials and experiments in animal, or veterinary, medicine.

What are new as investigative tools to many veterinarians, however, are the various retrospective approaches that have been developing recently for epidemiological research. Even given the possibilities inherent in veterinary medicine for the direct prospective experiment, difficulties are often encountered in hypothesizing candidate determinants for complex diseases, or in studying multiple, interacting determinants. These problems strongly recommend an initial retrospective approach to many animal disease problems. Added to these considerations are such practical factors as time and the often-prohibitive costs of prospective studies on adequately sized populations of animals.

ADVANTAGES AND DISADVANTAGES OF CASE-CONTROL VERSUS COHORT STUDIES

The case-control type study offers several advantages to the investigator:

(1) Since it makes use of preexisting data, it is relatively inexpensive to perform. This is a distinct advantage with diseases that are relatively rare, such as various types of cancer, where the cohorts required for prospective study would be very large.

(2) For the reason just mentioned, it can be performed quickly.

(3) Both of these facts make it particularly useful for the initial testing of hypotheses regarding possible disease determinants.

(4) It requires smaller numbers of subjects than a prospective study, and, therefore, is suitable for studying rare diseases.

The principal disadvantages of the case-control study are:

(1) Questions arise as to the representativeness of the case and the control, or comparison, groups. It is frequently impossible to know whether there have been some systematic losses among case or comparison groups, thereby leading to a sampling bias.

(2) Much greater difficulty arises in distinguishing between direct cause and effect associations and associations that are indirectly caused or that result from common causes or some other mechanism.

(3) Information may be incomplete (related to (1)).

(4) Unless it makes use of the entire population of sick and well animals, it yields only relative risk estimates that are not usable for the study of disease incidence.

Particularly important is that in situations of diseases of low incidence, the case-control approach may be the *only* study approach feasible. For example, say that carcinoma of the eye in a population of grade Hereford cattle with pigmented eyelids occurred with a frequency of 10/100,000 and among similar cattle with nonpigmented eyelids at a frequency of 100/100,000. A case-control study with 100 cases of ocular carcinoma and 100 controls would probably reveal a statistically significant increased risk. On the other hand, follow-up cohorts of 4000 cattle with pigmented eyelids and 4000 with nonpigmented eyelids would fail to detect a significant difference. Problem 11 verifies this important point.

Problem 11. Population size for prospective and retrospective studies

Consider the following diagram for a cohort-study framework, using the data given on bovine ocular carcinoma.

	Cases	Noncases	
Pigmented eyelids	.0001n	.9999n	n
Nonpigmented eyelids	.0010n	.9990n	n
	0.0011n	1.9989n	2n

Under the previous assumptions of n randomly selected cattle with pigmented eyelids, you would expect $0.0001n$ with cancer eye; and of n with nonpigmented eyelids, you expect $0.0010n$ with cancer eye.

Now use chi-square, say at the 1% level of significance, to calculate n for a prospective (cohort) study. Carry out this calculation.

Suppose you reverse your thinking, and consider cattle having cancer eye. It is apparent from the assumptions (including implicitly an assumption that the prevalence of pigmentation in eyelids of cattle is 50%) and from the first part of this problem that about 10 of 11 cattle with cancer eye should have nonpigmented eyelids, and among cattle without cancer eye about half should have nonpigmented eyelids. From this, you can diagram the plan for a case-control study, as follows.

	Cases	Controls	
Pigmented eyelids	.0909n	.5002n	0.5911n
Nonpigmented eyelids	.9091n	.4998n	1.4089n
	n	n	2n

Assuming there has been no selection bias against survivorship in either cases or controls, how many cattle would you need in a case-control study to detect a difference that you could call significant, say, at 1%?[1]

The preceding examples illustrate that, in planning a cohort study, we aim at equal numbers of individuals with or without the attribute, and we must have prior knowledge (assumption) about the expected incidence of disease in the two groups in order to design the study.

The general design can be expressed as in the following diagram

	Cases	Non-cases	
Attribute absent	aN	(1–a)N	N
Attribute present	bN	(1–b)N	N
	(a+b)N	(2–a–b)N	2N

In this example, a = 0.0001 and b = 0.001.

In planning a case-control study, we aim at equal numbers of cases and non-cases (controls) and we must have prior knowledge (assumption) about the proportion in each group that has the attribute.

The general design becomes

	Cases	Controls	
Attribute absent	aN	bN	(a+b)N
Attribute present	(1–a)N	(1–b)N	(2–a–b)N
	N	N	2N

In this example, a = 0.909 and b = 0.5002.

Study of multiple determinants

Another considerable advantage of the retrospective approach is the ability to quickly and simultaneously examine a number of possible disease determinants.[2] This procedure is particularly useful to identify candidate determinants of importance and to expose *leads for fuller investigation*. Some of the multivariate analytical methods that may be suitable for such a study are introduced in Chapter 13.

Problem of representative nature of data

One major difficulty with retrospective studies is their tendency to confound factors associated with *becoming a diseased or disease-free animal*, a case or control, with factors associated with the presence or absence of a disease. This problem is particularly apparent when cases and controls are derived from hospital, diagnostic laboratory, or similar populations where such factors as admission and referral policies

and economic status of animal owners may influence the availability of either or both classes of subjects. The influence of such confounding factors is lessened where retrospective studies are carried out in specific herd populations or in similar relatively controlled population groups.

For chronic diseases in which prevalence data (existing cases) are used, other confounding differences are introduced. These differences are associated with a disease's duration and are unrelated to increased or decreased risk of acquiring the disease. Incidence data (newly diagnosed cases), therefore, generally are preferable for retrospective studies.

Because of these problems of representativeness of the groups being compared, epidemiologists must interpret the results of case-control studies conservatively; that is, they must require not only statistically significant associations between disease frequency and the alleged disease determinant, but also medically *important* differences in the frequency of disease occurrence. As mentioned earlier, relative risk and attributable risk calculations and repetitions of studies in other settings can help in deciding whether such frequency differences are medically important. Again, the real problem in interpretation of a study's results often lies in its design (Chapter 5).

SELECTION OF COMPARISON GROUPS FOR CASE-CONTROL STUDIES

Choice of the comparison group is more difficult than choice of the case group in retrospective studies. Not only must each of the cases and controls selected be as representative as possible of the cases and unaffected animals in the general population at risk, but also it is important to case-control studies *that the means for recording responses from or otherwise observing each group be of similar quality*. This latter consideration has been discussed already in Chapter 5. These problems are most evident when using hospital, diagnostic laboratory, or similar data as the source of cases.

For hospital studies, for example, a comparison sample drawn from the "community" population may be more representative of that universe than a group of "hospital controls." On the other hand, response data obtainable for controls selected from the hospital environment usually are of the same quality as those for the cases. This feature may render hospital data the superior control choice. Hospital controls certainly provide the more accessible control group, and data collection from the hospital almost always is cheaper. Choices in case-control studies then really are four: (1) good data, good group; (2) good data, not so good group; (3) not so good data, good group; and (4) not so good data, not so good group. Although situation (1) is the most preferable, in retrospective studies dependent on hospital or similar sources for cases, the choice is often the difficult one between situations (2) and (3). The important point is that *all* available comparison populations be considered in detail before deciding on a study design, with selection of the one that meets the requirements best. Sometimes, for example, both hospital and community comparison groups could be used and the most conservative results accepted.

The *matching* of controls and cases often is a desirable practice if one suspects that, in addition to the hypothesized disease determinant, presence (or absence) of disease may be influenced by age, sex, breed, or some other matchable characteristic. This need for matching is illustrated in the ocular carcinoma example that follows. The canine bone sarcoma studies described later in this chapter also illustrate how unclassifiable data pertaining to cases or controls in retrospective studies should be classified in the analysis in such a way as to oppose the hypothesis of association being tested. A number of other points just discussed also are illustrated in that more detailed example. Epidemiologists contemplating retrospective studies of the case-control type are advised to consult the literature for more detailed discussions of some of the preceding problems.[3]

Occasionally *preexisting* data also may be used for a prospective-*type* cohort study. This approach is especially acceptable if the data are available for the entire population in which the disease events are taking place. It requires that knowledge of presence or absence of the hypothesized determinant be available for some point in time prior to occurrence of the disease event noted. An example of this type of situation is given next, and another occurs in Chapter 12. First, the more usual retrospective situation is described.

Squamous cell carcinoma in cattle

Suppose a veterinarian is responsible for the health of a Hereford herd. He maintains complete vital statistics and autopsy records. Included are photographs of each *sick* animal in the herd. Referring to these data, for 1974, he had 40 cases of ocular squamous cell carcinoma. He is interested in using these data to study an hypothesized association between occurrence of this tumor and nonpigmented eyelids. By examination of their photographs, he

can determine whether each of these animals with carcinoma, as well as *all other sick animals* in this herd, had nonpigmented eyelids. These data are expressed as in Table 11–1; that is, 600 animals were sick for *any* cause in 1974, 40 of them with carcinoma and 560 with all other diagnoses (i.e., without carcinoma).

Notice that from these data he cannot calculate the incidence of carcinoma given presence or absence of pigmentation because he does *not* know the distribution of eyelid pigmentation in the *total* noncarcinomatous population of this herd. The question these data do permit is that of *proportional* morbidity; that is, given *all* ill animals, what proportion had carcinoma? In addition, there is the "noncausal" question of association; given carcinoma, what is the conditional probability that these animals had nonpigmented eyelids? He is really interested in another question; given nonpigmented eyelids, what is the conditional probability that these animals will develop carcinoma? For this reason, in retrospective studies (unless there is access to the total population and *prior* knowledge of presence or absence of the factor in all individuals in this whole population, as in John Snow's study on the districts of London served by both water companies) one cannot address the question of a possibly causal association between an hypothesized factor and a disease.

The data in the preceding fourfold table can be analyzed statistically, however, *if* one knows that the "control" or comparison group available (i.e., the animals that were sick in 1974 from all diagnoses *other* than ocular carcinoma is *representative* of the entire population of animals free of ocular carcinoma, particularly if ocular pigmentation is distributed among cattle with other diagnoses than ocular carcinoma as it is in the general carcinoma-free herd population. This situation probably would be true unless another disease occurring fairly frequently during 1974 also was associated with pigmentation of the eyelids, *or* the three groups (cases, controls, entire population) differed appreciably according to some other factor related to ocular carcinoma (e.g., age). If neither of these latter circumstances occurred, the veterinarian could analyze the preceding data by calculating the *odds ratio* as an approximation of the relative risk and determing its statistical significance (p. 18). At this point, look at page 17 for other

Table 11–1.   Hypothetical Occurrence of Nonpigmented Eyelids in Herd of Hereford Cattle According to Whether They Had Experienced Ocular Squamous Cell Carcinoma or Some Other Illness During 1974

	Ocular Carcinoma	All Other Sick Animals	
Nonpigmented Eyelids	38	462	500
Pigmented Eyelids	2	98	100
	40	560	600

types of findings that might increase one's belief in the possible causal nature of statistically valid associations evident from studies such as the preceding one.

A SECOND SITUATION. There might often be circumstances when, for the general situation described previously, the disease seems to be associated too with some factor other than nonpigmentation of the eyelid, a factor that might be nonuniformly distributed in the ocular carcinoma and control groups. As stated, age might be such a factor, especially in this instance where there is reason to believe that the mean age of the ocular carcinoma group might be higher than for the control group. In that case, one could select *paired* controls from the control group for *each* ocular carcinoma case, which would be matched by age. Suppose the first ocular carcinoma case for 1974 was illness record number 1221, and the age of this animal was six years. The age-matched control would be selected by looking first at the next consecutive case 1222, say, a screwworm-infected animal three years old. This age is not the one needed. Animal 1223 is a 10-year-old animal with mastitis, but number 1224 is another six-year-old animal treated for a wire wound. Animal 1224 is the matched control for ocular carcinoma animal 1221. The same matching procedure is followed for the next carcinoma case; animal 1532, 10 years old, and its situation. Then use the formula for relative risk analysis given on page 180.

Often it is not possible to match exactly by age. In such cases, use intervals of age; for example, match each case by an animal whose age was within a year or two for adults and within three to six months for yearlings and heifers.

A THIRD SITUATION. Now suppose that the situation with this same Hereford herd is such that there are photographs of *all* animals in this herd (the population at risk), whether sick or not, and that they can be classified *for some point in the past*, say, at the beginning of 1974, as having pigmented or nonpigmented eyelids. One then could follow these animals and see which developed ocular carcinoma in 1974. These total preexisting data are displayed in the fourfold table (Table 11–2). Using the beginning of the 1974 year as the starting point, one now can ask the prospective questions of these already existing data; that is, given an animal in the cohort with nonpigmented eyelids, what is the conditional prob-

ability of development of ocular carcinoma; and given an animal in the cohort with pigmented eyelids, what is the conditional probability of development of ocular carcinoma? Note that the answers to these questions $38/5000 = 0.76\%$ and $2/1000 = 0.2\%$ are the year's *incidence rates* for ocular carcinoma in the groups with nonpigmented and pigmented eyelids. One then can calculate a relative risk and determine whether the difference between these probabilities is statistically significant.

Next come the analytical methods that might have been applied in these situations.

RELATIVE RISK AND ODDS RATIO

Analytical studies, including prospective and case-control studies, are conducted to determine the strength of the association, if any, between a factor and a disease. Suppose that each individual in a large population has been classified as + or − according to some hypothesized etiologic factor, and + or − according to the disease state under study. The disease state may refer to incidence or prevalence, depending upon the particular study, or may refer to death or other terminal or dichotomous states such as successful impregnation of heifers or delivery of a live foal by mares. For convenience of presentation, incidence of disease will be chosen.

Such categorizations can be summarized by using proportions of the *total* population.

Disease

		Present (+)	Absent (−)	Total
Factor	Present (+)	P_1	P_2	P_1+P_2
	Absent (−)	P_3	P_4	P_3+P_4
	Total	P_1+P_3	P_2+P_4	1.0

If the proportions, P_i, are known, as they should be in a thorough prospective study of the entire population, any association between factor and disease could be measured by the ratio of risks (the relative risk), in this situation the incidence of the disease among animals having the factor divided by the incidence among those not having the factor.

Table 11–2.   Hypothetical Occurrence of Nonpigmented Eyelids in Entire Herd of Hereford Cattle According to Whether They Had Experienced Ocular Squamous Cell Carcinoma During 1974

	Ocular Carcinoma	All Other Animals	
Nonpigmented Eyelids	38	4962	5000
Pigmented Eyelids	2	998	1000
	40	5960	6000

$$\text{Ratio of risks} = \frac{P_1/(P_1+P_2)}{P_3/(P_3+P_4)} \text{ or } \frac{P_1(P_3+P_4)}{P_3(P_1+P_2)}$$

Another statistical measure of risk expresses the ratio of the odds:

$$\text{Odds ratio} = \frac{P_1/P_2}{P_3/P_4} \text{ or } \frac{P_1 P_4}{P_2 P_3}$$

Although both ratios are legitimate statistical entities, of interest in themselves, under certain special conditions they are quite similar in value. If the disease under study is not very common (i.e., $P_1 \ll P_2$ and $P_3 \ll P_4$), then $P_2 \doteq (P_1+P_2)$ and $P_4 \doteq (P_3+P_4)$, and

$$\frac{P_1(P_3+P_4)}{P_3(P_1+P_2)} \doteq \frac{P_1 P_4}{P_3 P_2}$$

Rare diseases are the very ones usually studied retrospectively, at least initially, so the odds ratio is often used in retrospective studies as an approximate measure of the relative risk of the disease.

One can replace the proportions P_i, just given, by frequencies a, b, c, d in a large study:

Disease

		+	–	Total
Factor	+	a	b	a+b
	–	c	d	c+d
Total		a+c	b+d	N

For most retrospective case-control studies, such as those carried out using hospital or laboratory data, the frequencies of b and d for the true population at risk are unknown. In other words, the actual communities or populations in which the illness cases *a* and *c* take place are not known. Therefore, incidence $\frac{a}{a+b}$ and $\frac{c}{c+d}$ cannot be calculated. However, a satisfactory approximation of relative risk can be obtained by substituting the frequencies a, b, c, and d in the preceding odds ratio, $(P_1 P_4)/(P_2 P_3)$, as

$$R_a = \frac{ad}{bc}.$$

Note that the odds ratio R_a is a satisfactory estimate of relative risk only when the disease studied occurs infrequently, that is, when P_1 and P_3 are small compared to P_2 and P_4.[4]

The relative risk can be *estimated* by this means from (1) a random sample of the population, (2) a prospective cohort study, or (3) a retrospective (case-control) study.

If R_a is approximately 1.0 it may be inferred that the factor under study is not likely to have influenced the disease. Deviations from 1.0 should be evaluated for significance, and this evaluation can be done conveniently using a logarithmic scale. The procedure follows:[5]

(1) Find $\log_e R_a$, where e = 2.71828. . . is the base for natural (naperian) logarithms.

(2) Find the variance of $\log_e R_a$ using the approximation

$$\text{var}(\log_e R_a) = \frac{1}{a} + \frac{1}{b} + \frac{1}{c} + \frac{1}{d}.$$

(3) Find the standard error of $\log_e R_a$:

$$\text{SE}(\log_e R_a) = \sqrt{\text{var}(\log_e R_a)}.$$

(4) Use normal theory to construct the appropriate confidence interval:

$$100(1-\alpha)\% \text{C.I.}: \log_e R_a \pm Z_{\frac{1}{2}\alpha} \text{SE}(\log_e R_a).$$

(5) Transform the confidence bounds for $\log_e R_a$ back to the original R_a scale.

(6) Check whether 1.0 has been captured in the interval in (5).

Consider the example:

Disease

		+	–
Factor	+	20	40
	–	5	20

$$R_a = \frac{(20)(20)}{(5)(40)} = 2.$$

(1) $\log_e R_a = \log_e 2 \doteq 0.693$

(2) $\text{var}(\log_e R_a) = \frac{1}{20} + \frac{1}{5} + \frac{1}{40} + \frac{1}{20} = 0.325$

(3) $\text{SE}(\log_e R_a) = \sqrt{0.325} \doteq 0.57$

(4) For 95% confidence limits of $\log_e R_a$, use Z = 1.96 to find

$$\log_e R_a \pm (Z) \; [\text{SE}(\log_e R_a)] = .69 \pm (1.96)(0.57)$$

$$= 0.693 \pm 1.117 = [-0.42, 1.81]$$

(5) For 95% C.I. of R_a, one has, by transforming, antilogs ($^-0.42, 1.81$) = [0.66, 6.11]

(6) Note that the confidence interval contains 1.0. Thus, these data show no significant association between disease and factor. It should be noted that step (4) already contained this result: $0 (= \log_e 1)$ was "captured" in the interval in (4).

If, as in studies of disease outbreaks, the assumption concerning the proportion of diseased or ill subjects, $(P_1 + P_3)$, fails, that is, the disease is *not* of rare occurrence, then one should use the exact, rather than the approximate, relative risk

$$R = \frac{P_1(P_3+P_4)}{P_3(P_1+P_2)}.$$

The estimate of the exact relative risk becomes

$$R_e = \frac{a(c+d)}{c(a+b)}.$$

As with the odds ratio (approximate relative risk), if R_e is approximately 1, the factor under study is not likely to have influenced the disease. Deviations from 1 should be evaluated for significance, and this evaluation also can be done conveniently using a logarithmic scale. The procedure follows, and is analogous to that for the odds ratio:

(1') Same as (1) using R_e.

(2') Find $var(\log_e R_e)$ using the approximation

$$var(\log_e R_e) = \frac{1}{a} + \frac{1}{c} - \frac{1}{a+b} - \frac{1}{c+d}$$

(3')
(4')
(5')
(6')
▶ Same as (3), ..., (6) on page 178, using R_e.

Note that this procedure cannot be used if either a or c equals 0, for there would be a 0 divisor in the computation of R_e, or in the computation of $var(\log_e R_e)$ in steps (2) and (2'). Normally one would not calculate both R_a and R_e. In retrospective studies, R_a is usually calculated. Here the calculation of R_e is simply used as an illustration.

For the data in the example given on page 178,

$$R_e = \frac{(20)(25)}{(5)(60)} = \frac{5}{3} = 1.67$$

(1') $\log_e R_e = \log_e(5/3) = 0.51282$

(2') $var(\log_e R_e) = 1/20 + 1/5 - 1/25 - 1/60 = 0.193333$

(3') $SE(\log_e R_e) = \sqrt{0.193333} = 0.44$

(4') For 95% confidence limits of $\log_e R_e$, one uses Z = 1.96

$$\log_e R_e \pm Z[SE(\log_e R_e)] = 0.51 \pm 1.96(0.44)$$

$$= 0.51 \pm 0.86 = [-0.35, 1.37]$$

(5') For 95% C.I. of R_e, one has, by transforming

antilog(-0.35, 1.37) = (0.71, 3.95)

(6') Note that the confidence interval contains 1.0. Thus, these data show no significant association between disease and factor. It should be noted that in step (4'), this result was already known: note that $0(=\log_e 1)$ was captured in (4').

It is worth noting that in this example,

$$var(\log_e R_e) = 0.193333 < 0.325000 = var(\log_e R_a).$$

This formula is a special case of the more general situation, which is that $var(\log_e R_e) < var(\log_e R_a)$. One might be tempted to conclude, therefore, that significance can be shown more easily in the exact case than in the approximate case. However, it is also true that the exact relative risk always lies closer to 1 than does the approximate relative risk. Thus, it may occur that the tighter confidence intervals associated with the exact case are offset by the closer proximity of R_e to 1. In the present example, regardless of the fact that R_e is nearer to 1 than is R_a, the confidence interval associated with the exact case is entirely nested within the confidence interval for the approximate case. Whether this will always be the case is at present unknown, and should be investigated case by case when doubt exists.

For samples of data where a or c equals 0, neither the odds ratio nor exact relative risk estimates can be made. Alternative strategies must be followed, including (a) increase the sample size, or (b) replace 0 by some small number (say 0.25) to get a crude guesstimate of the variance, or (c) use chi-square.

Chi-square test for association between disease and hypothesized determinant

As indicated previously, the chi-square test for association is also a common test used in retrospective studies:

$$\chi^2_{(1)} = \frac{(ad-bc)^2 N}{(a+b)(a+c)(b+d)(c+d)}$$

For the data in the preceding example

$$\chi^2_{(1)} = \frac{[(20)(20) - (40)(5)]^2(85)}{(60)(25)(60)(25)}$$

$$= 1.51$$

Since 1.51 < 3.84, the critical value of chi-square for one degree of freedom, at the 5% level of significance, one would conclude that there is little or no evidence of an association between the factor and the disease.

This example illustrates the use of two statistical procedures for evaluating possible association between a factor and a disease. Normally, two such analyses would not be performed. However, it is possible that, of two persons examining the same data, one might choose to use the odds ratio approximation to relative risk and the other might choose the chi-square test for association. Except in borderline cases, both tests should lead to the same conclusion. Where one test might indicate a significant association and the other barely rejects the notion of a significant association, a fundamental question concerning the use of these tests may be apparent. However, the fundamental question is not so much "Which test do I use?" as "How well do these data represent the real disease-factor situation?" Where one test indicates significance yet the other may not, it is likely that the probabilities, i.e., the p-values or levels of significance, are small and similar for both tests.

Relative risk of ocular carcinoma among cattle with nonpigmented eyelids

To illustrate the use of relative risk, see the bovine ocular carcinoma examples beginning with the third situation on page 177. From the data on the total Hereford population provided in that fourfold table, one can calculate the actual relative risk,

$$R = \frac{\text{Incidence given nonpigmented eyelids}}{\text{Incidence given pigmented eyelids}} \text{ or}$$

$$\frac{38/5000}{2/1000}$$

The example shows that the risk of acquiring ocular carcinoma, given nonpigmented eyelids, is 3.8 times greater than that for pigmented eyelids.[6]

For the situation illustrated in the first approach, however, where there is only a sample of the total carcinoma-free population, that is, other *diseased* animals without ocular carcinoma, one can calculate (from the data in the fourfold table) an approximate relative risk by using the odds ratio

$$R_a = \frac{ad}{bc} \text{ or } \frac{(38)(98)}{(462)\ (2)} = 4.03$$

Thus, the probability of having nonpigmented eyelids in animals with ocular carcinoma is estimated as being 4.0 times greater than in animals without ocular carcinoma.[7]

Finally, for the situation illustrated in the second situation, where *a control animal* from the sick population sample is *matched by age* for each of the cases of ocular carcinoma, the result is the special situation indicated by the general case that follows:[8]

Cases of ocular carcinoma in pairs matched by age

Comparison individuals in pairs matched by age		Factor	
		Present	Absent
	Present Factor	r	s
	Absent	t	u

In the example, r = number of pairs in which both have the factor, u = number of pairs in which both lack the factor, s = number of pairs where cases do not have the factor and controls do, and t = number of pairs where cases have the factor and controls do not. In such a matched study, the estimated relative risk can be calculated by the formula

$$R_e = \frac{t}{s}$$

If these matched pairs in the example were distributed as

Cases

Matched comparison Factor individuals		Factor		
		Present	Absent	
	Present	1	10	11
	Absent	39	30	69
		40	40	80

the estimate of R would be $\frac{39}{10}$ = 3.9. McNemar's test for sample proportions which are *not* independent can be used for calculation of chi-square. Ties are eliminated, and only those pairs with discrepant results are considered.

$$\chi^2 = \frac{[(10-39)-1]^2}{10+39} = 16$$

Problem 12.   Disease outbreak on a mink ranch

Review again the outbreak investigation described in Chapter 3.

Using the data available, calculate the relative risks for each feedstuff.

Calculate the statistical significance of the relative risk values for liver and vegetable fat.

ATTRIBUTABLE RISK

Relative risk with respect to a certain exposure factor can be defined as the ratio of disease incidence among exposed individuals to the incidence among individuals not exposed to the factor; attributable risk is the *difference* between these incidence rates. For example, if the incidence of congenital malformations in lambs from ewes fed *Veratrum californicum* was 876 per 1000 per year, and 6 per 1000 among lambs from similar ewes not fed the plant, the risk *attributable* to *V. californicum* would be the difference or 870 per 1000 lambs per year. The attributable risk suggests the medical *importance* of the association being studied. This concept is well illustrated by the data in Table 11–3 on risks attributable to heavy cigarette smoking from case-control studies of deaths from pulmonary carcinoma and cardiovascular disease in man. Some deaths from both causes occur in nonsmokers. However, while cigarette smoking increases the risk of dying from pulmonary carcinoma by 32.4 times and the risk of dying from cardiovascular disease only 1.4 times, more cardiovascular disease deaths each year are attributable to smoking than are pulmonary carcinoma deaths. Thus, while the association with smoking is much stronger in pulmonary carcinoma, the association in cardiovascular disease is the more important one from the public health standpoint.

SECOND STAGE RELATIVE RISK

Situations commonly occur in which more than one causal variable or candidate disease determinant is apparent (or definitely exists). To control the confounding effects of one of the possible multiple determinants, say A or B, during the analyses, one can, for example, do rate adjustment for A or B, calculate A- or B-specific rates, or match individuals for A or B between the test and comparison populations. However, to help determine whether A and/or B actually are related causally to the disease in question, one may perform a second stage relative risk, that is, set up a fourfold table for relative risk in which one of these variables is "controlled."

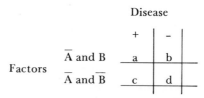

Conversely, one may wish to consider the risk when two factors act concurrently. The disadvantage of second stage relative risk is rapid loss of data.

Problem 13 is based upon data in the feedlot problem outlined in Chapter 3.

Problem 13. Epidemic of feed-borne disease in a feedlot

EXPOSE ONLY ONE QUESTION IN THIS PROBLEM AT A TIME.

An attack rate table for this feedlot cattle population, based upon feeds fed, is given in Table 11–4.

From these data, which feed or feeds would be suspect as the possible vehicle?

If one feedstuff is strongly suspected but one or two others cannot be completely ruled out (suppose batches of more than one feedstuff have been contaminated or only one of several batches of one feedstuff), what might you do?

Calculate the relative risks for cottonseed hulls, tankage, and beet molasses.

Reexamine your feed data (see the note for Chapter 6) and sort out the common feeding by pen of these three feeds and the places these three feeds each were fed independently of another. The distribution of deaths and populations by lot was shown in the note for Chapter 7.

Now what might you do in the way of analysis?

Carry out the appropriate second stage relative risk analyses and state your conclusion about the contaminated feed or feeds.

Problem 14. Breed association with canine epilepsy

Consider again the hypothetical canine epilepsy data from the records of a veterinary school clinic (p.

Table 11–3.   Relative Risk and Attributable Risk Estimated from Case-Control Studies of Lung Cancer and Coronary Heart Disease in Smoking and Nonsmoking British Males (Adapted from Doll, R., and Hill, A.B. 1964. Br. Med. J. 1:1399-1410, 1460-1467.)

Cause of death	Death rates per 1000 British males		Relative risk	Attributable risk
	Smokers	Nonsmokers		
Lung cancer	2.27	0.07	32.4	2.20
Cardiovascular disease	9.93	7.32	1.4	2.61

83), and note some of the possible sources of bias with respect to the breed distribution in this hospitalized group of cases. Recall that, of cases of epilepsy retrieved from these records, 20% were dogs of breed X and 28% were dogs of breed Y. Suppose you wished to carry out a retrospective case-control study using these data.

Consider the disease sample first. Are these dogs likely to be *all* the dogs with epilepsy in the *general* dog population of the community served by this clinic?

If not, are they typical or representative of this total number? For instance, are they representative of cases of epilepsy brought to small private practices in the population area, do they represent those not brought to a veterinarian at all? If they might not be representative cases, why?

Are any of your cases referral cases? If so, what might that imply?

Next, consider the breed distribution in your *case* population. Do you know that it does not resemble the breed distribution of dogs in your *total* hospital record population for this same time period? Do either of these distributions resemble the breed distribution in your *community* population of dogs? If not, what things might make them different? (In this connection, reread portions of Chapter 9 for a general discussion of host factors and their distribution.)

With these considerations in mind, design a case-control study for investigation of an hypothesized association between (predisposition to) canine epilepsy and breeds X and Y. Identify your data sources and create appropriate data for the case and comparison populations you would prefer to use, and fully describe these case and comparison groups. Indicate the ways in which you might reduce various biases in their composition, and then identify any possible biases that still remain. Carry out appropriate analyses of your hypothetical data and state your conclusions.

Problem 15.   Completing study of botulism epidemic on a mink ranch

Referring back a few pages, complete your analysis of data from this epidemic in mink using second stage relative risk.

After carefully reviewing the process of feed preparation on the mink ranch, it was found that three bags of liver were utilized during the epidemic period. One bag was for the rations of groups 1, 2, 3, and 4; a second for rations of groups 5, 6, 7, 8, and 9. Parts of a third bag were used for the remaining groups.

Differences in morbidity and mortality in the five categories of mink could be attributed to the vaccination status of these mink.

The presence of botulinum toxin was demonstrated by injecting extracts from gastric contents of dead mink into susceptible mice and subsequently typing with specific antisera.

Isolation of *Clostridium botulinum* was attempted in vain.

In summary, this example on a mink ranch illustrates a typical outbreak investigation—the type of problem often faced by veterinarians.

Multiple comparison problem in case-control studies

In the simple situation of a homogeneous population of cases and controls, presumably alike in all

Table 11-4.   Death Rates Among Feedlot Cattle by Feeds Consumed During Point Epidemic of Pesticide Poisoning

	Eaten			Not eaten		
Feed	Total cattle*	No. dead	Rate (%)*	Total cattle	No. dead	Rate (%)
Barley	42,000	3305	7.9	0	0	0
Wheat	20,100	1263	6.3	21,900	2042	9.3
Sorghums	23,900	2638	11.0	18,100	667	3.7
Beet molasses	5400	1270	23.5	36,600	2035	5.6
Dried beet pulp	13,300	1053	7.9	28,700	2252	7.8
Cottonseed cake	19,300	1920	9.9	22,700	1385	6.1
Tankage	5900	1907	32.3	36,100	1398	3.9
Sorghum fodder	13,200	2003	15.2	28,800	1302	4.5
Cottonseed hulls	15,600	3256	20.9	26,400	49	0.2
Sorghum silage	21,500	2583	12.0	20,500	722	3.5
Hay	42,000	3305	7.9	0	0	0

*These populations and rates reflect the risk in terms of the number of animals present and alive on the day preceding the outbreak.

characteristics except the one under investigation, the outcome of the study can be represented by a single contingency table as in the earlier examples. In the perhaps more common situation in which a number of recorded variables may be associated with the disease under study, the procedure applied should permit a factor to be tested, with control for the presence and absence of other factors. Statistical procedures for factor control and various approaches in calculation of risk have been developed; and an example of applying the procedures in a study of the feline urological syndrome has been published recently.[9]

The following example illustrates the principles in factor control. The reader should check the references in note 3 for more complete information. This example is hypothetical and refers to the earlier discussion of epilepsy in dogs (see Chapter 5). Assume that a case-control study with a proper control group has been carried out, with the resulting data shown in Table 11–5. It is now possible to calculate the risk associated with breed X.

To calculate approximate relative risk (R_a), form two columns of derivative computations from Table 11–5.

$\dfrac{AD}{T}$	$\dfrac{BC}{T}$
$\dfrac{(1)(5)}{(9)}$	$\dfrac{(2)(4)}{(9)}$
(10)	(11)
2.560	1.628
7.969	1.922
0.867	1.284
1.685	1.574
7.631	1.888
0.854	1.570
21.566	9.866

$$R_a = \Sigma(AD/T)/\Sigma(BC/T) = \frac{21.566}{9.866} = 2.19$$

It should be pointed out that there are other approaches for calculating relative risk in this situation. The choice depends on the circumstances of the study, and the reader can check the references in note 3 for details.

Total discrepancy is calculated from Table 11–5 as

$$Y = \Sigma(AD/T) - \Sigma(BC/T) = 21.57 - 9.86 = 11.71$$

To calculate chi-square, one needs the following derivative computations that are also based on the data in Table 11–5

		V(A)
$\dfrac{(3)(7)}{(9)} = (12)$	$\dfrac{(6)(8)}{(9)} = (13)$	$\dfrac{(12)(13)}{(9)-1.0}$
2.068	400.068	1.764
2.953	727.953	2.596
1.417	351.417	1.233
1.889	347.889	1.595
3.257	479.257	2.734
1.715	381.715	1.471

$$\chi^2 = (|Y| - 0.5)^2 / \Sigma V(A)$$

$$\chi^2 = (11.71 - 0.5)^2 / 11.393 = 11.03 > 9.21 \ (\alpha = 0.01)$$

Thus we find evidence that breed X is associated with the occurrence of epilepsy. The interpretation of this association is another matter. The reader will observe that the association between breed X and epilepsy in the present data is caused by an increased risk in breed X in the age group 1 through 3 years. The interpretation of this factor requires investigation of how case and control groups were assembled, the possibility of lower incidence of other diseases in

Table 11–5.   Cases of Canine Epilepsy and Control Animals by Breed, Sex, and Age (hypothetical data)

Age	Cases			Controls			Cases and controls		
	Breed X A (1)	Other breeds B (2)	Total N_1 (3)	Breed X C (4)	Other breeds D (5)	Total N_2 (6)	Breed X M_1 (7)	Other breeds M_2 (8)	Total T (9)
Males									
<1 year	3	15	18	51	401	452	54	416	470
1-3 years	9	27	36	59	734	793	68	761	829
>3 years	1	13	14	40	351	391	41	364	405
Females									
<1 year	2	13	15	50	348	398	52	361	413
1-3 years	9	18	27	60	485	545	69	503	572
>3 years	1	14	15	50	381	431	51	395	446
Total	25	100	125	310	2700	3010	335	2800	3135

breed X compared to other breeds, and other parameters.

SUCCESSIVE APPROXIMATIONS

At several points in this book, it has been indicated that epidemiological studies often take the form of a series of successive approximations. The current discussion of the retrospective epidemiological approach to learning about diseases provides a good point to illustrate this statement more fully while recapitulating a number of important concepts and cautions presented so far. It should be pointed out with respect to the studies cited in this example that they *each* did contribute to the understanding of the question addressed, and each was fairly typical of problem approaches at the time they were performed.

Bone sarcoma in dogs

Suppose you are an epidemiologist concerned with comparative studies on cancer in lower animals, and one particular problem of interest to you is bone sarcoma in dogs. In your review of the literature, you find several interesting reports. The first is concerned mostly with the pathology of a small series of cases of canine bone sarcoma, and the second with clinical aspects and pathology of a larger case series. Both papers contain statements about the frequency distribution of bone sarcomas in heavy versus light breeds of dogs. Examine these reports.

Study A is a report of 20 consecutive cases of canine bone sarcoma seen in a veterinary school clinic

in a two-year period.[10] The descriptive data from this paper on age, sex, and breed of dogs are given in Table 11–6.

These data on breed were not expressed as rates, and no data were presented in this paper for the distributions of this host variable either in the hospital population studied or in the universe population of dogs served by this hospital.

From these data and their review of several other cases from the literature, the authors of this study concluded that "this tumor most often affects dogs of the large breeds, and in particular the Great Dane."

Study B was a more elaborate study of the 130 cases of bone sarcoma seen in dogs during a 10-year period in another veterinary school clinic.[11] Frequency distributions of the bone sarcoma cases were given by age and breed (Fig. 11–2 and Table 11–7), and comparison data for breed were given for a total of 3773 consecutive canine admissions to this hospital for all causes during one of the study years (Table 11–7). Of 122 dogs with bone sarcoma for which sex was recorded, there were 69 males and 53 females.

The "great majority" of these bone sarcoma cases were said to have been referrals. Distributions of the breeds of dogs in the community population served by this clinic were not provided.

From their data, these authors made the following statements about age, sex, breed, and size of dogs with respect to bone sarcomas:

(1) "The average age of ... dogs with osteo-

Table 11–6.   Age, Sex, and Breed of 20 Hospitalized Dogs with Bone Sarcomas in Study A[10]

Dog no.	Age	Sex	Breed
1	12	M	Boston terrier
2	4	F	Great Dane
3	4	?	Great Dane
4	4½	M	Irish setter
5	8	F	Irish setter
6	Young	?	Spaniel
7	12	F	Shepherd
8	3	F	Bull terrier
9	4	F	Doberman pinscher
10	6	M	Terrier
11	5	M	Collie
12	9	M	Collie
13	10	?	Boxer
14	5½	M	Greyhound
15	6	F	Saint Bernard
16	9	M	Great Dane
17	4	M	Pointer
18	11	M	Greyhound
19	12	M	English setter
20	Aged	?	Cocker spaniel

sarcomas was 7.3 years .... The significance of age statistics is doubtful in a series in which there are many breeds of dogs with widely differing life expectancies." (There was no reference cited nor data given in this paper on life expectancies of dogs of different breeds in general, but the average ages of the four most frequently affected breeds in this reported series of cases was stated nevertheless as: St. Bernard 6.2 years, Great Dane 6.5 years, boxer 7.3 years, and Irish setter 8 years.)

(2) For the series there was "a male to female ratio of 1.3:1.0."

(3) "It is well known that osteosarcoma in dogs is primarily a disease of large dogs."

The proportions of dogs of three breeds in the hospital population and the bone sarcoma series then were compared as follows: Boxers, which comprised 8.0% of the hospital population, accounted for 24.6% of the bone sarcomas; Great Danes 0.8% of the hospital population and 17.0% of the sarcoma series; and St. Bernards 0.15% of the hospital population and 7.7% of the sarcomas. "From these figures it would appear that the St. Bernard and Great Dane have the greatest predisposition to osteosarcoma."

Although the authors of study B did not cite it, data from another published study of canine lymphomas in New Jersey might have been of interest in connection with study B.[12] These data included (1) the distribution of dogs by breed in the urban areas of New Jersey adjacent to Philadelphia, and (2) the distributions of dog breeds by median age and percentage 10 years of age and older in New Jersey, e.g., for terriers with median age 5.0 years and 17.8% age 10 or older, and collies with median age 2.4 years and 5.4% age 10 or older.

From another later paper in the literature, you become aware of the data given in Table 11–8.[13]

Study C was based upon a *postulated* excess frequency of bone sarcoma cases among larger breeds of dogs in the United States.[14] Before he carried out this study, its author reviewed the aforementioned reports and stated "unfortunately, lack of information regarding the breed or body-size composition of the canine population at risk has precluded meaningful interpretation. . . ." He adds "there would seem to be no valid data in support of any assumption to the effect that canine clinic populations represent a valid sample of the population at risk. Consequently, while it is assumed the proportion of large dogs represented among cases is excessive, it has not been possible to confirm this assumption and quantitate any existent relationship between body size and occurrence of bone sarcoma."

Study C was designed to test the hypothesis that large dogs are subject to an excess risk of primary bone sarcoma. It utilized clinical data received upon request from 14 institutional veterinary hospitals (mostly university hospitals) in the United States and Canada. These data were obtained *before* the existence of the Veterinary Medical Data Program (Chapter 14). Data used were abstracted from the records of a total of 404 canine primary bone sarcoma cases. Ninety-four percent of these diagnoses had been confirmed by histopathology or radiology. Distribution of these cases by weight class is given in Table 11–9. All breeds were apportioned to these classes; e.g., Great Danes and St. Bernards were classified as "giant" breeds (80 lbs. or over) and boxers as a "large" breed (40 to 80 lbs.). The hypothesis to be examined was that the frequency of primary bone sarcoma in dogs is a function of body weight.

Comparable breed data were not obtainable at that time for the *total* hospitalized dog populations of

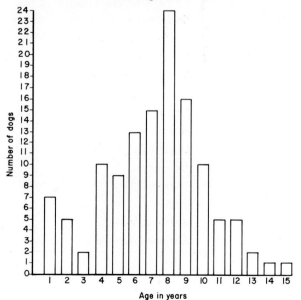

Fig. 11–2. Age distribution of dogs with bone sarcomas in study B (from Brodey, R.S., Sauer, R.M., and Medway, W.C. 1963. Canine bone neoplasms. J. Am. Vet. Med. Assoc. 143:471).

Table 11–7.   Breed Distribution of 130 Hospitalized Dogs with Bone Sarcoma and 3773 Consecutively
Admitted Dogs with All Diseases in Study B[11]

| No. dogs | | |
Bone sarcoma	All illnesses	Breed
32	325	Boxer
22	33	Great Dane
10	6	Saint Bernard
9	37	Irish setter
7	188	Collie
4	217	German shepherd
3	30	English setter
3	36*	Golden retriever
3	45	Doberman pinscher
2	48	Springer spaniel
2	23	Pointer
2	149†	Standard poodle
2	42	Dalmatian
2	0	Labrador retriever
2	0	Chesapeake Bay retriever
1	0	English bulldog
1	30	Weimaraner
1	0	Miniature poodle
1	132	Dachshund
1	0	Greyhound
1	0	Foxhound
1	0	Afghan hound
1	0	Giant schnauzer
1		Boxer–English bulldog
1		Chow–shepherd
1	1326	Setter cross
2		Unidentified large breed (50 lbs.)
8		Mixed breed (30–40 lbs.)
4		Mixed breed (15–25 lbs.)
0	431	Cocker spaniel
0	258	Fox terrier
0	109	Beagle
0	100	Boston terrier
0	88	Chihuahua
0	35	Pekingese
0	31	Spitz
0	29	Shetland collie
0	25	Manchester terrier
130	3773 Total	

*All retrievers
†All poodles

Table 11–8.   Breed Distribution in Two Hospitalized Canine Populations and Those of Adjacent Communities[13]

Breed	Purebred population (%)			
	Michigan State University Veterinary Clinic	Lansing, Michigan	University of Pennsylvania Veterinary Clinic	New Jersey
Poodle	15.1	5.3	5.6	1.1
German shepherd	10.2	2.6	8.1	7.0
Dachshund	9.1	6.6	4.9	2.9
Cocker spaniel	5.4	19.9	16.1	16.0
Beagle	5.3	12.0	4.1	8.0
Collie	4.7	3.4	7.0	8.8
Boston terrier	3.0	3.5	3.7	2.1
Boxer	2.9	2.9	12.2	7.7
Chihuahua	1.7	2.9	3.3	1.2

these 14 institutions, nor did census data for the total dog population of the United States exist. Data for "normal" dog populations actually used for comparison with cases in this study were dog licensure records from 12 different U.S. communities (Table 11–10). The author of this study stated that "non-licensure was assumed to be a randomized variable." These 12 dog population samples represented large and small, as well as urban and rural communities, and in total comprised 123,123 dogs, which then were distributed by weight class (Table 11–10).

The analytical method employed by this author was that of the odds ratio or approximation of relative risk. From the studies already cited, he had reason to hypothesize that the frequency of bone sarcomas is greater in large dogs. His 12 "normal" dog populations differed from one another in distribution of dogs by weight class (Table 11–10). This author performed a number of analyses using different ones of these comparison populations and all in combination. He often grouped dogs as giant-large or medium-small. He weighted his study against his hypothesis by classifying all dogs of unknown breed in his *case* group as medium-small and all dogs of unknown breed in his *comparison* population as giant-large.

This author concluded from his approximate relative risk values (e.g., R_a for giant dogs at least 61 times that for small dogs) that "larger canine breeds are subject to excess risk of primary bone sarcoma . . . [and that this] is characteristic of the larger breeds as a group rather than of one or several particular breeds."

His preliminary analysis on limited data also suggested the possibility that there is some increased risk of cancer *other* than bone sarcoma among larger breeds of dogs and he viewed this hypothesis as a possibly confounding factor in his study.

Since the time when study C was performed, and partially because of it, the U.S. National Cancer

Institute's Veterinary Medical Data Program was developed for 14 participating U.S. and Canadian veterinary colleges. Review the description of that program in Chapter 14. Your study will utilize this computerized clinical data bank for the period March, 1964, through May, 1973.[15]

In your study (D), you find that a diagnosis of osteosarcoma in 303 dogs has been confirmed histologically in 13 of 14 institutions for the period of this study. These cases comprise 3.4% of all confirmed canine tumors. For the osteosarcoma cases, 248 of the 303 are distributed among 40 purebreds. The distribution of these cases by breed, age, and sex is shown in Table 11–11.

Data for two possible comparison groups are available to you: (1) the clinical population of dogs (minus the cases) from these same institutions for the same time period as the cases, and (2) all dogs with histologically confirmed tumors (minus the cases) for the same time period as the cases.

You counted each dog only once—the first year it was brought to the participating institution for any reason; and repeat visits by the same dog in subsequent years were not counted. This clinical dog population consisted of 292,116 dogs brought at least once to these 13 veterinary clinics during the approximately nine-year study period. The clinical dog population is categorized by age, breed, and sex in Table 11–12, and the 8,802 dogs of the confirmed tumor cases (not bone sarcoma) are categorized similarly in Table 11–13.

Problem 16. Retrospective approaches for identifying determinants of diseases of unknown etiology.

Comment as meaningfully as you can upon (1) the appropriateness of the design of the preceding studies A, B, and C; (2) the sources of possible errors (biases) in each; (3) the way in which these biases might have been avoided in each study; (4) possible analyses that

Table 11–9.   Distribution of Canine Bone Sarcoma Cases by Age Interval and Weight Class in Study C[14]

Weight class	No. cases per age interval*										Unknown	Total
	<1	1–2	3–4	5–6	7–8	9–10	11–12	13–14	15–16	17>		
Giant		4	9	23	17	6					2	61
Large	2	36	25	37	53	64	33	12	1		9	272
Medium			4	4	3	9	4	3			2	29
Small		2		4	5	4	4	2		1	1	23
Unknown	1	1	2	1	1	7	3	2			1	19
Totals	3	43	40	69	79	90	44	19	1	1	15	404
Percentage of total†	0.8	11.1	10.3	17.7	20.3	23.1	11.3	4.9	0.3	0.3		100.0

*Age intervals indicate completed years.
†Based on total of 389 cases of known age

Table 11–10.   Distribution of Normal Canine Population Samples by Weight Class[14]

Sample source and year	Total licensed population	Sample size (% of total)	Breed specified*					Crossbreds or unknown*					Totals*					
			Giant	Large	Medium	Small	Total	Large	Medium	Small	Unknown†	Total	Giant	Large	Medium	Small	Unknown	Total
Ottawa Co., Mich.‡—1963	7400	49.8	0.46	30.00	25.06	9.74	65.26	4.96	3.55	6.40	19.83	34.74	0.46	34.96	28.61	16.14	19.83	100.00
Norfolk Co., Mass.—1963	29,275	20.8	0.82	25.92	20.27	9.02	56.03	7.01	3.51	2.28	31.17	43.97	0.82	32.93	23.78	11.30	31.17	100.00
Lansing, Mich.—1963	7800	50.2	0.03	20.40	34.96	17.42	72.81	2.37	2.76	4.60	17.47	27.20	0.03	22.78	37.72	22.01	17.47	100.01
Ingham Co., Mich.§—1963	8700	49.1	0.21	32.81	27.17	11.04	71.24	5.45	3.77	3.25	16.30	28.76	0.21	38.26	30.94	14.29	16.30	100.00
East Lansing, Mich.—1963	1281	100.0	0.39	25.37	32.94	13.04	71.74	1.41	2.19	2.42	22.25	28.26	0.39	26.78	35.13	15.46	22.25	100.00
Grand Haven, Mich.—1963	440	100.0	0	18.86	28.86	20.68	68.41	4.77	6.82	2.73	17.27	31.59	0	23.64	35.68	23.41	17.27	100.00
Hudsonville, Mich.—1963	176	100.0	0.57	11.93	37.50	9.09	59.09	10.80	0	13.07	17.05	40.91	0.57	22.73	37.50	22.16	17.05	100.00
Holland, Mich.—1963	1411	100.0	0.21	16.44	30.97	24.38	72.01	2.41	3.69	6.02	15.88	27.99	0.21	18.85	34.66	30.40	15.88	100.00
Kent Co., Mich.¶∥—1962	6000	56.0	0.48	27.67	26.47	10.15	64.77	4.44	5.51	4.02	21.26	35.23	0.48	32.10	31.98	14.18	21.26	100.00
Grand Rapids, Mich.—1963	6000	38.0	0.44	17.94	26.80	18.38	63.55	3.16	3.60	3.73	25.96	36.45	0.44	21.10	30.39	22.11	25.96	100.00
Franklin Co., Ohio*—1963	44,640	18.9	0.40	16.61	25.10	15.67	57.78	4.91	4.85	3.18	29.27	42.22	0.40	21.52	29.95	18.85	29.27	100.00
Licking Co., Ohio—1962	10,000	43.1	0.26	20.62	28.37	10.84	60.08	6.45	5.15	4.02	24.29	39.92	0.26	27.07	33.53	14.86	24.29	100.00
Combined samples	123,123	32.2	0.40	23.13	26.68	13.19	63.40	4.90	4.09	3.80	23.82	36.60	0.40	28.03	30.77	16.98	23.82	100.00

*Figures represent percentage of respective population samples.
†Including poodles and schnauzers not specified as to type
‡Excluding cities of Holland, Grand Haven, and Hudsonville
§Excluding cities of Lansing and East Lansing
¶Excluding city of Grand Rapids
#Including city of Columbus

the authors might have done; and (5) any stated conclusions of the authors.

Make your own conclusions from each of these studies as they were conducted.

Identify the hypotheses suggested by the *results* of each study.

If you think these studies addressed questions of importance from the standpoint of comparative medicine, discuss these questions in some detail.

Using the data given previously and in Tables 11–11 to 11–13, design a case-control study, indicating clearly your hypotheses. Carry out all desirable calculations. State your conclusions and recommendations for any further investigations. (Weight ranges for dog breeds are available from breed and kennel club publications).

FURTHER APPROACHES

Other particularly useful techniques for carrying out retrospective epidemiological studies are those that permit the simultaneous analysis of large numbers of variables, some or all of which may act as important determinants of the frequency of occurrence of a disease, determinants of the rates of

Table 11–11. Age, Breed, and Sex Distribution of Canine Osteosarcoma Cases from 13 Institutions for Study D, 1964-1973[15]

Breed	Sex	Age group (years)					Total
		0-1	2-3	4-7	8-10	>10	
Boxer	M	0	1	1	2	4	8
	F	0	0	0	1	1	2
Collie	M	1	0	0	1	5	7
	F	0	0	3	2	2	7
Doberman pinscher	M	1	0	1	0	1	3
	F	1	1	3	0	2	7
German shepherd	M	3	6	6	8	3	26
	F	6	0	4	7	4	21
Great Dane	M	0	3	2	0	0	5
	F	1	1	6	1	1	10
German shorthair pointer	M	0	0	2	1	1	4
	F	2	0	0	0	0	2
Standard poodle	M	0	0	1	2	1	4
	F	1	0	0	0	0	1
Golden retriever	M	3	0	0	2	4	9
	F	1	3	0	2	2	8
Labrador retriever	M	0	0	3	4	2	9
	F	0	0	0	1	2	3
Saint Bernard	M	1	1	10	7	0	19
	F	0	0	11	8	0	19
Irish setter	M	0	4	3	0	0	7
	F	1	2	2	2	2	9
Other purebreds	M	5	5	6	7	9	32
	F	2	3	5	9	7	26
Unspecified purebred	M	1	0	7	3	2	13
	F	0	0	5	5	2	12
Mixed breed	M	2	1	2	6	4	15
	F	1	0	4	2	8	15
All breeds	M	17	21	44	43	36	161
	F	16	10	43	40	33	142
Total		33	31	87	83	69	303

The specific breeds listed are those having at least five cases of canine osteosarcoma. "Other purebreds" refers to a group of other specific breeds, each of which has less than five cases.

Table 11–12.   Age, Breed, and Sex Distribution of Total Canine Clinical Population of 13 Institutions Supplying Data for Study D, 1964-1973[15]

Breed	Sex	Age group (years)					Total
		0-1	2-3	4-7	8-10	>10	
Boxer	M	688	294	409	413	299	2103
	F	552	328	348	362	306	1896
Collie	M	2963	734	646	414	290	5047
	F	3201	875	893	422	336	5727
Doberman pinscher	M	1220	377	234	123	47	2001
	F	1103	351	276	142	50	1922
German shepherd	M	7499	2555	1929	1110	462	13,555
	F	6360	2344	1905	1025	440	12,074
Great Dane	M	1243	368	240	93	10	1954
	F	955	324	182	62	12	1535
German shorthair pointer	M	646	290	249	165	97	1447
	F	604	55	61	41	32	793
Standard poodle	M	762	363	348	296	206	1975
	F	716	388	367	231	178	1880
Golden retriever	M	929	386	269	130	91	1805
	F	781	390	254	134	76	1635
Labrador retriever	M	2362	864	688	367	228	4509
	F	1988	823	552	286	201	3850
Saint Bernard	M	1803	595	295	84	14	2791
	F	1550	575	325	88	8	2546
Irish setter	M	1644	502	325	127	103	2701
	F	1717	602	312	130	82	2843
Other purebreds	M	24,787	12,523	11,638	7822	5094	61,864
	F	25,558	13,733	13,481	8397	5902	67,071
Unspecified purebred	M	3461	836	1280	446	276	6299
	F	3273	1290	891	488	306	6248
Mixed breed	M	20,955	5596	4098	2391	2254	35,294
	F	21,938	6252	4716	2921	2929	38,756
All breeds	M	70,962	26,283	22,648	13,981	9471	143,345
	F	70,296	28,330	24,563	14,729	10,858	148,776
Total		141,258	54,613	47,211	28,710	20,329	292,121

The specific breeds listed were selected to correspond to those listed for the distribution of the cases of canine osteosarcoma in Table 11–11. The total given here for reference population excludes those dogs of unknown sex and age.

progress in disease control efforts in different areas, or determinants of other characteristics. Multivariate techniques for these purposes, which permit a more natural holistic approach rather than a piecemeal approach to multicausal problems, are introduced in Chapter 13.

In summary, descriptive epidemiological studies yield hypotheses to investigate and often *identify* possibilities for retrospective observational (case-control) studies, or nature's "experiments." The analytical strategy in such investigations commences with the definition and selection of the actual population groups (cases, controls) to be compared, and continues with the analysis of the data.

Table 11–13.   Age, Breed, and Sex Distribution of All Microscopically Confirmed Canine Tumors Other Than Osteosarcoma from 13 Institutions for Study D, 1964-1973[15]

Breed	Sex	Age group (years)					Total
		0-1	2-3	4-7	8-10	>10	
Boxer	M	17	15	69	94	120	315
	F	5	12	44	77	90	228
Collie	M	9	6	25	46	50	136
	F	5	5	17	36	44	107
Doberman pinscher	M	11	6	19	14	10	60
	F	10	15	16	16	15	72
German shepherd	M	22	39	81	90	71	303
	F	28	27	76	94	46	271
Great Dane	M	10	17	16	7	3	53
	F	5	12	19	14	8	58
German shorthair pointer	M	2	2	6	25	29	64
	F	3	5	11	29	28	76
Standard poodle	M	1	3	11	25	42	82
	F	3	5	13	37	41	99
Golden retriever	M	5	4	19	22	42	92
	F	2	4	13	28	23	70
Labrador retriever	M	7	9	35	47	50	148
	F	2	2	21	47	34	106
Saint Bernard	M	8	18	29	16	0	71
	F	5	12	19	21	1	58
Irish setter	M	8	10	13	13	20	64
	F	8	9	11	22	18	68
Other purebreds	M	87	132	334	591	825	1969
	F	69	112	397	744	1091	2413
Unspecified purebred	M	15	12	29	37	8	101
	F	13	9	41	46	71	180
Mixed breed	M	65	41	102	164	330	702
	F	47	41	101	208	439	836
All breeds	M	267	314	788	1191	1600	4160
	F	205	270	799	1419	1949	4642
Total		472	584	1587	2610	3549	8802

Chapter 12

COHORT STUDIES

ANOTHER important aspect of the analytical or mathematical approach to epidemiology is the general area of prospective studies. Prospective studies, also known as cohort or follow-up studies, derive their name from the fact that some characteristic (or maneuver) is used to define the population groups, and these groups (cohorts) then are followed, awaiting the onset of a disease or some other response. At this point, the reader may want to review the relevant sections of Chapter 5.

Prospective studies are designed primarily to test an hypothesis or several specific hypotheses. Almost all vaccine trials, drug trials, and other so-called clinical trials are population-based follow-up studies of this type.

In their diagnostic use, cohort studies are longitudinal studies of groups of animals identified in some way other than by exhibiting the disease whose etiological determinants are under investigation. For example, in a cattle feedlot study of shipping fever, cohorts might be identified by such candidate determinants as (1) mode of transport to the feedlot (rail versus truck); (2) distance traveled to the feedlot (less than 100 miles, 100 to 300 miles, more than 300 miles); (3) age at arrival at feedlot (less than six months, six to nine months, more than nine months); (4) various combinations of (1) to (3); or (5) other factors.

TYPES OF COHORT STUDIES

For the sake of simplicity, reference in this chapter is to cohort studies on possible disease determinants. Two general types of cohort studies are of interest. The first type concerns a general population of animals, or some readily accessible part of that population, divided into study groups. The second type relies on the use of a study group presumably exposed to some specific risk factor, or otherwise at particular risk of acquiring some disease.

The first type of study requires that a general population be separated into two or more groups according to level of exposure to one or more factors,

in this case hypothesized determinants of an observed frequency of a disease, a reaction to a particular test, or other characteristics. For example, in a cohort study of the influence of environmental and host factors on the frequency of development of antibodies to *Anaplasma marginale* in cattle in California, cohorts from a general cattle population might be defined in terms of elevation above sea level of the home ranch, sources of replacement calves and heifers, breed, various management practices, or contact with ticks and other vectors. Naturally, more specific criteria for cohort designation could be developed to attempt to answer specific questions of interest.

The second type of cohort study, follow-up of a special risk group, often presents a major problem in trying to identify appropriate nonexposed groups. Suppose the selected population is one of horses observed through descriptive studies to be at apparent high risk of developing disease XYZ, a disease of unknown etiology. Moreover, the descriptive studies have suggested several possibly causal variables or candidate determinants, one of them R. One could examine this high risk population by selecting from it all horses with R (one cohort) and all without R (the other cohort), or random samples of each, and then compare them for future occurrence of XYZ. This study is conducted just like the study from a general population. Suppose, on the other hand, one wishes to follow up the survivorship of horses that have been exposed to high, but not immediately fatal, levels of lead, as might occur in animals grazing near a lead smelter, animals whose normal grazing area is alongside a heavily traveled highway, or animals grazing on pasture having soil with relatively high lead content. To conduct such studies satisfactorily, defining nonexposed or lower level of exposure groups whose survival experience can be compared with the special exposure groups presents difficulties not unlike those considered with respect to comparison groups in the preceding chapter (see also the discussion of *group* in Chapter 5).

As suggested by the preceding examples, the distinction between these two types of cohort studies is not always clear-cut. For example, follow-up studies of a group of horses exposed to lead as a result of automobile-induced pollution might be interpreted as either type of study, because one might compare its survivorship with that of some *other* comparison group (cohort), *or* one might divide and group it into different subgroups (cohorts) based on, say, grazing distance from the highway, prevailing wind direction, or some other less-direct candidate determinant than lead *per se*.

In summary, several types of cohort studies could be attempted. It is possible, for example, to make use of:

(1) Whole "communities," e.g., all horses in a certain locale versus horses in some other geographic location.

(2) Populations defined by occupation (or activity), e.g., racing horses versus pleasure horses versus breeder horses.

(3) Populations determined by self-selection, e.g., horses owned by various groups of owner volunteers. (Self-selection produces results of questionable reliability, but may be used in providing clues for the more definitive studies that may and should follow.)

(4) Genetically defined populations; e.g., the extensive breeding programs in the horse-raising industry provide opportunities for outstanding cohort-type studies. (It is surprising that relatively little use has been made of such study situations.)

As suggested already, not only might such categorizations each be conceived as representing different "general" populations from which cohorts exposed to different levels of some factor of interest could be identified, but also each of the above categories could itself be thought of as being a cohort in some more encompassing population or "universe" of horses. For example, "horses' usual activity" (racing versus pleasure riding versus stud farm use) might be the factor one wants to explore as a determinant of the frequency of a particular disease. If one were to undertake that particular study, a number of possibly confounding factors such as age, breed, and sex (including castrate-intact) might operate.

In this connection, refer to the discussion at the beginning of Chapter 2 about what populations a veterinarian might be concerned with in his practice. The comments about what constitutes the general or special risk populations, or cohorts, address the same point. All will depend upon how far a veterinarian's practice permits him to generalize a particular study's findings, e.g., to one herd of cattle, to all cattle in his county or practice area, to the cattle population of a state or country, or to "cattle," period.

Therefore, confusions in terminology may easily arise in the design of cohort studies, and alternative approaches to cohort selection reflect the same considerations of stages and strata as were discussed in Chapter 5 with respect to sampling generally.

General population studies

No matter how a general population group is identified, data are required to define various subgroups or cohorts by level of exposure to the factors (e.g., hypothesized disease determinants) under investigation. These several exposure groups then are compared with respect to occurrence of the disease or other event being investigated, attention being paid to possible effects of other factors not being studied, such as the respective age, sex, or breed composition of the cohorts (as in the horse activity example mentioned). If dissimilarities between cohorts exist in any of these factors, further consideration must be given to study design; and/or allowance must be made for such differences in the analyses of the study data (e.g., various additional categorizations or matching of individuals in the former case, or analysis of covariance; use of age, breed, sex specific rates, or some other appropriate statistical tools for the latter).

Origin of the factor

Two possibilities are recognized with respect to the factor (viz., disease determinant being studied). In one, the level of factor occurs independently of the investigator's actions. He merely identifies it. In the other, the investigator himself introduces the factor to be examined. This latter is the case in most so-called clinical trials, e.g., a vaccine trial. This latter type of study has all the characteristics of an experiment while the first is a type of observational study. Some additional comments on differences between these study possibilities preface Chapter 11. These remarks might be reread at this point.

Blind studies

In attempting to eliminate various forms of bias from prospective studies, they often are carried out "blind." In other words, the *assignment* of animals to the study cohort and the comparison cohorts is not based on subjective judgment. Rather, the epidemiologist is unaware of which animals represent which group. Various ways to accomplish this result include the assignment of numbered animals using a table of random numbers, alternate assignment, or a variety of other approaches. The code indicating the assignment is kept from the investigator until the study is completed. In the "clinical trial" type of study, further precautions are taken to see that the test preparations and the placebos also are identified by code numbers but otherwise are indistinguishable.

When the investigator himself also judges the response of the individual animals, blind assignment of animals to the cohorts assures that the *assessment* is blind as well. When, however, another observer is assessing, or aiding in assessment of the study's results, this additional assessor must also be unaware of which animals are in the study cohort and which are in the comparison cohort or cohorts. In human medicine, the patient himself may fulfill this assessor role; in veterinary medicine, it is often the animal owner or caretaker. When this additional assessment precaution is taken, the study is said to be conducted "double blind."

FOLLOW-UP OF COHORTS

Whether the cohort study is of the general population or of a special risk group, follow-up of the selected individuals frequently presents difficulties. Study animals may, for example, die of causes unrelated to the factor of interest, owners may become bored with the follow-up routines, animals (or owners) may move to other communities making follow-up excessively expensive and time-consuming, or owners may refuse to continue to participate.

The sources of information about the cohorts' experiences should be reliable, revealing the great majority of cases of the disease (or other event) actually occurring in each cohort. Death, as an index of outcome, may be useful in some insidious and often fatal diseases such as cancer; but it is generally too crude an index to be of value in the follow-up of milder or more acute diseases, or those with well-defined onsets. Because of the limitations of death as an index of disease, follow-up studies often must rely largely on periodic examinations of the study subjects. Unfortunately, such procedures also have disadvantages since, as the duration of the study increases, the individuals remaining in the study may become increasingly self-selected (or owner-selected), and diagnosis of outcome may become confounded with exposure class because observations may not remain independent. Every effort should be made to reduce such self-selection and to understand its effects (e.g., by comparing subjects who continue with those who do not continue to participate in the study), and finally to eliminate bias by making diagnoses as nearly "blind" as possible. Considering the broad spectrum of problems commonly associated with self-selection, the follow-up of cohorts must be as comprehensive as possible.

Several follow-up situations may exist, as for example in vaccine trials, in which the investigator may wait for natural exposure of his vaccinated and nonvaccinated cohorts; or, in situations of an infection of relatively low incidence, he may choose to "challenge" the cohorts with the agent directly.

Individual clinical trials often are designed so that their results are generalizable only to the herd in which they were carried out. Confidence that such results may apply more generally can be heightened by repetition of the trial in a number of other herds.

Again, one's willingness to accept the results of the trial as representing some fairly general pheonomena would depend upon whether the sample of herds used for the trial series was merely a convenience sample or a random sample.

ANALYSIS OF DATA

The analysis of data from cohort studies is essentially a derivation and comparison of rates of a specified outcome among the cohorts being studied. Such rates can be compared among various exposure groups of the general population; or they can be compared by calculating an expected number of cases, based on general population data, and comparing it to the particular cohort of interest.

In calculating the rates to be compared, some suitable denominator should be used, e.g., person-years of risk, dog-months, mouse-weeks, or whatever is appropriate in terms of species and time periods. The major analytical difficulty in such "individual-times" is that the resulting rates may be troublesome to test statistically.

When basing conclusions upon animals that have been successfully followed up, one assumes too that the condition of being followed up is not related to the characteristic (or factor) being studied or to the outcome being observed, such as survival of animals or onset of the particular disease.

A particularly useful statistical tool in cohort studies is the follow-up life table. (Current life tables were discussed in Chapter 5.)

Construction of follow-up life table

Suppose that 166 cattle were treated for leukemia, as in the following hypothetical table, and 27 died within the first year of follow-up, four were sold ("lost"), and two died of causes unrelated to leukemia. In the usual situation in veterinary medicine, one cannot obtain such a large number of diseased animals at one time; but as the disease cases appear in this study population, one can include them in the study.

Assume that among animals lost to follow-up and those dying from causes unrelated to the disease under study, each animal has been observable for *half* the year. Then, among the 166 animals starting the study and the six removed, one will have accumulated 163 animal-years of exposure [166-(1/2)(6)]. In this way, one can build up the cohort life table illustrated in Table 12–1. There may be animals, as under column (5), that were added to the study so recently that they have not yet been observed for the full five years. Their survivorship experience can be taken into account by having this additional category in the follow-up life table.

Columns (1), (2), and (7) are self-explanatory, and columns (3), (4), and (5) can be used to designate

Table 12–1.   Construction of Follow-up Life Table of Cattle Undergoing Experimental Therapy to Alleviate Leukemia (hypothetical data).

Year after treatment	No. alive at beginning of year	No. lost to follow-up during year	No. dying of causes unrelated to therapeutic regimen	No. alive observed for only part of the year	No. exposed to risk of dying during the year	No. dying during the year (due to leukemia)	Proportion dying during the year	Proportion surviving the year	Proportion surviving from start of treatment to start of xth year
	O_x	$_nW_x$	$_nD_x$	$_nS_x$	$_nR_x$	$_nd_x$	$_nq_x$	$_nP_x$	P_x
(1)	(2)	(3)*	(4)	(5)	(6)*	(7)	(8)	(9)	(10)
0	166	4	2	0	163	27	0.166	0.834	1.000
1	133	3	2	2	129.5	18	0.139	0.861	0.834
2	108	2	0	7	103.5	10	0.097	0.903	0.718
3	89	3	1	12	81	8	0.099	0.901	0.649
4	65	0	3	13	57	3	0.053	0.947	0.585
5	46	1	2	10	39.5	1	0.025	0.975	0.554
									0.540

*Columns 3, 4, and 5 are included to illustrate the possibility of specifying in detail certain kinds of losses to follow-up; e.g., deaths due to accidents may be excluded from numbers of individuals dying during the time interval.

Column 6 = column 2 − 1/2 (losses to follow-up) = column 2 − 1/2 (columns 3+4+5)

Column 10 for year i is (column 10 for year i−1) x (column 9 for year i)

various types of withdrawals or durations of participation in the study. In column (6),

$$_nR_x = 0_x - 1/2[_nW_x + _nD_x + _nS_x].$$

The proportions in columns (8) and (9) are obtained in the usual way from columns (6) and (7), with

$$_nq_x = \frac{_nd_x}{_nR_x}, \text{and } _nP_x = 1-_nq_x.$$

The proportion surviving from the start of treatment, column (10), is created by consecutive products of proportions in column (9):

$$P_0 = 1.0.$$

$$P_1 = (_nP_0) = 0.834 \text{ in the example.}$$

$$P_2 = (_nP_0)(_nP_1) = (0.834)(0.861).$$

In general,

$$P_x = (_nP_0)(_nP_1) \ldots (_nP_{x-1})$$

$$= (P_{x-1})(_nP_{x-1}).$$

The five-year follow-up survival rate in this cohort is approximately 0.554 = 55.4%. Other interesting details also can be perceived in such a cohort life table, e.g., the changing pattern for $_nP_x$, and the losses to follow-up.

The standard error of the proportion surviving, P_x, can be calculated using the formula

$$SE(P_x) = P_x\sqrt{\sum \frac{_nq_x}{_nR_x - _nd_x}}$$

where the sum extends from x=0, the initiation of follow-up, through the interval prior to that containing P_x. In the example, the standard error of P_3 is

$$SE(P_3) = 0.649 \left\{ \frac{27}{(163)(136)} + \frac{18}{(129.5)(111.5)} + \frac{10}{(103.5)(93.5)} \right\}^{1/2}$$

$$= (0.649\sqrt{0.003498})$$

$$= (0.649)(0.059)$$

$$= 0.038$$

One can now construct confidence intervals in the usual way. If, as would be the case in a therapeutic or other trial, another follow-up group exists in the study, one can test whether it represents a significantly different survivorship.

As mentioned in Chapter 5, life table techniques may also be applied in veterinary medicine to problems concerned with reproductive life or certain other sequences of events that are of epidemiological interest.

Problem 17. Construction of follow-up life table for dairy calves.[1]

Suppose that you have a herd health contract with a dairyman with a 200-cow milking herd and that, during the last year, 100 live heifer calves were born. Twenty of these died in their first five weeks of life. Of these 20, eight died during the first week of life, seven during the second week, three during the third week, one during the fourth week, and one during the fifth week.

Express this herd's neonatal mortality pattern in terms of a life table.

Survivorship curves

Survivorship curves are related to life tables, but in this graphic type of description of age specific mortality in a population, ℓ_x, the number living at a given age is plotted against age (x). Different forms of such curves are encountered (Fig. 12–1). In curve I in Figure 12–1, deaths occur more frequently in older individuals; in curve II, a constant number die per unit of time; in curve III, the age specific death rate is constant (when the ℓ_x scale is logarithmic, this curve is a straight line); and in curve IV, deaths occur more frequently in young individuals. Survivorship curves also may be plotted as probability of surviving against age, as for monkeys in Figure 12–2. These data are related to those in the accompanying life table on monkeys (Table 12–2) born in the California Primate Research Center.[2]

Other statistical tests

Some prospective cohort studies may require the use of relative risk. If so, one should use the actual relative risk ratio (R_e), for it is unlikely that the odds ratio would provide a suitable estimate of the risk ratio.[3]

The chi-square test for association also is applicable in prospective studies. These subjects were discussed in some detail in Chapter 11.

Problem 18. Alternative approaches to a vaccine trial.[4]

During 1974, several clients of a veterinary practitioner (Dr. A) suffered exceptionally heavy losses from calf diarrhea. The age of onset was about one week, and the attack rate was approximately 90%. The diarrhea-related mortality rate up to 21 days of age varied from 20 to 35% of calves born on individual farms. Good sanitation combined with antibiotic and electrolyte therapy seemed to have little effect on the course of the disease.

A majority of the dead calves were necropsied. Usually there were no gross lesions other than the ones associated with dehydration and diarrhea. Bacteriological examination of spleen and liver specimens from these calves usually produced negative results, which could be attributed to the fact that all affected calves had received antibiotics. Some sick and moribund calves were euthanized in order to collect additional laboratory specimens. Many appropriately collected intestine samples were positive for a virus ("X") using a fluorescent antibody test. Apparently healthy calves in these herds were not examined microbiologically.

Arrangements were made with a commercial laboratory to run prospective field trials in three of these herds using an experimental oral modified live virus "X" calf diarrhea vaccine. The initial field trial protocol called for a double-blind experimental design using 60 to 100 calves per trial. The vaccine-to-placebo ratio was 3:1. Each dose of vaccine was number coded. When a calf was vaccinated, usually within a few hours after birth, the vial number and calf's ear tag number were recorded. All treatments and responses to treatments were recorded for the first 21 days of each calf's life. Fecal samples were collected and frozen when any calf developed diarrhea. These samples were taken as soon as possible after the problem was observed. All dead calves less than 21 days of age were necropsied, and ligated

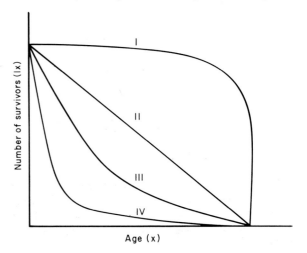

Fig. 12–1. Survivorship curves.

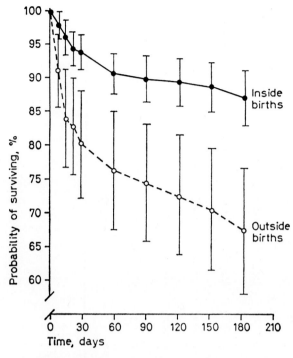

Fig. 12–2. Survivorship curves for 270 *Macaca mulatta* infants born in indoor cages and 105 *M. mulatta* infants born in outdoor cages at the California Primate Research Center, 1970-1972. Nonoverlapping 95% confidence intervals indicate statistical significance at the 5% level (from Hird et al,[2] S. Karger AG, Basel).

sections of intestine were collected and frozen. At the completion of the trial all specimens were sent to the laboratory. The results of this trial, which lasted from October to November, 1974, are shown in Table 12–3. Apparently, this trial was carried out in the face of an epidemic of calf diarrhea.

Following this trial, one client (Herd 1) elected to continue to use this vaccine, without placebo, for further experimentation during November and December. An odd-even day vaccination schedule was used. Calves born on even days were vaccinated, while calves born on odd days were not. One hundred calves were included in each group (Table 12–4).

Following this alternate-day vaccination experiment, every calf on this farm (Herd 1) was vaccinated (for approximately two months, January and February, 1975) before Dr. A unintentionally ran out of vaccine. Following this unfortunate incident, a total of 77 calves were unvaccinated before vaccine was again available, at which time vaccination of every calf was resumed. The morbidity and mortality experience of these calves also was followed (Table 12–5).

Some veterinarians who examined Dr. A's data differed in their conclusions regarding evidence for or against this vaccine's efficacy. One veterinarian, for example, while acknowledging that there probably were seasonal differences in calf mortality levels in their practice area, suggested that the data based upon historical controls in Table 12–5 represented a preferred type of trial for a live virus vaccine and concluded that this vaccine was, in fact, efficacious. Other veterinarians strongly disagreed.

(1) Comment in detail upon the merits and limitations of the design and conduct of these three successive forms of cohort trials for a modified live virus vaccine. What biological factors must be considered? What questions may arise in carrying out such tests in the face of an epidemic? Is any other information desired?

(2) What conclusions, if any, would you reach from the data presented in Tables 12–3 to 12–5? Are there other things not mentioned previously that you would wish to know?

(3) How would you have field tested this live virus vaccine?

Problem 19. Prospective cohort trial on a dairy farm[5]

UNCOVER ONE QUESTION AT A TIME.

Suppose the owner of a large dairy farm milking about 2000 cows became a new client for your herd health plan practice. He outlined initially his peri- and neonatal routines with calves (and dams). Most of these procedures sounded reasonable. However, your preliminary observations quickly indicated that the stated routines were not being followed consistently. Therefore, two veterinary student clerks employed in your practice were instructed to keep a detailed log of procedures actually followed on this farm on a 24-hour basis for two weeks. Among their findings were the following:

No one person had overall responsibility for the calves, and orders frequently were changed or countermanded. Of 10 calves born on a typical day, only three were born in the calving barn; the others were

Table 12-2.   Follow-up Life Table Showing Survivorship for 361 Male *Macaca mulatta* Infants and 376 Female *M. mulatta* Infants Born at California Primate Research Center, University of California, Davis, 1968-1972 (from Hird *et al*; S. Karger AG, Basel[2])

Beginning of interval days (x)	No. alive at beginning of interval (o_x)		No. withdrawn from study during the interval ($_nW_x$)		No. dying during the interval ($_nd_x$)		Probability of dying during the interval ($_nq_x$)		Probability of surviving during the interval ($_np_x$)		Probability of surviving to beginning of interval (survivorship) (P_x, %)		Standard error of P_x SE(P_x)	
	Male	Female	Male	Female	Male	Female	Male	Female	Male	Female	Male	Female	Male	Female
0	361	376	12	11	23	20	0.0648	0.0540	0.9352	0.9460	100.0	100.0	–	–
8	326	345	1	1	10	11	0.0307	0.0319	0.9693	0.9680	93.5	94.6	1.30	1.17
15	315	333	0	0	1	1	0.0032	0.0030	0.9968	0.9969	90.6	91.6	1.55	1.45
22	314	332	1	0	6	2	0.0191	0.0060	0.9809	0.9940	90.4	91.3	1.57	1.47
29	307	330	6	2	7	10	0.0230	0.0304	0.9770	0.9696	88.6	90.7	1.69	1.51
60	294	318	8	7	6	5	0.0207	0.0159	0.9793	0.9841	86.6	88.0	1.82	1.70
91	280	306	4	4	3	4	0.0108	0.0132	0.9892	0.9868	84.8	86.6	1.92	1.78
122	273	298	5	4	3	3	0.0111	0.0101	0.9889	0.9899	83.9	85.5	1.98	1.85
153	265	291	1	1	3	5	0.0113	0.0172	0.9887	0.9828	83.0	84.6	2.03	1.90
184	261	285									82.0	83.1	2.07	1.96

Table 12-3.   Results from Double-Blind Trial of Experimental Modified Live Virus Vaccine "X" Against Calf Diarrhea in Three Southern California Dairy Herds, October-November, 1974[4]

Herd	Treatment	No. calves	A.R. (%) up to 21 days of age	Cause-specific death rate (%) up to 21 days of age
1	Vaccine	75	93	16
	Placebo	25	84	12
2	Vaccine	75	88	20
	Placebo	25	96	28
3	Vaccine	68	73	4.5
	Placebo	22	73	0

dropped in the dry cow corral. No effort was made to see that these latter calves nursed their dams before they were moved into the calf-raising barn. Times during which dams and calves actually remained together varied between 1½ and 42 hours. Calves born in the calving barn sometimes were given pooled colostrum, sometimes whole milk, sometimes a polyvalent immune serum. Navels were swabbed with 7% iodine with about the same regularity as colostrum feeding. Stomachs usually were palpated before calves were moved from the calving barn to the calf-raising barn.

Calves were raised on milk-replacer, the amount given varying according to who was doing the feeding. The teats on all the feeder buckets were slashed, and calves frequently coughed and choked during feeding.

Different antibiotic combinations were given by the calf raiser to virtually all calves with little regard for dosage, periodicity of treatments, or completion of courses. Syringe and needle hygiene were minimal and inconsistent. Calves received *Pasteurella* vaccine whenever about 40 calves *about* 30 days of age accumulated. Dehorning paste also was applied at that time.

The owner was willing to acknowledge that actual calf-raising procedures probably deviated substantially from the routine he believed was followed; but he was not convinced of the value of several well-established procedures you had recommended as the result of these observations. Particularly he doubted the need for *early* colostrum feeding and navel disinfection in preference to use of a polyvalent hyperimmune serum that he had been purchasing for some time. Therefore, you decided to carry out a prospective trial of these alternative procedures, as the first of an eventual series of such trials that, you assumed, would result from your overall program of surveillance and retrospective studies then in progress on this farm.

Design in all details a prospective trial for this farm to compare an early colostrum feeding and prompt navel disinfection regimen with use of the polyvalent serum.

The farm routines were such that, of necessity, the cohorts of calves used in this trial were composed of calves that actually differed as follows:

Cohort I. Fed colostrum and navel disinfected by a veterinary student within six hours of birth; not

Table 12-4.   Results from Trial* of Experimental Modified Live Virus Vaccine "X" Against Calf Diarrhea in Herd 1 in Southern California, November-December, 1974[4]

Treatment	No. calves	A.R. (%) up to 21 days of age	Cause-specific death rate (%) up to 21 days of age
Vaccinated	100	90	10
Not vaccinated	100	90	15

*Calves born on even-numbered days were vaccinated; those born on odd-numbered days were not.

Table 12–5.   Results from Study of Experimental Modified Live Virus Vaccine "X" Against Calf
                Diarrhea in Herd 1 in Southern California, February-March, 1975[4]

Treatment	Time period	No. calves	A.R. (%) up to 21 days of age	Cause-specific death rate (%) up to 21 days of age
Every calf vaccinated	Early Feb.	77*	38	0
No calves vaccinated	Late Feb.	77	51	0
Every calf vaccinated	Early Mar.	77*	25	0

*The compiler of these data included only the last 77 calves vaccinated before the vaccine supply ran out and the first 77 vaccinated when vaccine was again available, presumably because 77 calves had not been vaccinated in the late February interval.

given serum but otherwise subjected to the "normal hit-and-miss" farm routine.

Cohort II. Given polyvalent immune serum by a veterinary student within six hours of birth; otherwise subjected to "normal hit-and-miss" farm routine.

Cohort III. Not given polyvalent serum or colostrum by a student but otherwise subjected to "normal hit-and-miss" farm routine. This group was the comparison or control cohort.

Every third calf born was allocated to each of these three cohorts. *All* calves were *observed* closely during the first six hours after birth to see which actually did receive prompt colostrum and navel dipping at the hands of the farm's calf-rearer. Results of this trial are shown in Table 12–6. Comment on the design of this trial.

Analyze the data and interpret the results. Summarize concisely the information you have derived

Table 12–6A.   Distribution of Calves by Management Procedure and Sex in Three Cohorts for Prospective Trial of Preventive Procedures in California Dairy Herd[5]

	Cohort I	Cohort II	Cohort III
Total calves	25	26	24
Sex of calves			
Males	12	12	12
Females	12	14	11
Unknown sex	1*	—	1*
Colostrum fed within 6 hours of birth	100%	48%	40%
Navel dipped within 6 hours of birth	100%	20%	28%
Birth required assistance			
No (natural birth)	17	18	16
Yes (dystocia)	8	8	7
Unknown	—	—	1

*Animals died during first day of life

Table 12–6B.   Distribution of Calf Deaths by Age for Three Cohorts in Prospective Trial of Preventive Procedures in California Dairy Herd[5]

Age group (days)	Deaths		
	Cohort I	Cohort II	Cohort III
1–7	1	5	5
8–14	1	0	1
15–21	5	1	5
22–28	0	2	1
29–35	0	2	3

from this trial and the expected effects of applying it in practice.

COHORT-TYPE STUDIES PERFORMED WITH EXISTING DATA

The principal disadvantages of prospective cohort studies generally are cost and time. Sometimes, however, *existing* data may be used to define a test cohort and a comparison cohort at some time in the past, and then the cohorts can be followed to determine their morbidity or mortality experience. If this is the case, a cohort study can be carried out retrospectively, quickly, and inexpensively. This approach has been touched upon briefly in the last chapter. Dairy Herd Improvement records or other long-term closed population records may provide sources of suitable data for such purposes.

The following example of this approach is from a study of mortality in California veterinarians.

Mortality in California veterinarians[6]

This study was carried out in 1963. The factor being examined in relation to cause specific mortality was the "occupation of being a veterinarian." The test cohort consisted of all 1725 white male veterinarians who were licensed to practice in California and were residing in California on January 1, 1950. This information was obtained from the State Board of Examiners in Veterinary Medicine. Other information about the individuals in the cohort, including type of practice, was obtained from the American Veterinary Medical Association Directory, local veterinary medical societies, and letters to veterinarians. This cohort was followed until December 31, 1962, and death certificates were obtained for the 148 veterinarians who had died during the study period. Causes of death were coded. Age specific overall mortality rates were calculated for the cohort using person-years; also calculated were cause specific rates and age specific rates by cause for malignancies (overall and by type), cerebral-vascular accidents, heart disease, accidents, and suicides.

The comparison population was all white California males for whom comparable 1960 mortality rates were calculated. (Using these latter rates as standard and the indirect method of age adjustment, expected numbers of deaths, standardized mortality ratios, and age adjusted mortality rates by the preceding causes were determined.) Comparisons of observed and expected deaths among veterinarians revealed a statistically significant decreased overall death risk and a decreased death risk from cerebrovascular accidents. There was a statistically significant increased risk of death from malignant melanoma of the skin and nonsyphilitic aortic and dissecting aneurysms.

SOME REMINDERS

Several important points are first mentioned in Chapter 5 and then illustrated in this chapter and the preceding one. The first point is that both case-control and cohort studies can be visualized and carried out at different population levels, using rather differently conceived units in identifying population samples or groups (as they are called in Chapter 5). For instance, groups to be compared are often made up of individual animals *per se*, such as groups drawn from the individual bulls in a large artificial insemination service; or the groups to be studied could be at the level of "natural groups of groups of individuals," such as groups of multiple-animal mouse cages in an experimental mouse colony. Similarly, the study groups could be broiler houses in a large broiler operation or groups of dairy farm units or herds from a two-county area or groups of counties in a state. In other words, study groups can comprise individuals, herds, or other units.

A second point is that, whatever the level of sampling represented in the identification of study groups intended for analytical studies, groups to be compared must resemble one another in every epidemiologically important regard except the characteristic being studied. Related to this point is the further necessity for the sample groups to be *representative* of the population, that is, unbiased. In addition, the "research instruments" used to detect the responses of interest (e.g., illness, presence of antibodies, and recovery) must be the same for both the study group and the comparison group, and they must be applied with equal thoroughness and skill.

Chapter 13

ANALYTICAL METHODS

THIS chapter briefly introduces some additional analytical methods that are especially suitable for the study of multiple variables. Their initial use often may be the identification (for further study) of candidate determinants of disease frequency. The methods are equally useful for conceptualizing the relationships between variables in complex disease processes (e.g., a "web of causation") and for predicting levels of disease occurrence or other factors.

MULTIPLE REGRESSION

The discussion of regression in Chapter 5 examined the relationship between the dependent (output) variable and the independent (input) variable. Many situations in veterinary practice provoke interest in the relationship between the dependent variable and a set of *two or more* independent variables. In these situations, multiple regression methods might be useful.

One might, for example, be interested in examining the possible causative influence of climatological variables on the neonatal death rate in calves. It is known that the neonatal death rate varies among farms, and by seasons within farms. By using a sufficiently large and detailed array of climatic and meteorological variables, it may be possible to identify particular climatological determinants of mortality in newborn calves for a given geographic region.

In another situation, a veterinarian may wish to be able to predict the value of the dependent variable at some future point in time; e.g., he may be interested in the frequency of disease following some particular combination of circumstances. A third use of multiple regression may be the examination of the influence of a variety of independent variables simultaneously, in order to understand the influence of any one of them, as, for example, their direct or indirect roles as disease determinants.

In general, the multiple linear regression approach is a relatively straightforward generalization of the methods used in simple linear regression. It is assumed that the independent variables, x_1, $x_2, \ldots x_r$, are known exactly, and y is a function of them. The relationship between an observed value of y and the input variables is specified by

$$y = A + B_1 x_1 + \ldots + B_r x_r + e$$

where e, the error term, follows a normal distribution with mean zero and variance σ^2, and the e's are independently distributed for different individuals.

It should be noted that, although the x_i's are called independent variables, they often are related and/or correlated. Because of this confusion in terminology, some authors[1] have recommended the use of the terms *predictor* or *explanatory* variables for the x_i's. The dependent variable, y, may be referred to then as the *criterion* variable.

As in simple linear regression, A is the y intercept. In multiple regression the B's are called partial regression coefficients. When these parameters are estimated, one obtains an equation of the form

$$y = a + b_1 x_1 + \ldots + b_r x_r.$$

The estimates, a, $b_1, \ldots, b_r$, can be obtained in several ways; but with the relatively widespread availability of computers, they are frequently obtained by matrix algebra.

Stepwise multiple regression

Many times in epidemiological studies, one has available a large number of possible explanatory (e.g., possible determinant) variables, some of which may be highly correlated with one another. With such a group of interrelated predictors, it may be difficult to interpret the meaning of the corresponding B's, the partial regression coefficients. For this reason, and also to reduce the number of predictor variables, some strategies have been developed by which the computer automatically selects a "best" subset of predictors. Unfortunately, the definition of *best* varies among computer programs commonly in use, and the criterion for optimality may be quite arbitrary.

One strategy for selecting an optimal subset of explanatory variables is called the *step-up* procedure. In this method, all the *r* simple linear regressions are tried, using only one predictor variable. The "best" of these is chosen, with "best" being defined generally as the simple regression having the highest sum of squares for regression. Following this selection, the remaining explanatory variables are each tried in conjunction with the one variable chosen initially, forming a set of r-1 two-variable regressions. Of these two-variable regressions, the one usually selected as best is the one adding the largest increment to the sum of squares for regression. The process continues in such a stepwise fashion, retaining all variables selected at any previous stage and appending, at each step, one additional variable to the set of predictors already selected. The step-up procedure is halted at that step in which the sum of squares for regression is not increased significantly relative to the residual sum of squares.

There also are *step-down* procedures. They begin with the regression of y on all explanatory variables, and selectively remove nonsignificant predictors in a stepwise fashion. The step-down procedure is halted when all the explanatory variables retained are significant, where "significant" has been defined in various ways for the various stepwise procedures being used.

It should be noted that, if one uses a step-up procedure to construct a regression equation for a particular set of data, and then also uses a step-down procedure to construct a regression equation, the variables retained in the two equations need not be the same. In other words, stepwise procedures need not yield the optimal solution; but, because of their ease of use and rapid calculation, they have become important tools in analytical epidemiology.

To suggest further the value of stepwise multiple regression, suppose there are 10 candidate predictor variables. There would be 10 regressions possible on single variables, 45 possible regressions using two predictors, 120 using three predictors, 210 using four, 252 using five, 210 using six, 120 using seven, 45 using eight predictors, 10 regressions using nine predictors, and the one equation using all 10 predictors. If one were looking for the optimal (in some sense) prediction equation, he would have to examine all $2^{10}-1=1023$ of these equations. In general, with n candidate explanatory variables, an "all regressions" strategy in searching for the equation would require examination of 2^n-1 equations. It is not surprising, therefore, that stepwise procedures using computers have been developed and are being used extensively.

Many existing computer programs for stepwise multiple regression have an added feature built in. For example, in a step-up procedure, at each step the computer program checks whether any one of the variables already selected for inclusion in the prediction set could safely be removed without significantly altering the remaining sets' ability to predict the criterion variable.

STUDY OF DAIRY CALF MORTALITY. The influence of meteorological factors on dairy calf mortality in Tulare County, California, was studied using a multiple regression procedure.[2] The predictor variables used are tabulated (Table 13–1). Due to the nature of the husbandry practices as well as the definite dry and wet seasons in Tulare County, separate analyses were made for these seasons. The results of the regression analyses (Table 13–2) indicated the predictive value of minimum and maximum daily temperatures as well as of various measures of

Table 13–1.   Monthly Weather Statistics Utilized in Study of Calf Mortality Rates in Tulare County, California (January 1, 1968 to June 30, 1973)[2]

Assigned symbol	Monthly weather statistic
T_M	Avg. daily maximal temperature
T_m	Avg. daily minimal temperature
T_A	Avg. daily mean temperature
T_F	No. degrees fluctuation ($T_M - T_m$)
T_{DP}	Avg. daily dew point
D_{32}	No. days $\geq 32°$ C
D_0	No. days $\leq 0°$ C
R	Rainfall (monthly total)
W	Avg. daily wind speed

Table 13–2. Summary and Stepwise Regression of Monthly County Calf Mortality Rates on Weather Data in Tulare County, California (1968-1973)^2

Weather statistic*	Apr. through Sept.			Oct. through Mar.			Nov. through Feb.		
	Summer Avg. temp (C.)	Correlation coefficient	Entry sequence†/ coefficient of determination (r^2)	Winter avg. temp (C.)	Correlation coefficient	Entry sequence†/ coefficient of determination (r^2)	Winter avg. temp (C.)	Correlation coefficient	Entry sequence†/ coefficient of determination (r^2)
T_M	31.1	0.395	3/0.319‡	16.8	-0.160	2/.135	14.1	-0.479	1/0.230‡
T_m	19.8	0.455	1/0.207‡	10.3	0.016	—	4.1	-0.249	6/0.440
T_A	22.7	0.415	2/0.299‡	11.1	-0.111	7/.393	9.1	-0.427	3/0.323
T_F	11.3	0.162	—	6.5	-0.291	1/.085	10.0	-0.468	—
T_{DP}	9.3	0.428	5/0.337‡	5.7	-0.025	6/.388‡	5.3	-0.310	5/0.407
D_{32}	16.3	0.312	4/0.335‡	0.5	-0.003	8/.398	0	—	—
D_0	0	—	—	3.5	0.203	3/.289‡	5.0	0.289	4/0.382
R	0.51	-0.089	—	4.1	0.287	5/.375‡	5.1	0.303	7/0.444
W	12.1	0.111	6/0.339	9.33	0.132	4/.344‡	9.2	0.458	2/0.308

*See Table 13–1 for definitions.

†Refers to the step number at which this variable entered the regression equation

‡Denotes significant F value (P≤0.05)

moisture and air movements. Most important, by examining the wet and dry months separately, the differential effects, by season, were noted.

These results show specifically that, for the summer months, the first five variables entered into the regression equation resulted in statistically significant increases in the coefficient of determination (r^2), to a maximum r^2 of 0.337. Thus, these five variables explained (or predicted) 33.7% of the summer monthly variation in calf mortality rates in Tulare County. Conversely, 66.3% of this mortality variance was *not* explainable by these weather variables.

Furthermore, Table 13–2 shows that the first variable entered into each of the three equations is that having the highest individual correlation with calf mortality (e.g., T_m for the summer). Note, however, that variable two and subsequent variables were not necessarily entered into the equation in descending order of their individual correlations with the calf mortality rate. The reason was explained in the introduction to this section.

The observed mortality rates (Fig. 13–1) in the Tulare study can be compared with the rates that were predicted (Fig. 13–2) by the multiple regression equations. For example, for the summer months (April to September), for this regression equation with the form

$$y = a + b_1x_1 + b_2x_2 + b_3x_3 + b_4x_4 + b_5x_5,$$

y would be the predicted monthly calf mortality rate, x_1 the first variable entered in the regression equation (T_m), x_2 the second variable entered (T_A), and so on to x_5, the fifth and last significant variable entered (T_{DP}). Using the values for a and b_i's for the equation obtained from the multiple regression analysis and inserting the appropriate monthly T_m, T_A, T_M, D_{32}, and T_{DP} values for x_1 through x_5, the predicted monthly calf mortality rates for each of the summer months are calculated (see Fig. 13–2). Although the predicted peaks and valleys in the rates are not as precipitous as those actually observed, the weather variables have predicted reasonably well the times at which high and low mortality rates should have been observed.

Again, what must always be borne in mind when using powerful tools such as stepwise multiple regression is that the various associations demonstrated by these analyses may not be causal ones, may reflect common causes, *or* may be indirectly as well as directly causal. Furthermore, because many of the independent variables examined may themselves be multiply correlated (as will be shown in matrices printed out by most multiple regression computer programs), some of the individual predictor values may be associated with the dependent variable through several pathways. For example, the first predictor variable entered in the calf mortality illustration (see Fig. 13–2) for the winter months

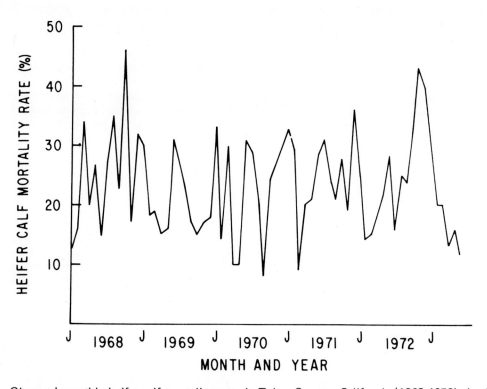

Fig. 13–1. Observed monthly heifer calf mortality rates in Tulare County, California (1968-1973). J = January.[2]

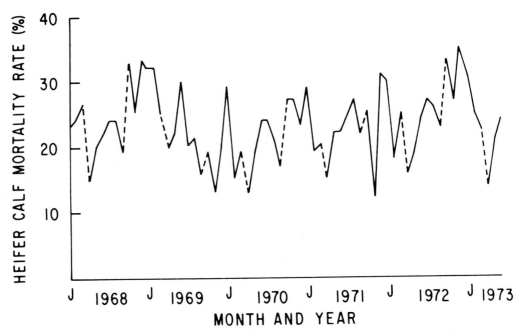

Fig. 13-2. Predicted monthly heifer calf mortality rates in Tulare County, California (1968-1973), calculated
during regression analyses. Dashes emphasize that data from winter and summer months were separately analyzed. J = January.[2]

(November to February) is T_M, average daily maximum temperature. This negative correlation with highest temperature reached in a day alone explains 23% of the variance in wintertime calf mortality rates. One might *reason* that this particular relationship exists overall through at least three main *paths* of action: (1) possible direct effects of cold temperature upon the calf, (2) possible effects of temperature on the transmission of infectious organisms (e.g., direct effect on the free-living survival of microorganisms) and (3) possible effects of cold on the calf tender (e.g., his reluctance to visit calves frequently in cold weather or to spend much time with them on each visit).

Attempts to identify and analyze such pathways, that is, to define a "web of causation," is part of a process of *causal modeling* called *path analysis*.

PATH ANALYSIS

In the words of workers with these techniques in the social sciences, causal modeling "attempts to explain empirical findings in a manner that reflects the total process which the researcher believes underlies the situation under study rather than just the bivariate relationships."[3] This analytical process often involves construction of model diagrams (Fig. 13-3) with calculation of appropriate *path coefficients*. These latter are the standardized regression coefficients when the independent variables are restricted to those that are considered to have a *prior* effect on the dependent variable. Hypothetical examples for weather and calf mortality are shown in Fig. 13-3, while modeling in general is discussed in Chapter 16.

Fig. 13-3. A partial causal model for calf mortality
in the wintertime, showing hypothetical
path coefficients.

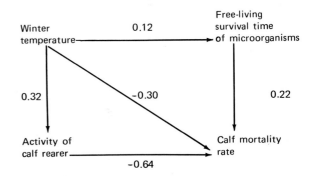

Path analysis adds an important dimension to the standard multiple regression techniques already illustrated. In stepwise multiple regression, epidemiological judgment is limited to the selection of the independent variables that are believed to influence a dependent variable, say, the level of calf mortality. In such studies one learns what correlates with what, which is helpful. Stepwise multiple regression indicates, first, which one of the independent variables is the best predictor of the dependent variable all by itself. Second, it reflects the proportion of the total variance of the dependent variable explained by the independent variables in the regression equation. Although one can visualize something of the nature of the relationships by observing the effects of omitting particular variables from the analyses, standard multiple regression techniques go little further than simply a descriptive or estimation model, one of whose principal uses may be to let one predict certain outcomes before they occur. On the other hand, one's real interest may be in causal relationships, of *how* certain independent variables relate to the dependent variable he is attempting to understand.

Path analysis, therefore, goes beyond standard multiple regression methods to approach the question of how each variable affects other variables in the system. Rather than having the computer decide, on purely statistical grounds, the order that independent variables enter the regression equations, path analysis lets one utilize his epidemiological knowledge and judgmental ability in sequentially ordering the variables in such a way as to resemble the relationships in nature that characterize his system. In other words, he constructs a causal model in which different paths of relationship are diagrammed by unidirectional arrows. Further, he can learn what portion of the total effect of one variable on another may be direct and what portion may be acting indirectly through another variable or variables. Finally, he can determine whether there may be other independent variables not visualized in his system that explain part of the variance of the dependent variable.

For each path in his model, he calculates a standardized numerical value, a positive or negative path coefficient which indicates that, if he were to change the antecedent variable by one standard deviation, he would change the variable at the end of a particular path by that portion of its standard deviation equivalent to the value of the particular path coefficient. This type of model lets him determine the likely effects of changing certain variables without actually carrying out such an experimental cohort study. For example, a causal model of calf mortality constructed by the path analysis of observational data might enable him to predict the effects upon calf mortality rates of increasing the percentage of calves that received adequate amounts of colostrum early enough. In Problem 19 in Chapter 12, you

saw that it would take considerable time and effort to obtain an answer to that particular question through a prospective cohort trial.

Path analysis has been little used for epidemiological studies; but its potential, in conjunction with other approaches such as factor analysis, is great. However, its application is dependent on one's ability to construct realistic path diagrams for his causal model.

The following illustration of path analysis is from a study of the epidemiology and control of hydatid disease in New Zealand.[4] A more detailed discussion of this tool is given in Nie *et al.*[3]

Determinants of prevalence level of *Echinococcus granulosus* infections in New Zealand

New Zealand is one of very few countries to successfully control hydatid disease. Preliminary to an attempt to understand variables within New Zealand that contributed locally to rapid and slow progress in control, an effort was made to understand why the precontrol program levels of *Echinococcus* prevalence in dogs varied considerably from one area of New Zealand to another.

Starting with some knowledge of the biology of the parasite, the epidemiology of the disease, and the patterns of animal husbandry in New Zealand, stepwise multiple regression methods were used in preliminary studies on hypothesized determinants of *Echinococcus* prevalence. From these preliminary analyses, several tentative causal models were constructed to indicate the modes of action—the pathways—of possible direct and indirect determinants of prevalence. One of these models for the North Island of New Zealand is shown in Figure 13–4. The variables used in this model were:

(1) Exogenous (predetermined) variables

Climate:　Mean daily maximum temperature in °C. for complete year

　　　　　Mean daily maximum temperature in °C. for hottest month only

　　　　　Mean daily % relative humidity

　　　　　Mean daily run of wind in kilometers

　　　　　Annual hours of bright sunshine

　　　　　Annual millimeters of rainfall

Altitude:　% of area above 300 meters

Soil:　% of surface soils of high porosity

Maori:　% of Maoris in the human population

Feral pigs:　Relative population density

Feral goats:　Relative population density

(2) Endogenous (dependent) variables

Pasture:　% of grazing area containing native unimproved grasses

% sheep farms:　% of farms obtaining at least 50% of their income from sheep production

Area per farm:　Mean grazing area in hectares per farm

Sheep per farm:　Mean number of sheep per farm

Sheep per hectare: Measure of relative sheep density
Rabbits: Relative population density
Dogs per farm: Mean number of working dogs per farm
Dogs per owner: Mean number of working dogs per working dog owner
Economics: % of rural male wage earners earning more than the median rural male income for New Zealand
Initial canine prevalence rate: % of fecal samples infected with *Echinococcus granulosus* during the first complete testing round (1959-1960)

The model shown in Figure 13–4 is simplified for clarity of presentation. Each variable enters the causal pathway as indicated by a unidirectional arrow leading from that variable. Once entered, the variable is considered to have an effect on *every other variable added subsequent to it,* except those exogenous (predetermined) variables on the extreme left of the model (i.e., climate, altitude, soil, Maoris, feral pigs, feral goats). No attempt is made to explain the variability in these exogenous variables.

Initially, the first path in the causal model is examined by regressing pasture on climate, altitude, and soil. From this multiple regression, path coefficients are obtained from each independent variable to the dependent variable, pasture. The next intervening variable in the model, % sheep farms, is now used as the dependent variable and is regressed on all prior variables (i.e., climate, altitude, soil, and pasture). This procedure is repeated, adding intervening endogenous (dependent) variables individually in sequence until the final "effect," initial canine prevalence rate, is added as a dependent variable. All the variables are present in this final multiple regression analysis; and a correlation matrix, showing the zero-order correlation coefficients for every pair of variables in the model is obtained.

A correlation coefficient expresses the degree of linear relationship between two variables and can be considered a measure of their *total association.* This total association is composed of a direct effect, indirect effects, and "spurious" effects. The *direct effect* of one variable on another is that effect which is not transmitted via intervening variables and which remains when all other variables have been held constant. It is measured by the path coefficient. The *indirect effects* are those that are transmitted through intervening variables; each is given by the product of the path coefficients in the appropriate indirect path. Finally, the *spurious effects* are those due to the joint dependence of the variables on common causes and correlations among the antecedent variables; they equal simply the correlation coefficient minus the direct and indirect effects.

Using the preceding method of decomposition of effects in path analysis, not only can important causal pathways in the model be identified, but also the effects of manipulation of individual variables can be estimated. Extracts from the data from the New Zealand study, given in Table 13-3, can be used to illustrate the utility of path analysis as an epidemiological tool. The total association between the variables in Table 13–3 and initial prevalence can be broken down as follows:

(1) Maori: completely due to a direct effect.

(2) Maximum temperature for year: due to a negative indirect effect mediated primarily through % sheep farms and counteracting positive "spurious" effects.

(3) % sheep farms: mainly due to a large positive direct effect and a small indirect effect via sheep per hectare.

(4) Sheep per hectare: due to a positive direct effect and large negative "spurious" effects.

From these examples, it can be seen that no other variables have any effect on the relationship between

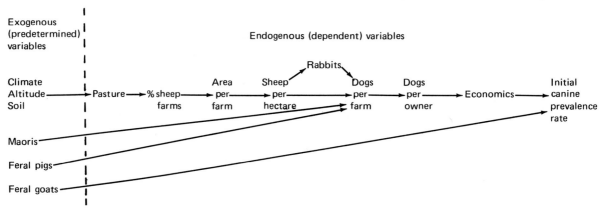

Fig. 13–4. Simplified causal model used for path analytic studies of variables responsible for differences in initial prevalence levels of *Echinococcus granulosus* in dogs among hydatid control districts of the North Island of New Zealand.[4]

Table 13-3.   Selected Path Analysis Data from Study of Variables Responsible for Differences in Initial Prevalence Levels of *Echinococcus granulosus* in Dogs Among Hydatid Control Areas on the North Island of New Zealand.[4]

Antecedent variable	Correlation coefficient with initial prevalence (r) (total effect)	Decomposition of correlation coefficient r		
		Direct effect or path coefficient (p)	Indirect effects (i)	"Spurious" effects (r−p−i)
Maori	0.46	0.46	−0.02	0.02
Temp. for year (max.)	−0.17	−0.05	−0.61	0.49
Sheep farms (%)	0.71	0.80	−0.21	0.12
Sheep per hectare	−0.50	0.33	−0.03	−0.80

Maoris and initial prevalence. In contrast, if % sheep farms were to be manipulated (e.g., by changing the pattern of livestock production in New Zealand), the indirect effect of "maximum temperature for year on initial prevalence" would be altered, and the magnitude of this alteration could be calculated. To control echinococcosis, the aims would be to maximize the negative direct and indirect effects on prevalence of *E. granulosus* and to minimize the positive effects. Path analysis provides a methodology whereby the effects of realistic manipulation of variables can be visualized.

FACTOR ANALYSIS

Factor analysis, another multivariate technique, is useful in explaining observed relations among a large number of variables in terms of simpler relations. In other words, it is particularly useful in studying the underlying structure of a set of data. In factor analysis, if two variables are measuring the same quantitative entity, these variables can be combined and studied together. Mathematically, factor analysis is useful in ascertaining the normal multivariate structure underlying a statistical universe that can be sampled with respect to numerous correlated variables.

As a statistical technique, factor analysis can be used to reduce large numbers of correlated variables to terms of a small number of uncorrelated variables. Naturally, these uncorrelated variables (called factors) are abstract hypothetical components. Factor analysis is a method for classifying variables or manifestations; and, in this statistical methodology, it is frequently desirable to group manifestations (variables) with respect to observed clusters of correlations existing among these manifestations. Each such cluster of closely correlated variables may be called a surface trait or syndrome, speaking nonmedically.

Factor analysis has particular appeal to epidemiologists because it is one of very few methods that facilitate assessing what would happen through manipulation or experimentation, when for various reasons manipulation is impossible. In particular, this method is useful in elucidating information from survey results preparatory to more detailed study. Factor analytic studies have been performed in several areas of biology, and social scientists have found this research methodology very productive. Because epidemiologists and veterinary practitioners often must deal with human variables (e.g., manager factors) as well as with strictly veterinary (i.e., animal or biomedical) variables, factor analysis is a particularly attractive technique. To illustrate the method, data from a survey of diarrhea in dairy calves have been factor analyzed.[5]

Diarrhea in dairy calves

Dairy farms in San Joaquin and Tulare counties in California were surveyed in June, 1969, attempting to ascertain whether various management factors may have been related to diarrheal problems in calves on farms in these counties. The questions considered to be critical (Table 13-4) and the correlations among answers are indicated in the tabulated material (Table 13-5). Results from preliminary analyses had indicated that the data from the two counties should be analyzed separately because of (1) differences in major causes of calf diarrhea between the two counties' farms, and (2) wide differences in management and husbandry practices between the two counties. In particular, the onset of diarrhea usually occurred at an earlier age in calves of San Joaquin County than in calves of Tulare County, vaccination practices and use of veterinary services differed among farms between the two counties, and feeding practices and general uses and procedures for medication differed between the two counties.

The results of factor analysis of the data from each county indicated that about 13 factors accounted for 80% of the "information" in the original 39 variables, or 21 factors accounted for about 95% of the total variance among farms in each county (Table 13-6). The *structure* of these factors (the hypothetical constructs) is usually interesting, so the pattern for

Table 13–4.   Variables (Questions) Used for Factor Analysis of Diarrhea in Dairy Calves (Data Collected from Farms in San Joaquin and Tulare Counties, California, June 1969)[5]

No.	Variables Grouping	Identification (and answers)
1	Seasonal problems	Winter (yes, no)
2		Spring (yes, no)
3		Summer (yes, no)
4		Fall (yes, no)
5		At what age is calf removed from dam?
6		Is colostrum fed to calves (yes, no)?
7	Calving site	Maternity stall (yes, no)
8		Corral (yes, no)
9		Field (yes, no)
10		Housing (type of pen) used for calf (coded)
11	Type of bedding used	Shavings (yes, no)
12		Straw (yes, no)
13		Sawdust (yes, no)
14		How frequently are pens cleaned (coded)?
15		How frequently are pens disinfected (coded)?
16		Is the temperature controlled where calves are housed (yes, no)?
17	Source of milk used to feed calves	Hospital string (yes, no)
18		Milk string (yes, no)
19		Replacer (yes, no)
20		Calf feeding (frequency per day)
21		Calf feeding device (automatic, bottle, bucket)
22*		Is milk warmed before it is fed to calf (yes, no)?
23		Is hot water used to warm milk (yes, no)?
24	Age at which calf has access to	Water
25		Grain
26		Hay
27		Treatment begun immediately (time)
28		Do you have a program of preventive treatment for diarrhea in calves (yes, no)?
29		Do you segregate sick calves from healthy calves (yes, no)?
30	Vaccination	IBR vaccine (yes, no)
31		BVD vaccine (yes, no)
32		Leptospirosis vaccine (yes, no)
33		Mastitis vaccine (yes, no)
34		Is cow fed grain before calving (yes, no)?
35		Is vitamin A additive used (yes, no)?
36		Are mineral additives used (yes, no)?
37		Is umbilicus treated (yes, no)?
38		Farm size in 1968 (by code 1, 2, 3, 4)
39†		Parainfluenza vaccine (yes, no)

*All Tulare County dairy farmers interviewed heat all milk that is to be fed to calves.

†Parainfluenza vaccine data used only for Tulare County analysis; only two San Joaquin farmers used parainfluenza vaccine.

the 13 most important factors is detailed (Table 13–7). This pattern, known as a factor matrix, is a table of coefficients expressing the relationship between the observable manifestations (variables) and the underlying factors. These coefficients, called factor loadings, express the correlations between the manifestations and the factors.

Careful study of these factor loadings (see Table 13–7) is informative, but can be very difficult. However, interpretation of factors and various interrelationships can be made more easily if the factor matrix is rotated so that (1) each column of the rotated matrix has at least as many loadings that are approximately zero as there are factors; (2) each row

Table 13–5.   Correlation Matrices in Factor Analysis of Calves in San Joaquin and Tulare Counties, California, 1970[5]

San Joaquin Data

Var. No.*	1	2	3	4	5	6	7	8	9	10	11	12	13	14	15	16	17	18	19	20	21	22	23	24	25	26	27	28	29	30	31	32	33	34	35	36	37	38
1	1.0																																					
2	-0.42	1.0																																				
3	-0.88	-0.06	1.0																																			
4	-0.42	-0.03	0.48	1.0																																	
5	-0.04	-0.02	0.05	-0.02	1.0																																
6	0.19	-0.08	-0.17	-0.08	-0.05	1.0																															
7	0.09	-0.04	-0.08	-0.04	0.09	-0.02	1.0																														
8	0.28	-0.18	-0.21	0.15	-0.01	0.11	-0.26	1.0																													
9	-0.19	0.15	0.14	-0.18	-0.06	-0.01	0.11	-0.60	1.0																												
10	-0.04	0.10	-0.01	-0.11	0.0	0.15	-0.15	-0.33	0.38	1.0																											
11	-0.04	0.15	-0.04	0.0	0.04	0.0	0.01	0.17	0.57	-0.28	1.0																										
12	0.01	-0.08	0.03	-0.08	0.07	0.01	0.22	0.02	0.06	-0.15	-0.32	1.0																									
13	-0.04	-0.07	0.09	-0.12	-0.15	-0.06	-0.10	-0.19	-0.15	-0.10	-0.32	-0.57	1.0																								
14	-0.21	0.45	0.0	0.07	0.0	0.14	-0.07	-0.24	0.10	0.23	-0.06	-0.14	-0.05	1.0																							
15	0.08	-0.16	0.0	0.15	0.16	0.03	0.04	0.16	0.05	-0.13	0.05	0.10	0.02	-0.29	1.0																						
16	0.18	-0.08	0.15	-0.08	-0.05	0.02	-0.26	0.04	0.29	-0.12	0.11	-0.15	0.08	0.30	0.07	1.0																					
17	-0.03	0.22	-0.03	-0.13	0.35	0.12	-0.26	0.04	-0.12	-0.22	0.06	0.19	0.16	-0.25	0.07	0.07	1.0																				
18	0.09	-0.26	0.03	0.10	-0.28	-0.01	-0.17	0.07	0.03	0.24	0.03	-0.24	-0.08	0.30	-0.21	-0.22	-0.47	1.0																			
19	0.04	0.18	-0.14	-0.15	0.01	0.19	0.22	0.01	0.36	-0.11	0.14	-0.24	0.05	-0.16	0.03	0.15	-0.14	-0.13	1.0																		
20	0.10	0.20	-0.09	-0.04	0.04	0.11	0.02	0.13	0.06	-0.02	-0.24	0.17	0.21	-0.04	0.16	0.06	-0.02	0.04	0.17	1.0																		
21	-0.23	0.10	0.20	-0.17	-0.06	0.12	-0.17	0.05	0.24	0.06	-0.07	-0.06	0.21	-0.01	0.02	0.03	-0.05	0.13	0.0	0.02	1.0																	
22†	-0.06	0.03	0.06	-0.06	0.03	-0.10	-0.06	0.14	-0.02	0.07	0.15	0.15	0.10	-0.02	0.15	0.16	0.17	0.10	0.0	0.02	-0.64	1.0																
23	0.27	-0.26	-0.16	0.16	0.10	0.02	-0.26	0.04	0.04	0.05	0.11	0.06	-0.15	0.07	0.06	0.08	0.08	-0.22	-0.17	0.07	0.04	0.04	1.0															
24	-0.21	0.16	0.15	0.10	0.10	0.19	-0.11	-0.15	0.16	0.0	0.06	-0.22	-0.11	0.16	0.22	-0.15	0.30	-0.19	0.23	0.18	-0.10	-0.09	0.26	1.0														
25	0.0	0.42	0.16	-0.05	-0.10	-0.01	-0.30	0.13	0.20	-0.19	-0.07	0.20	-0.10	0.28	0.28	-0.41	0.05	0.20	0.31	0.13	0.0	0.13	0.13	0.12	1.0													
26	0.24	0.10	-0.03	0.02	0.03	0.14	0.07	-0.02	0.07	0.06	0.06	0.08	0.07	0.05	0.43	-0.33	0.17	0.05	0.0	0.05	-0.17	0.20	0.07	0.17	0.11	1.0												
27	0.18	-0.32	0.19	0.12	-0.16	-0.01	-0.08	0.01	0.01	0.01	0.01	-0.19	0.27	-0.13	0.06	0.13	0.08	-0.18	0.24	-0.05	-0.22	0.11	0.32	0.24	0.23	-0.02	1.0											
28	-0.10	-0.16	-0.28	-0.20	0.19	0.09	0.01	0.13	0.11	0.12	0.01	-0.11	0.17	0.11	0.13	0.11	-0.18	0.08	-0.15	-0.10	-0.10	-0.23	0.16	0.14	-0.05	0.10	0.23	1.0										
29	0.42	-0.35	0.19	-0.35	0.05	0.09	0.26	0.38	0.16	0.12	-0.02	0.08	0.02	0.0	0.0	0.07	0.05	0.08	0.0	0.02	0.14	0.30	-0.08	0.30	0.02	0.05	0.59	0.18	1.0									
30	0.23	-0.16	-0.28	-0.16	0.0	0.27	0.26	0.38	0.16	-0.05	-0.13	0.0	0.0	0.0	-0.29	0.26	0.07	0.22	0.16	0.16	-0.17	-0.06	-0.16	-0.17	-0.12	0.22	0.13	0.32	0.32	1.0								
31	0.04	0.04	-0.16	0.04	0.08	0.22	0.22	0.05	0.11	0.04	0.04	0.15	0.19	0.13	0.17	0.17	0.15	0.31	0.13	0.19	0.34	0.15	0.10	0.13	0.09	0.29	-0.11	0.07	0.31	0.58	1.0							
32	-0.01	0.08	-0.13	-0.03	0.08	-0.13	0.12	-0.11	0.23	-0.08	-0.11	-0.08	-0.13	0.10	0.22	0.28	-0.09	-0.11	-0.19	0.20	-0.08	-0.27	0.18	-0.04	0.13	0.18	0.24	0.02	0.23	0.52	0.33	1.0						
33	0.14	0.22	0.16	0.08	-0.03	-0.13	0.12	-0.27	-0.07	0.14	0.01	-0.09	-0.19	-0.13	0.28	0.31	0.15	-0.27	0.13	0.13	0.34	-0.07	0.10	0.0	0.12	0.31	0.24	0.04	-0.07	-0.08	-0.14	0.13	1.0					
34	-0.09	-0.10	0.04	-0.13	0.26	-0.07	0.11	-0.07	0.11	0.01	0.01	-0.19	-0.12	-0.09	0.05	-0.20	-0.10	-0.20	-0.12	-0.11	0.15	0.0	-0.10	-0.10	0.0	-0.11	0.04	-0.02	0.0	-0.20	0.24	0.04	-0.13	1.0				
35	0.18	-0.08	-0.13	-0.08	-0.12	-0.23	0.15	-0.25	0.16	0.01	0.15	0.09	0.06	-0.21	0.06	-0.20	-0.03	-0.17	-0.15	-0.15	0.06	0.10	0.30	-0.14	0.09	-0.25	-0.29	-0.04	0.23	0.15	0.17	-0.25	-0.22	-0.15	1.0			
36	-0.07	-0.11	-0.04	-0.12	-0.13	-0.22	0.16	-0.22	0.16	-0.07	-0.07	-0.16	-0.21	-0.14	-0.11	0.15	-0.03	0.18	0.15	0.07	-0.18	0.10	-0.04	0.06	0.13	-0.40	-0.16	-0.04	0.32	0.23	-0.16	-0.07	-0.40	-0.06	0.55	1.0		
37	0.12	-0.18	-0.04	-0.04	-0.18	-0.22	0.15	-0.25	0.15	0.04	0.04	-0.18	-0.05	-0.05	0.15	0.16	-0.17	0.36	0.36	0.17	0.0	0.05	0.29	0.01	0.13	0.29	0.05	0.05	0.26	-0.16	-0.04	0.05	-0.08	-0.01	0.43	0.61	1.0	
38	-0.06	0.12	0.0	-0.08	-0.04	-0.28	0.16	-0.29	0.16	0.11	0.11	-0.12	0.01	0.04	-0.02	0.03	0.02	-0.07	0.21	0.0	0.03	-0.07	-0.02	-0.02	0.21	-0.20	-0.01	-0.01	-0.07	-0.16	0.10	0.12	-0.02	-0.38	0.16	0.12	0.21	1.0
39†																																						

Table 13–5.   Correlation Matrices in Factor Analysis of Calves in San Joaquin and Tulare Counties, California, 1970[5]   (Continued)

Tulare Data

Var. No.	1	2	3	4	5	6	7	8	9	10	11	12	13	14	15	16	17	18	19	20	21	23	24	25	26	27	28	29	30	31	32	33	34	35	36	37	38	39
1	1.0																																					
2	-0.24	1.0																																				
3	-0.57	-0.06	1.0																																			
4	-0.24	-0.03	0.42	1.0																																		
5	-0.18	-0.18	0.15	0.06	1.0																																	
6	-0.24	-0.03	-0.06	-0.03	-0.18	1.0																																
7	0.23	-0.06	-0.13	-0.06	0.13	-0.06	1.0																															
8	-0.06	0.10	0.08	0.10	-0.42	0.10	-0.54	1.0																														
9	-0.02	-0.09	-0.03	-0.09	0.40	-0.09	0.01	-0.74	1.0																													
10	0.02	-0.13	0.25	0.08	-0.13	0.08	-0.05	-0.03	0.12	1.0																												
11	0.14	-0.07	-0.17	-0.07	0.17	-0.07	0.56	-0.36	0.10	0.22	1.0																											
12	-0.23	0.16	0.39	0.16	0.0	-0.16	-0.17	-0.19	-0.30	-0.43		1.0																										
13	0.29	-0.07	-0.17	-0.07	0.12	-0.15	0.10	0.03	-0.19	0.03	0.05	-0.09	1.0																									
14	-0.33	0.06	0.14	0.06	-0.27	0.47	0.09	0.04	0.27	0.05	0.04	0.0	-0.21	1.0																								
15	-0.07	-0.13	0.19	-0.13	-0.03	-0.13	-0.11	0.09	0.04	0.11	0.27	0.0	-0.19	-0.19	1.0																							
16	-0.01	-0.05	0.17	-0.05	0.11	-0.05	0.19	-0.16	-0.23	0.19	-0.03	0.14	-0.03	-0.06	-0.02	1.0																						
17	-0.02	-0.28	-0.12	0.10	0.19	-0.07	0.10	0.01	0.21	0.03	-0.07	0.10	-0.05	-0.07	-0.04	-0.05	1.0																					
18	-0.04	0.15	0.04	-0.18	-0.19	-0.04	0.01	-0.12	0.19	0.10	-0.04	0.24	0.0	0.0	0.09	0.24	-0.54	1.0																				
19	0.18	-0.08	-0.18	-0.08	0.49	-0.08	0.06	-0.15	0.0	-0.05	0.07	-0.02	0.11	0.06	-0.13	-0.05	0.10	-0.23	1.0																			
20	-0.24	-0.03	-0.06	-0.03	-0.08	-0.03	-0.15	0.09	-0.26	0.21	0.30	-0.06	-0.05	-0.26	0.31	-0.18	0.47	-0.16	-0.08	1.0																		
21	0.15	0.09	0.03	0.09	-0.13	0.03	-0.30	-0.01	-0.08	0.21	0.08	0.24	0.07	0.04	0.04	0.07	-0.33	0.10	-0.18	-0.30	1.0																	
23†	0.19	-0.18	0.04	0.15	-0.04	0.15	-0.04	-0.11	0.13	0.02	-0.19	0.07	0.10	0.10	0.02	0.05	0.06	0.12	-0.06	-0.12	0.15	1.0																
24	0.20	0.14	-0.31	-0.26	0.15	-0.10	0.05	0.08	-0.16	-0.11	0.05	-0.19	-0.02	0.01	-0.13	-0.06	-0.01	-0.06	0.01	0.15	0.04	0.09	1.0															
25	-0.01	0.08	-0.06	-0.13	-0.05	0.13	0.24	-0.13	0.03	-0.05	0.10	0.08	0.18	0.06	0.03	0.24	0.19	0.04	0.03	0.19	0.17	0.13	0.34	1.0														
26	0.03	0.26	-0.16	-0.28	-0.07	0.08	0.21	-0.20	0.07	-0.07	0.03	-0.07	0.17	0.24	0.17	0.01	-0.03	0.13	0.01	-0.03	-0.08	-0.20	0.07	0.07	1.0													
27	-0.16	0.04	0.09	-0.15	0.13	0.04	0.13	-0.20	-0.14	0.03	0.10	-0.14	-0.06	-0.22	-0.06	0.28	-0.05	0.03	0.04	-0.11	-0.11	-0.21	-0.11	-0.11	-0.02	1.0												
28	0.26	0.13	0.0	0.13	-0.08	0.13	-0.08	0.28	-0.16	-0.08	0.21	-0.09	-0.24	-0.09	0.11	-0.24	-0.36	-0.24	-0.03	0.03	0.06	0.03	-0.28	-0.11	-0.04	0.05	1.0											
29	0.24	0.06	-0.08	-0.42	-0.38	0.06	0.13	0.09	-0.15	-0.04	0.10	0.05	0.11	-0.20	0.10	0.17	0.11	-0.04	-0.02	0.15	0.15	-0.19	0.09	-0.11	-0.11	-0.09	-0.16	1.0										
30	0.15	0.11	-0.07	0.07	-0.24	0.11	0.23	-0.18	0.11	-0.03	0.02	0.0	-0.01	-0.04	0.06	-0.05	0.24	-0.04	-0.03	0.30	0.0	0.18	0.36	0.06	0.0	-0.20	-0.08	0.26	1.0									
31	0.03	0.13	0.08	0.10	-0.20	0.08	0.07	-0.26	0.08	0.07	0.14	-0.06	0.28	-0.17	0.24	0.01	0.01	-0.03	-0.03	0.23	0.05	0.03	-0.13	0.05	-0.10	0.02	0.09	0.23	0.07	1.0								
32	0.07	0.10	-0.11	0.09	-0.05	0.10	0.02	-0.05	0.07	0.02	0.23	-0.01	0.30	-0.10	0.13	0.06	0.28	-0.09	-0.03	0.36	-0.07	0.18	-0.06	0.06	0.02	0.07	0.32	0.24	-0.08	0.43	1.0							
33	0.20	0.10	-0.06	-0.05	-0.10	0.11	-0.10	-0.02	-0.05	-0.10	0.09	0.14	0.23	-0.13	0.18	0.07	0.02	-0.05	-0.15	0.18	0.05	0.13	-0.17	-0.02	0.09	0.02	0.24	0.24	0.11	0.04	0.19	1.0						
34	0.15	-0.10	-0.13	-0.10	0.23	0.23	0.18	-0.28	0.37	-0.28	0.23	-0.20	0.07	0.09	-0.28	0.36	0.31	0.31	0.36	-0.16	0.19	-0.24	-0.06	-0.02	0.24	0.02	-0.13	0.28	0.41	0.24	0.25	0.05	1.0					
35	0.05	-0.13	-0.06	-0.06	0.20	-0.12	-0.12	0.22	-0.15	-0.14	0.01	0.0	-0.06	-0.01	0.25	0.02	0.05	0.09	-0.20	-0.31	0.09	-0.24	0.04	0.04	0.03	0.17	0.28	0.13	0.01	-0.05	0.25	-0.10	-0.20	1.0				
36	-0.23	0.48	-0.12	-0.13	0.23	0.20	0.23	-0.25	0.22	-0.14	0.30	-0.06	-0.01	-0.06	0.02	0.25	-0.32	-0.27	-0.20	0.23	-0.12	-0.24	0.04	0.03	-0.06	0.17	0.28	0.01	-0.05	-0.23	-0.10	0.09	-0.21	0.07	1.0			
37	-0.11	0.23	-0.12	-0.06	0.03	0.23	0.48	-0.25	-0.21	-0.06	-0.01	-0.06	-0.16	0.07	0.22	0.02	-0.01	0.45	0.23	-0.22	-0.01	0.06	0.23	-0.06	-0.13	0.25	0.30	0.19	0.25	0.09	-0.01	0.27	0.20	0.48	0.11	1.0		
38	0.23	-0.11	-0.13	-0.11	-0.32	0.17	-0.25	0.13	-0.21	-0.13	0.16	0.21	0.07	-0.44	0.18	-0.07	-0.27	-0.27	-0.22	-0.04	0.36	0.06	-0.06	0.23	0.28	-0.06	0.30	0.19	0.11	0.53	0.55	0.49	0.11	0.39	-0.02	0.21	1.0	
39*	-0.04	-0.16	-0.06	-0.06	0.17	0.06	0.17	0.02	-0.03	-0.13	0.02	0.21	-0.27	0.03	-0.07	0.21	0.03	-0.04	-0.04	-0.16	-0.09	0.22	-0.02	-0.14	-0.06	-0.01	0.01	-0.16	-0.10	-0.01	0.53	-0.01	0.11	-0.15	0.20	0.01	0.03	1.0
Var. No.	1	2	3	4	5	6	7	8	9	10	11	12	13	14	15	16	17	18	19	20	21	23	24	25	26	27	28	29	30	31	32	33	34	35	36	37	38	39

*See Table 13-4 for identification of variables.
†Variable 39 was not used for San Joaquin data; variable 22 was not used for Tulare data.

Table 13–6. Latent Roots (Eigenvalues) for Principal-Components Factor Analysis of Data Collected from Dairy Farms in San Joaquin County and Tulare County, California, June 1969[5]

	San Joaquin County			Tulare County	
Root no.	Latent root	Cumulative proportion of total variance	Root no.	Latent root	Cumulative proportion of total variance
1	4.35	0.115	1	4.34	0.114
2	3.71	0.212	2	4.08	0.222
3	3.24	0.297	3	3.19	0.306
4	3.06	0.378	4	2.84	0.380
5	2.67	0.448	5	2.19	0.438
6	2.09	0.503	6	2.12	0.494
7	1.92	0.554	7	2.08	0.549
8	1.84	0.602	8	1.70	0.593
9	1.69	0.647	9	1.65	0.637
10	1.63	0.690	10	1.56	0.678
11	1.45	0.728	11	1.44	0.716
12	1.30	0.762	12	1.32	0.751
13	1.25	0.795	13	1.23	0.783
14	1.08	0.823	14	1.11	0.812
15	1.00	0.850	15	0.93	0.837
16	0.78	0.870	16	0.87	0.859
17	0.69	0.889	17	0.78	0.880
18	0.57	0.904	18	0.75	0.900
19	0.57	0.919	19	0.58	0.915
20	0.54	0.933	20	0.54	0.929
21	0.45	0.945	21	0.50	0.942
22	0.35	0.954	22	0.41	0.953
23	0.33	0.962	23	0.39	0.963
24	0.30	0.970	24	0.30	0.971
25	0.26	0.977	25	0.26	0.978

has at least one loading equal to or approximately zero; (3) for each pair of factors, there will be several variables (manifestations) with nonzero loadings in one factor but not in the other; (4) for every pair of factors within the factor matrix, there will be very few variables with nonzero loadings in both factors; and (5) if more than three factors occur, a large proportion of the variables should have negligible loadings on any pair of factors.

These criteria require as many pure variables as possible in the rotated factor matrix, and have been built into most computer programs used for factor analysis.[6] The rotated factor matrices for San Joaquin and Tulare data are given in Table 13–8. Looking for common elements among the observable manifestations within each hypothetical factor, ro-

tated factors in San Joaquin's data were labeled as source of milk, vaccination and antibodies, season of birth I, calving site I, season of birth II, diet/feed additives, calf feeding practices, calving site II, food temperature, pen disinfection, vaccination II, housing/temperature, and bedding. The structure of factors in the Tulare data also indicated the importance of vaccination practices, source of milk fed to calves, calving site, season of birth, bedding, calf-dam interactions, housing temperature, vaccination and antibodies, housing and bedding, pen cleaning, and treatment of infected calves. These analyses, based on the results of surveys, indicated a need for further studies on the use of vaccines, in the control of dehydration, and management aspects of diet, hygiene, and housing.

Table 13–7.   Principal Factor Pattern* (Data Collected from 33 Farms in San Joaquin County and 38 Farms in Tulare County, California)[5]

San Joaquin County

Category	Variable†	I	II	III	IV	V	VI	VII	VIII	IX	X	XI	XII	XIII
Season	1	47		-56		-53								
	2	-43	34		-35									
	3			44	77									
	4			45	42	-36								
	5		-33								32		33	
Calving site	6			-35				46		-46	40			
	7			-37					61		-32			
	8	63		55										
	9	-34			-34		43			41				
	10	-49							-39					
Type of bedding	11			31	67				-32					
	12	-35		-41	-47									-35
	13				-45							-36		55
	14	-55						-49	-34					
	15	42									59			
Source of milk for calves	16	30			41				30				-58	
	17	-36		-38				-44	-32					
	18	42	-32	46			-41							
	19						46			-42				
	20	38	39				-34	-37			-41			
Age at access to	21	-45			44		30							
	22		-31		-31			-42					-44	
	23		-38		-39		-42			-39				
(Water)	24			62	-50									
(Grain)	25	-46				-52				-31				
(Hay)	26	41				-35								
	27		-37	-42							31			
	28	39			-48	38								
	29		-37	-50										35
Vaccination	30	51	56	-31										
	31	38	43				34			31				
	32		49							-30				
	33		51			-49								
	34				32	42		-43						
Feed additives	35		-73								-34			
	36		-69				45							
	37	57	-42				39							
	38			33					-38			-54		

Table 13–7.   Principal Factor Pattern* (Data Collected from 33 Farms in San Joaquin County and 38 Farms in Tulare County, California)[5] (Continued)

Variable[†]		I	II	III	IV	V	VI	VII	VIII	IX	X	XI	XII	XIII
								Factor						

Tulare County

	Variable	I	II	III	IV	V	VI	VII	VIII	IX	X	XI	XII	XIII
Season	1		-43	43	-50									
	2								-35	52				
	3			-52	33		32							
	4			-48					37					-46
	5	-55	34		34			39						
Calving site	6		34					-52			-39			
	7	-48						-47						
	8	65		-38										
	9	-47		38				32						31
	10			33							-63			
Type of bedding	11	-32	-37	45	32									
	12			-74										
	13			33					36	31				31
	14		64					-35						
	15		-31		31							30		32
Source of milk for calves	16						61	33	-33					
	17	-50	37		-30	41			30					
	18		-55		40									
	19			46		52		42						
	20		57				-42							
Age at access to Water Grain Hay	21		-49			-41							43	
	22													
	23				-45	-41	-35							
	24		-32									47		
	25	47					-41					-33		
	26					48	-36							
	27				49				-33				40	
	28		-54										-43	
	29		-33				45		-39					
Vacci- nation	30	-63	-37	-33										
	31	-59	-35							35				
	32	-47	-42	-54										
	33					41		37		39				
	34	-57									-42			
Feed additives	35	39	-36		38					48				
	36				54			-50	36					
	37	40			35	44								
	38		-67								-43		30	30
	39	-51		-40										

*Factor loadings are coefficients expressing the correlation between factors and variables constituting them. Only factor loadings numerically greater than 0.30 are used, but decimal points have been dropped. Other researchers also have used 0.30 as the cutoff value for reporting factor loadings, usually to simplify the structure of the tables used for such reporting. Some cutoff value is necessary for simplification (and significance); 0.30 has been used by others, and pragmatically, a sample of 38 pairs of observations requires an observed coefficient of correlation approximately 0.3 to call it significant at P = 0.05 level.

†See Table 13-4 for identification of variables.

Table 13–8.　　Rotated Factor Matrices, 13 Factors* (Data Collected from 33 Farms in San Joaquin County and 38 Farms in Tulare County, California)[5]

Variable No.†	I	II	III	IV	V	VI	VII	VIII	IX	X	XI	XII	XIII
					Rotated factor								
					San Joaquin County								
1			-29	10	-92								
2		89			11								
3			-14		95								
4				20	42	-14				13			
5	-15					-11	11						
6		87			-12	-18			15			-12	-15
7							93			-11		-11	
8				66	-20	16		-29	13			-17	-14
9				-93				-17	11				
10	-10			-22								12	
11				27		26	10	-30	10				-45
12				-15		-10		10				12	
13		-11											96
14	-12		23						-18	-14		13	
15									-12	92			
16	11				-12							-92	-11
17	-85	-10	11			11			14	-13	-11	13	-10
18	36	-25	-21			19	-27	-40	-18		20	-15	-12
19		11	11										
20				16			-88						16
21	-13				17		84					-16	
22†	12	-13							-91				
23	12	13	-10		-17				-12				10
24	26			-20	13			-22	-18			32	14
25		19			-11	-22	15			-19			
26					-22					17			
27			-13						-19				
28		13			17		-23		-10		-13	12	
29	-12		-13	-18	-34	30			21				
30	-19	24			-19	-22	-16	-13			-45		
31		10						-12			-19		
32											-95		
33	-10	-23		-20	-13	-28	-50	-12	22	26			-14
34	-19				10								
35		-14		14	-18	66		10			20		-13
36					11	89	16						
37	12	14				74				12		-13	
38		-15				11		-15					
39‡													

Table 13–8. Rotated Factor Matrices, 13 Factors* (Data Collected from 33 Farms in San Joaquin County and 38 Farms in Tulare County, California)[5] (Continued)

Variable No.[†]	Rotated factor												
	I	II	III	IV	V	VI	VII	VIII	IX	X	XI	XII	XIII
						Tulare County							
1				−74	−25	15			−15				16
2					94								
3				89		−10		−12					
4	−10			23									−23
5		12	35	18			−32	−19	−11	−27		19	−31
6	10												
7	−12		23	−18		−15	−58		11				
8	13		−90				19						
9			86			13	17						
10								13		−96			
11			13			−11	−18			−11			
12	−12	11	−12	24	13	−42			−15	23		25	
13	13			−14	94							−11	
14		14	22	17	−11						25		−11
15		−11		11									
16			−13				12	−92		14			
17	−10	34			−16								−14
18		−89										15	
19		15	14	−12					−20			−13	
20	19	12	22										−22
21			10										
22[‡]													
23	−15				−11		11					−11	
24				−15				11		15		−10	
25	24		−11			−18	26	14	11				
26			−14		14		14						
27		−12	11			−12						94	
28	−14	−49		−14	13	−13		30	−18	−18			
29													89
30	−84				10								
31	−89		12					−16					
32	−55	−18			11	−19	−11		−21				
33							11		−95				
34	−26		21										
35		−12	−14	−11	33					−15			−13
36				17	−10		−84	16	14				
37		−15	−11										
38		−27	−19	−14	−13			14	−22			28	17
39[†]	−73	17			−21	−16	−11	12		12			

*Only factor loadings, fr, for which |fr| ≥ 0.10 are listed, illustrating that the criteria of Thurstone[7] are satisfied. Decimal points have been omitted. Loadings express the correlation between rotated factors and observable variables.

[†]See Table 13-4 for identification of variables.

[‡]Variable no. 22 was not used for Tulare data; variable no. 39 was not used for San Joaquin data.

Some of the potential usefulness of factor analysis for epidemiological studies may be easier to visualize from a somewhat simpler example. This illustration uses data from the study of determinants of different initial levels of *Echinococcus granulosus* in dogs in geographic areas of New Zealand, a study referred to earlier in the discussion of path analysis.[4]

Climate and prevalence of *Echinococcus* in New Zealand

Among the exogenous (predetermined) variables used in an effort to explain district-to-district variations in precontrol prevalence of *E. granulosus* in dogs were six weather variables: (1) mean daily maximum temperature for all the year in $^\circ$C. (Temp y), (2) mean daily maximum temperature for the hottest month only in $^\circ$C. (Temp m), (3) mean annual hours of bright sunshine (Sun), (4) mean annual rainfall in mm (Rain), (5) mean daily percent relative humidity (RH), and (6) mean daily run of wind in km (Wind). For 27 hydatid control districts on the South Island of New Zealand, the means and standard deviations of these variables were:

	Mean	Standard deviation
Temp y	16.0593	1.0412
Temp m	22.6037	1.4012
Sun	1976.8519	229.7244
Rain	882.2593	436.7037
Relative humidity	75.3704	4.0302
Wind	218.5556	72.9638

These variables were highly correlated (Table 13-9).

Table 13-10 shows by factor analysis that about 80% of the variance among districts could be accounted for by uncorrelated "factors" 1, 2, and 3. Using these three factors, a factor matrix was printed out to show the structure of each in terms of the original six weather variables (Table 13-11). Orthogonal (right angle) rotation of this matrix, as explained previously, permits easy identification of common factor loadings (Table 13-12). Thus, factor 1 consists largely of Temp y, Temp m and Sun (now designated "heatness"), factor 2 mostly of Rain and Relative humidity ("wetness"), and factor 3 mostly

of Wind. The clustering of these variables on a two-dimensional printout is shown in Figure 13-5.

The utility of factor analysis may be in the fact that "it seeks conclusions by statistical finesse rather than by manipulative control."[7] As an epidemiological tool, it is eminently useful in providing clues for the kinds of studies (manipulative control) that are likely to answer some important and complex etiological questions. Further discussion of this method is given by Nie *et al.*[3]

DISCRIMINANT ANALYSES

Discriminant analysis, another method for multivariate analysis, also is valuable in many epidemiological study situations. For certain uses, it can be visualized as a generalization of a t test. Suppose that there are k classes of individuals, with n_i individuals in the *i*th group, and r measurements have been obtained on each individual. For example, suppose that one is studying the determinants of lamb mortality, the r measurements being birth weight of the lamb, date of birth (relative to some reference date, e.g., July 1), age of the ewe, minimum temperature in the 24 hours preceding birth, and maximum temperature. Suppose also that there are four groups of interest: (1) lambs that died before leaving the lambing barn (age < two days), (2) lambs surviving two days, but not more than seven, (3) lambs dying from eight to 28 days of age, and (4) those surviving more than 28 days. If one constructs a rule so that for any new lamb born into such a population, he could "predict" to which group it would belong, he would be constructing a *discriminant function*. The most common discriminant functions are *linear* discriminant functions.[8]

The linear discriminant function has the form:

$$Z = B_1 x_1 + B_2 x_2 + \ldots B_r x_r.$$

If there are only two groups, then an individual is assigned to one group if that individual's calculated value of Z is less than the discriminating value Z_0. If the individual's value is $Z > Z_0$, that individual is assigned to the other group.

Table 13-9.	Correlation Coefficients Between Exogenous Predetermined Variables in Study of *Echinococcus granulosus* Prevalence in Dogs in New Zealand[4]

	Temp Y	Temp M	Sun	Rain	Relative Humidity	Wind
Temp Y	1.00000	0.72693	0.29359	0.11902	–0.18600	–0.02571
Temp M	0.72693	1.00000	0.50559	–0.19085	–0.58734	–0.14437
Sun	0.29359	0.50559	1.00000	–0.04773	–0.47777	–0.01339
Rain	0.11902	–0.19085	–0.04773	1.00000	0.41653	–0.17101
RH	–0.18600	–0.58734	–0.47777	0.41653	1.00000	0.15832
Wind	–0.02571	–0.14437	–0.01339	–0.17101	0.15832	1.00000

Table 13-10.   Latent Roots (Eigenvalues) for Principal-Components Factor
Analyses of Data on Prevalence of *Echinococcus granulosus*
in Dogs in New Zealand[4]

Factor	Eigenvalue	Variation (%)	Cumulative (%)
1	2.48603	41.4	41.4
2	1.29933	21.7	63.1
3	1.01895	17.0	80.1
4	0.72408	12.1	92.1
5	0.33200	5.5	97.7
6	0.13961	2.3	100.0

If the set of discriminators consists of two variables, x_1, x_2, the problem of discriminant function construction is to find a line on the x_1, x_2 – plane so that all points on one side of the line are said to belong to one population and all points on the other side belong to the second population. Naturally, more than two variables can be used as the set of discriminators, but the geometric interpretation would be somewhat more complex.

Diarrhea in dairy calves

One may, for example, be interested in identifying candidate causal variables for the frequency level of a particular disease. If he took the principal factors identified in the illustration of factor analysis in the farmer survey of calf diarrhea in San Joaquin County, California[5] (see the previous study), he could use them to construct the discriminant function that would best distinguish between farms in San Joaquin County with "high" incidence (49% or greater) and those with "low" incidence (less than 25%) of diarrhea in calves. Table 13-13 shows that 31 of the 38 farms (82%) could be correctly classified as high or low incidence using only 13 factors.

Brucellosis in Ontario

For another use, in a two-county area of Ontario classified since 1961 as a Brucellosis Certified Area,[9] one might be interested in attempting to explain the occurrences of infection on certain farms. A study was carried out to examine several categories of variables that might discriminate between infected farms (N = 46 in the two-county area) and noninfected farms (N = 86, chosen at random from a list of all of the two counties' noninfected farms).

Table 13-14 shows the results of discriminant analyses (mean value of x_i's for the two groups and the order in which they were entered into the discriminant function) employing one set of the variables examined. Note that in such an analysis, values such as 0, 1 are assigned to dichotomous data, as explained in Chapter 5. Using the first six variables in Table 13-14, 100 of the 132 herds (70 of 96 uninfected; 30 of 46 infected) could be correctly categorized as infected or noninfected. The addition of other variables made no further contribution to this categorization.

Table 13-11.   Factor Matrix Using Principal Factors from Study
of Data on Prevalence of *Echinococcus granulosus*
in Dogs in New Zealand[4]

	Factor 1	Factor 2	Factor 3
Temp Y	0.66587	0.49664	–0.38663
Temp M	0.92130	0.14124	–0.08619
Sun	0.70323	0.01128	–0.05948
Rain	–0.28547	0.85515	–0.04283
Relative humidity	–0.77027	0.37342	–0.29760
Wind	–0.15657	–0.40234	–0.87641

Table 13–12.   Rotated Factor Matrix from Study of Prevalence of
Echinococcus granulosus in Dogs in New Zealand[4]

	Factor 1	Factor 2	Factor 3
Temp Y	0.87456	0.26052	0.08244
Temp M	0.89961	-0.23154	-0.11520
Sun	0.65219	-0.26296	-0.06082
Rain	0.04535	0.87736	-0.20683
Relative humidity	-0.48224	0.71791	0.27090
Wind	-0.03207	-0.06712	0.97415

Fig. 13–5. Plot of rotated matrix for weather variables in an *Echinococcus* prevalence study, showing their clustering as "factors."[4]

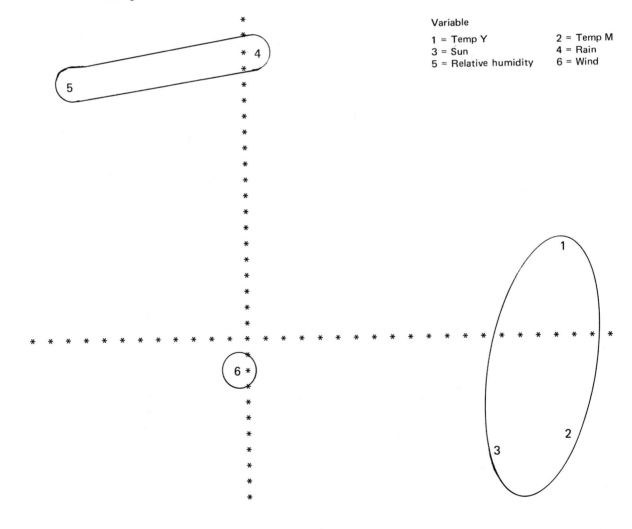

Variable

1 = Temp Y	2 = Temp M
3 = Sun	4 = Rain
5 = Relative humidity	6 = Wind

Table 13–13.   Discriminant Analysis on Basis of Principal Factors in Study of Diarrhea in Dairy Calves (San Joaquin County, California, June, 1969)[5]

Statistical Classification	No. farms with serious problems (49 to 100% incidence)	No. farms with few problems (less than 25% incidence)	Total
13 Principal Factors			
Very serious	13	4	17
Not serious	3	18	21
Total	16	22	38

Classification ratio: (13 + 18)/38 = 31/38

Table 13–14.   Results of Discriminant Analysis Between Brucellosis Case Herds and Control Herds in Two Ontario Counties, Canada, 1974–75[9]

Step No.*	Variable	Cases (N = 46) Mean ±	Controls (N = 86) Mean ±	Overall Mean
1	No. reactor herds within 2 miles	1.35 ± 1.4	0.43 ± 0.6	0.75
2	Exposure rating (contact with other cattle)	3.28 ± 0.9	2.77 ± 1.0	2.95
3	Herd type	2.41 ± 0.9	2.62 ± 0.7	2.55
4	Percent susceptibles vaccinated	16.50 ± 21.7	26.77 ± 27.3	23.19
5	History of previous reactor	1.67 ± 0.5	1.60 ± 0.5	1.63
6	Stabling type	1.65 ± 0.5	1.51 ± 0.5	1.56
7	Herd registration	1.98 ± 0.1	1.90 ± 0.3	1.92
8	Herd size	59.80 ± 40.5	50.27 ± 43.8	53.59
9	Control herds within 2 miles	0.89 ± 1.1	0.85 ± 0.9	0.86
10	Use of maternity pens	2.13 ± 0.5	2.20 ± 0.8	2.17
11	Insemination method	2.35 ± 0.8	2.41 ± 0.8	2.39

*Refers to step at which variable entered the discriminant function.

Part 4

SPECIAL OBJECTIVES

*"A system that isn't innovating
is a system that is dying"*
John W. Gardner

Chapter 14

EPIDEMIOLOGICAL INTELLIGENCE

THE general ideas of surveillance and intensive follow-up were introduced in Chapters 1 and 3. While the first of these approaches calls for the setting up of a multifaceted, long-term disease intelligence system intended for some directed action, the latter approach involves provision for more flexible and focused efforts of relatively short duration. In practice, these two avenues for epidemiological intelligence complement one another. In other words, data from the intensive follow-up of a case or an outbreak of disease provide valuable surveillance information *per se*, while the continuous aspects of surveillance programs yield the individual reports of cases and outbreaks, which are followed up intensively. In this chapter, surveillance is considered in somewhat greater detail, particularly with respect to its potential for further application in the public and private practice of veterinary medicine.

SURVEILLANCE

As the term is used in epidemiology, surveillance means an active intelligence and accounting process intended to continuously monitor the overall disease and health status of a population or group of populations. It is the organized mechanism that enables government agencies responsible for animal disease control to "keep their finger on the pulse of their 'patient'." It is similarly applicable to herd-health types of private veterinary practice (see Chapter 17). This surveillance process has several recognized components: (1) the collection of data; (2) the collation and analysis of data; and (3) the expression, interpretation, and prompt dissemination of disease intelligence information to all those who need to know.

COLLECTION OF DATA

Potentially useful data about animal diseases are available from a variety of sources. Some of these sources are detailed in this chapter, but discussion first focuses on the very important prerequisite questions of animal identification, disease nomenclature, and disease classification as they bear upon surveillance data collection. Other considerations relating to data availability and quality, for example, herd records systems and problem-oriented medical record systems, are discussed later in the chapter.

Animal identification

A critical *key* to the development of sophisticated systems of epidemiological surveillance in veterinary medicine is broad application of practical methods for identification of individual livestock. Some methods used for marking and identifying wildlife were mentioned in Chapter 4. The problem of identifying livestock is a somewhat different one.

In the past, livestock identification was undertaken largely on a herd basis, to show ownership in general and to deter theft in particular. Owners sometimes further identified animals *within* a herd to indicate their breeding status. Individual identification within herds also has been used to indicate animals that have been tested as part of some mass testing or similar specific disease control effort. Less frequently, animals have been identified to enable them to be traced back to farm of origin from a slaughterhouse or other point of destination, as in the M.C.I. program against brucellosis in the United States (see Chapter 3). Occasionally, very progressive farmers or others may have identified stock in order to carry out experimental trials, for example, comparisons of different feeding regimens.

Various methods have been used to identify individual livestock. In some animal-centered societies, and for small herds generally, the detailed physical appearance of each animal may be known to its owner. Other methods in common use include (1) firebrands; (2) coded patterns of notches cut in ears, horns, and wattles; and (3) paint marks, the latter, for example, to indicate the breeding status of sheep. Less used forms of identification include ear tags, tail tags, back tags, neck chains, freeze brands, tattoos, and other markers.

Ideally, some of the characteristics of a system of animal identification, to be epidemiologically useful, would be that the chosen system provide positive identification for the life of the animal, that it be a numerical system suitable for computer input, that it be applicable to large populations (for nationwide or even international use), and that it be as tamper-proof as possible. Other important considerations would include readability at a distance, ease of application, low cost, lack of damage to the animal, and overall acceptability to livestock owners and private veterinary practitioners (e.g., suitable for within-herd needs for identification). The identification systems now used most widely for epidemiological purposes are those based upon various inserted ear tags, glued-on back tags (Fig. 3–2 as used by the U.S. Department of Agriculture), and tattoos, including slap-tattooing of swine.[1]. Each of these systems has certain disadvantages, most of them obvious.

Of possibly great future value are electronic identification systems, which are in various stages of development. One attractive system with interesting possibilities depends upon the subcutaneous implantation in an animal of an inexpensive solid-state "transponder" measuring about ¼ inch on a side. This implant is preset with a coded identification number that can be read at a distance of 10 feet or less by a portable electronic "interrogator." The sole source of power is in the interrogator, which can feed identification data directly into a computer. This particular system has an additional value in that it also can read an animal's body temperature with considerable precision.

A variety of outstanding epidemiological advantages would result, from the large-scale adoption of an electronic system for livestock identification. One obvious use for a remote reading system would involve placing interrogators in all sales yards or other livestock congregation and dissemination points to scan the identification numbers of animals passing through. These data with dates and lot numbers could be fed into a computer. In any instance in which a diseased or infected animal of interest was diagnosed (e.g., in the slaughterhouse, on a farm, in a sales yard), not only could its total movement (see Fig. 3–1) be traced by retrieval of its identifying number and the associated data, but also all animals it could have contacted could be determined, and, if necessary, they also could be traced to their destinations.

An important prerequisite to implementation of any efficient animal identification system is the full support of livestock producers. The distinct economic advantages of such a system (with possibilities for improved surveillance) and the secondary benefits to the farmer from its adoption must be made very clear. Livestock producers' inherent suspicion and inability to comprehend long-range advantages to themselves or the nation already have been recognized as formidable barriers (in several countries) to initiation of universal livestock identification. For example, initial cattle industry support for the M.C.I.

system of cattle identification and traceback in the United States required a tacit understanding that the surveillance capability that it allowed would *not* be used to diagnose diseases other than brucellosis.

Farmers must be convinced that the long-term *economic* benefits of *knowing* what diseases their animals have or are at risk of acquiring are far greater than any short-term costs that may result from detection of individual affected animals. This is a situation *par excellence* for the types of combined epidemiologic-economic studies introduced in Chapter 15, and it also suggests that veterinary services collaborate with individuals qualified in anthropology and related social sciences.

Disease nomenclature and classification

Similar prerequisites for data collection and analysis aspects of surveillance are reliable diagnoses and adoption of a consistent system for disease nomenclature. To permit computer processing of disease data, an additional requirement is a numerically coded classification of diseases.

The closest thing to an internationally accepted disease nomenclature and classification code in veterinary medicine is the *Standard Nomenclature of Veterinary Diseases and Operations*, known also by the acronym S.N.V.D.O.[2] This publication was developed in 1964 by the Epizootiology Section of the National Cancer Institute of the U.S. Public Health Service. (A revised version appeared in 1966.) S.N.V.D.O. is used by veterinary schools in the United States and Canada, and is accepted by the World Health Organization as the basis for a clinical data collection program for other countries.

The S.N.V.D.O. coding system consists of two four-digit series (0000-0000) indicating the topographic designation in the first instance and the etiologic designation in the second, as follows.

Topographic Classification

0000 Body as a whole
1000 Integumentary system
2000 Musculoskeletal system
3000 Respiratory system
4000 Cardiovascular system
5000 Hemic and lymphatic system
6000 Digestive system
7000 Urogenital system
8000 Endocrine system
9000 Nervous system
X000 Organs of special sense

Etiologic Classification

0000 Genetic and prenatal influence
1000 Lower plant organism (fungi, bacteria, rickettsiae, viruses)
2000 Animal parasites (protozoa, metazoa)
3000 Intoxication

4000 Trauma or physical agent

5000 Secondary to circulatory disturbance

5500 Secondary to disturbance of innervation or of psychic control

6000 Static mechanical abnormality due to unknown cause

7000 Disorder of metabolism, growth, or nutrition

8000 New growths

9000 Unknown or uncertain cause with the structural reaction manifest; hereditary and familial diseases of this nature

X000 Unknown or uncertain cause with the functional reaction alone manifest; hereditary and familial disease of this nature

Y000 Unknown cause

As examples, rabies is coded 0100-1817 and parathyroid hyperplasia 8200-9430. Uses of S.N.V.D.O. for the Veterinary Medical Data Program are indicated on page 187.

S.N.V.D.O. is still in its early stages of development. Similar human nomenclatures and classifications have been revised and improved many times over a period of decades, but they still are subject to periodic revision. If there is a lesson to be learned from experience with human disease classification systems, it is that it would be the greatest folly in veterinary medicine for competing and noncompatible classification systems to be developed by diagnostic laboratory personnel and other users of clinical and diagnostic records solely to suit special use. Rather, all prospective users of such a nomenclature and classification should participate in S.N.V.D.O.'s future revisions so that the whole system (or *compatible* portions, simplifications, or extensions of it) is developed, thus assuring its more universal adoption and use.

S.N.V.D.O. was patterned after the American Medical Association's *Standard Nomenclature of Diseases and Operations.* Both this publication and the World Health Organization's *Manual of the International Statistical Classification of Diseases, Injuries and Causes of Death (International Classification of Diseases)* are used widely in human medicine. Veterinarians making use of human hospital data, as for example in studies of zoonotic infections or animal-induced injuries, need to be familiar with both of these publications, as well as with the U.S. Public Health Service's version of the latter publication, which is adapted for indexing hospital records. Of similar interest to veterinarians concerned with surveillance is the American Medical Association's *Current Medical Terminology.*

Surveillance data sources

Despite the fact that effective surveillance could provide the foundation for many aspects of veterinary service in the future, there does not seem to be any existing large-scale disease surveillance system, in veterinary medicine or public health, that begins to draw upon the full range of potential sources of useful intelligence information. The possibilities considered in this chapter are merely illustrative of, but are in no sense an exhaustive catalog of, the types of data available or of potential sources of data.

MORTALITY REGISTRATION. Registrations of human deaths with government agencies, particularly when cause of death is more or less accurately determined, provide a valuable continuous source of epidemiological data for public health agencies. No such death registration systems exist generally in veterinary medicine, although in some countries periodic livestock censuses and surveys usually include questions yielding mortality data suitable for analysis. Such is the case, for example, in Canada. Sometimes, it may also be possible to insert such questions into one-time censuses or surveys being conducted for other purposes. Routine mortality data also are obtainable in herd-health type veterinary practices and from intensive follow-up studies of outbreaks and other sources.

In addition, some types of general mortality data for a species or breed could be obtained from breed registries, the records of some herd improvement schemes, and a few specific population-based disease registries or large closed population studies. Life tables and other summaries derived from these data sources may indicate general patterns of death risk, more rarely of cause-specific death risks, for populations of particular species. Little surveillance usage has yet been made of possible mortality data sources in veterinary medicine.

Canadian animal mortality report. Since 1951, the Bureau of Statistics of Canada has included in its semiannual livestock survey questions about animal deaths. Together with the census information provided by the same survey, these data could be a useful part of an overall disease surveillance effort for Canada. Although a cumulative analysis of this material was published by the Economic Branch of the Canada Department of Agriculture in 1969,[3] that analysis was not undertaken with epidemiological surveillance in mind and, therefore, has relatively little value for the purpose.

Nevertheless, it contains suggestions, for example, of seasonal patterns for the crude death rates of Canadian cattle and sheep, though not for swine. It would appear, too, that there have been secular trends upward in crude death rates for both cattle and sheep, and downward for swine, during the 17-year observation period reported. Such interpretations would definitely depend upon knowledge that changes in method or thoroughness of reporting, or other factors, had not occurred during that same period.

ON-GOING MORBIDITY INCIDENCE REPORTING. As indicated in Chapter 3, reporting of disease incidence to government agencies has provided the backbone for public health, but not for veterinary, disease intelligence efforts. Some of the reasons were given. The respective epidemiological merits of morbidity incidence and prevalence data *per se* are discussed in Chapter 5.

There are a number of possible sources of disease incidence data in veterinary medicine; and, in the United States, several of the individual states' veterinary agencies over the years have adopted a variety of systems in some attempt to obtain incidence data.[4] Most of these state systems have been based upon voluntary reporting of cases of specific diseases by private veterinary practitioners. The results have varied. Incidence reporting by practitioners in veterinary and in human medicine invariably suffers overall from the unreliability of many diagnoses, particularly those for which laboratory confirmation may be lacking. Incompleteness of reporting also is a difficulty, and the full cooperation of reporters is rare. For a few very important animal diseases, such as rabies, where reporting by practitioners has been made legally mandatory, cooperation often is more satisfactory. Some individual states have obtained generally improved practitioner participation through such devices as routine telephone inquiries of delinquent reporters and efforts to tie reporting cooperation to requirements for continuing licensure of practitioners.

Other specific measures to improve practitioner reporting have been demonstrated in a few disease registries. For example, the Alameda and Contra Costa counties (California) Animal Tumor Registry has, since 1963, obtained very complete reporting of suspected dog and cat tumors from veterinary practitioners in those counties by providing them in return a free histopathological diagnostic service. Government laboratories could offer similar free or partially subsidized services in general or for specific disease categories in return for the appreciable surveillance benefits. Another special device effectively utilized by the U.S. Public Health Service's Center for Disease Control, and perhaps applicable in selected veterinary situations, has been the encouragement to report suspected exotic or *unusual* diseases by making available, as an advertised service to reporting physicians, certain unlicensed drugs otherwise unobtainable in the United States for treatment of reported, laboratory-confirmed cases of those diseases.

Experience suggests that practitioner cooperation is greatest when they receive for their efforts prompt reports of total surveillance data in forms clearly useful to them. The quality of morbidity data obtained from private food-animal practitioners is immeasurably improved when practitioners assist their clients in maintaining suitable records.

Herd record-keeping for surveillance purposes in private and public veterinary practice.[5] The population unit of primary concern in both public and private practice of veterinary medicine in economically well-developed countries is increasingly coming to be the individual "farm" or enterprise population of animals. These population units are frequently of considerable size. Managers of such animal enterprises usually maintain some form of records, most often for production purposes. Some commonly recorded production indices, such as production of milk or eggs, may themselves be sensitive indicators of clinical or subclinical illness. Vital statistics and reproduction records also possess preventive medical value.

Quite frequently in some countries, livestock producers are enrolled in organized record and test systems for monitoring and stimulating production. This practice is particularly common in the dairy industry. In the United States, for example, the number of dairy cows covered by one or more organized record systems considerably exceeds 3 million. Under auspices of the National Cooperative Dairy Herd Improvement Association are several distinct programs: (1) the official Dairy Herd Improvement Program, which covers about 2.1 million cows in 34,000 herds; (2) the owner sampler dairy record-keeping program, which includes an additional 900,000 cows in 23,000 herds; and (3) the Dairy Herd Improvement Registry Program, with 230,000 cows in 4,000 herds. Increasingly, such programs are based upon data storage and processing by electronic computer with frequent and detailed printouts supplied to enrolled producers and with opportunities for variable data inputs by management, which may allow for optional forms of data processing and analysis.

Individual herd surveillance programs serve a dual function. Herd-health-type veterinary practitioners require for their own purposes disease recording and analysis systems that can respond quickly to their needs. At the same time such individual farm-unit surveillance systems can provide valuable inputs of data about animal wastage for larger-scale government surveillance efforts. The components of an individual farm-unit surveillance system resemble those for a national system, and depend on collection of all types of available disease information on the individual farm by veterinarians and owners. Their ultimate form of expression should be in cost-benefit terms. Clearly, the missing ingredient in many herd health programs up to now has been sufficient epidemiological input, particularly an input in which the concepts of surveillance and intensive follow-up have been extended to include assessment of the impact of diseases on animal production and its economic return.

For example, a dairy herd record-keeping system adequate for these dual surveillance purposes probably would include:

(1) Provision for animal identification with recording of detailed information on each animal (e.g., age, breed, sex, and specified traits).

(2) Basic descriptive data on the whole farm operation and herd. These data might include: (a) a statement of objectives for the enterprise as defined by the owner; (b) an explicit account of the management system used, and (c) identification of important characteristics such as herd population density and possible stress factors, a history of past herd problems (medical as well as managerial), and such baseline laboratory data as can be provided.

(3) A recording system for reproductive performance, other vital statistics, production data, morbidity data (including diagnostic, prophylactic, and therapeutic procedures), changes in management practices, and other changes or unusual events of possible epidemiological importance.

(4) Market and other information required to assess the economic impact of disease and disease management methods.

(5) An appropriate format for the prompt presentation of analyzed data and recommendations to the producer-owner.

As already mentioned, organized programs that employ herd record-keeping systems exist for different animal industries in several countries. However, most of these systems are oriented entirely towards the collection and analysis of production statistics. Some such systems do provide space for recording health data, but until now few attempts have been made to use such data to evaluate the effects of disease on production. Similarly, little epidemiological use has been made of the production-type information being gathered by such systems.

There are a number of possible reasons for these past oversights. Because most existing herd record-keeping systems are for production data, and quantitative data on the effects of disease and health upon production are not well known, most sponsoring organizations have not encouraged the collection of health data and have seemed content to use illness only to explain or adjust erratic production figures. In addition, some farmers are reluctant to record health observations because they lack confidence in the value of their own clinical observations, because they want to believe that diseases do not occur on their farms with any frequency, because they do not want other farmers, government officials, or the public to know they are having disease problems, or because they believe diseases do not appreciably influence production even if they do occur. Many farmers accept a given level of disease as normal. Finally, the veterinary profession has not convincingly demonstrated to many farmers the usefulness of complete herd health records and the economic returns associated with different on-farm herd health systems or control systems for specific diseases.

As indicated, improved herd records as part of herd health programs could also improve the quality of state morbidity reporting systems. Some details of two U.S. state veterinary practitioner incidence reporting systems are given next.

Colorado State Animal Disease Reporting System. Initiated in 1952, this was the first animal morbidity reporting system in the United States to be organized on a statewide basis. Unlike some other state programs that were developed administratively as part of agriculturally based veterinary services, the Colorado program was set up by the veterinary public health section of the State Department of Health.

The stated objectives of the Colorado reporting system are:

(1) To maintain an up-to-date list of veterinary practitioners.

(2) To determine the incidence and distribution of animal diseases.

(3) To provide data useful to the establishment of disease control programs.

(4) To observe seasonal trends in the occurrence of diseases.

(5) To determine research needs.

(6) To provide statistics on animal diseases to interested individuals and agencies.

(7) To observe outbreaks and to initiate field investigations.

All veterinary practitioners licensed to practice veterinary medicine in Colorado are invited to participate in this program, in return for which they receive both monthly and annual morbidity summaries. Each month, all currently licensed practitioners receive in the mail a double postcard, one half of which merely lists the 51 animal diseases currently reportable in Colorado and briefly explains the program, while the other half, which is to be torn off and returned, provides spaces to note the species involved and numbers of cases (and/or herds) for 17 of these diseases. Information is solicited also on vaccinations for encephalitis, rabies, and distemper; and additional space is provided for reporting other diseases. Suspected rabies reports are required immediately by telephone. About 350 practitioners receive these cards. In 1955, the percentage reporting each month varied between 44 and 54%, and, in 1973, between 34 and 41% of practitioners returned their cards.

All reported data are coded for disease, animal species, reporting practitioner, and reporting county; the data are then computer-processed. Monthly summary reports returned to collaborators and those others with a need to know include separate tabular presentations of large animal and small animal data by disease and county, with cumulative statistics given for "total cases (herds) this month," "total cases (herds) this year," and "total cases (herds) this time last year." In addition, each four-page monthly report contains one or more narrative news items of interest to reporting practitioners.

The annual reports follow the same general format, but are somewhat more detailed and provide additional information of interest on diseases of relatively infrequent occurrence, current data on animal populations, as well as other information of interest to practitioners, e.g., the locations of poison control centers.

A somewhat different reporting approach based upon sampling has been instituted in the state of Minnesota.

Minnesota disease reporting system.[6] This incidence reporting system was developed in 1971 by the Infectious Disease Committee of the Minnesota Veterinary Medical Association, and implemented through cooperation with the Minnesota Livestock Sanitary Board, government district veterinarians, private veterinary practitioners, and farmers. A sample of farmers report monthly to their veterinary practitioner the number of animals that become ill with any of a number of diseases listed on a supplied reporting card. The total populations of animals of each species present on the farm are also reported, permitting the calculation of incidence rates. There is no reporting of outcome of cases of disease or monetary cost of treatments.

The veterinary practitioner forwards the information based on these farmers' reports through the district veterinarian to the Minnesota Livestock Sanitary Board. The collected disease data are analyzed at the Computer Center of the University of Minnesota and expressed as incidence rates per 1000 animals of the various species. An incidence report is published every three months.

The sample of reporting farmers is obtained by a multistage cluster sampling procedure. An equal number of veterinary practices is sampled in each district of the state, and an equal number of farms is sampled for each practice. Because these districts were created on the basis of approximately equal numbers of livestock, this sampling is fairly uniform throughout the state. The participating veterinarians were selected randomly from lists of all practitioners in each district. Each selected practitioner then submitted a list of clients that he felt would report (a source of recognized bias); and from each practitioner's list, 10 clients were selected.

Based upon a predetermined level of change in disease incidence to be detected by this program, the number of participating farms should be about 500 in this Minnesota program and the number of participating veterinarians about 50. The actual participation in 1973-74 was 182 farms and 23 veterinarians. These low figures reflect a problem that affects all disease reporting schemes, namely, fading enthusiasm.

The Minnesota system is rationally designed, inexpensive to operate, and no doubt potentially valuable. The interest of farmers and veterinary practitioners in disease reporting systems will undoubtedly increase considerably as the collected data are utilized to obtain information that can be used directly by farmers and practitioners. While general incidence reporting schemes such as these can provide *one* very useful source of surveillance data, they cannot in themselves provide the sole basis for a modern and comprehensive disease intelligence system.

In addition to general reporting by individual veterinary practitioners, another potential source of animal disease case incidence reports for the United States and Canada is the so-called Veterinary Medical Data Program, which routinely collects and stores on computers clinical data from large institutional veterinary hospitals. To date these data have been used almost exclusively for case-control type epidemiological studies rather than as an input into surveillance systems. Since these data are derived from hospitalized populations that contain a high proportion of referred patients, they probably reflect disproportionately low or high frequencies of particular diagnoses. This consideration, however, does not negate their potential surveillance value.

Prerequisites for good data programs based upon institutional clinics are good-quality clinical records and qualified abstracters of diagnoses and other epidemiologically relevant data. One system highly recommended to meet this first prerequisite of suitable records is the problem-oriented approach advocated by Weed.[7]

Problem-oriented medical records. Anyone who has attempted to use medical records from human hospitals or large veterinary hospitals for epidemiological purposes knows the distressingly poor and inconsistent quality of most of these data. It is an encouraging sign, therefore, that a *system* of problem-oriented medical record keeping, advocated initially as a means to improve patient care and medical education, is seeing wide adoption both in human medicine and in veterinary medicine. For, although its partisans have not stressed the fact, this new system also improves immeasurably the usefulness of medical record data for epidemiological surveillance and research. As the system's author has noted, "if communities were the size of cells and if hospitals, pharmacies, laboratories, patients, and physicians were the size of subcellular particles, no doubt they would be the subjects of a great deal of research." We can do no more than echo this opinion and our belief that wider use of a consistent system of problem-oriented medical records will favor conduct of more population-based research in the future.

Basically the problem-oriented record system consists of four parts. The first is a *Data Base* for each patient consisting of the following elements: (1) chief complaint, (2) patient profile, (3) present illness or illnesses, (4) past history and systems review, (5) physical examination, and (6) baseline laboratory examination. This Data Base is followed by a *Problem List*, an *Initial Plan* and, finally, *Progress Notes*.

From the epidemiological point of view, these components of the patient's record would include the following features:

Data Base

Chief complaint. In veterinary medicine, this item would be the animal owner's concise statement of just *why* he sought veterinary assistance for his animal.

Patient profile. This section is more or less the equivalent of a complete *epidemiologic* history of the individual patient, with description of all host and environmental (including potential agent) factors associated with the patient and its normal activities, exclusive of the patient's medical history *per se*.

Present illness or illnesses. This topic covers symptomatic and objective evidence concerning, as appropriate, either the undiagnosed condition for which the patient is presented for veterinary care, or similar information about possible relapse from or continuation of a previously diagnosed condition.

Past history and systems review. This area comprises a definite series of logically arranged questions for each system involved, based on use of *standard* printed questionnaires. (The reader is referred to the cited reference for suggestions and details.)

Physical examination. The examination is a complete and consistent process. As in the epidemiologic and medical history sections, it should be ascertainable from the record exactly what information was sought and what was not sought; that is, the record is clear about whether a certain finding was negative or merely was not ascertained.

Baseline laboratory examination. The record specifies precisely what tests were ordered.

Problem List.

This part is the core of the problem-oriented medical record. It begins with a numbered *index list* of *all* of the patient's past and present medical problems, with the highest possible level of diagnostic precision. The reference cited includes detailed suggestions on the organization of this Problem List. In brief, problems are identified, for example, as primary, secondary, predisposing, or contributory; as active, inactive, or resolved; and as minor or temporary. This list, which is of great epidemiological value, is subject to revision and modification; but it always supplies the *key or index to the actions taken or recommended and the results obtained.*

Initial Plan.

Following the numbers of the Problem List, the plan for *each* problem is developed separately with respect to further diagnostic efforts required and/or its management. The process for ruling out possibilities in a differential diagnosis is stated clearly, with the specific tests and results required to rule out any particular diagnostic possibility. For example, the logic of each sequential battery of tests proposed should be indicated in a simple flowchart. Similarly, treatments proposed are described in detail, and instructions for the animal's owner are precisely specified.

Progress Notes.

Given an adequate Problem List and Initial Plan, fully dated Progress Notes may consist initially of little more than results or data produced. Again, these notes are keyed to the Problem List. They provide specific feedback links to the individual problems and the individual plans of action. All new data should be properly integrated into these notes, not just stapled into the record; and the significance of each new datum *must* be commented upon. Plans should be modified accordingly and *each* problem eventually resolved in some acceptable fashion. Were clinical records more generally of this quality, clinical data retrieval systems such as the one described next would have even more surveillance and research value than at present.

The second prerequisite for epidemiological use of an institutional record abstracting and retrieval system, as described next, is employment of qualified abstracters. The potential problem of this practice is illustrated by the experience of one of the authors. His attempt to retrieve diagnoses of human hydatid disease from 800,000 computerized California human hospital records in 1970 yielded 72 cases coded as hydatid disease. However, follow-up showed that only two of these cases actually were hydatid disease, the remaining 70 hospital records having been cases of hydatidiform moles and ovarian hydatids of Morgagni miscoded by abstracters.

Veterinary Medical Data Program. This ongoing data collection program for institutional clinics in North America is based upon the *Standard Nomenclature of Veterinary Diseases and Operations*. It was begun by the U.S. National Cancer Institute in 1964; and by 1974, over 1 million medical case records from 13 cooperating veterinary colleges were available on magnetic tape for epidemiological use. The type of case abstract card used for this program is shown in Figure 14–1. An illustrative problem, based upon this data source, is given in Chapter 11.

A similar program, also based upon the S.N.V.D.O. code, is operated by the Veterinary Public Health Unit of the World Health Organization for institutional clinics outside North America. Further potentially valuable sources of both morbidity *and* mortality data are public and private diagnostic laboratories.

VETERINARY MEDICAL CASE ABSTRACT

Batch ________ Page ________

Patient Number ________ Discharge Date ________ Owners Name ________

Batch ________ Page ________

Institution	Patient Number	Date of Discharge (Mo. Day Year)	Length of Stay (Days)	Attending Clinician	Sex	Species	Breed Code
1 2	3 4 5 6 7 8	9 10 11 12 13 14	15 16	17 18	19: 0 – Litter, 1 F, 2 FS, 3 FU, 4 – M, 5 – MC, 6 – Other/unk	20: 0 Bovine, 1 – Equine, 2 – Porcine, 3 Ovine, 4 Caprine, 5 Other LA, 6 Canine, 7 Feline, 8 Avian, 9 Other SA	21 22 23

DISCHARGE STATUS (24)
0 – Alive
1 Died Necropsy
2 Died No Necropsy
3 Euthanasia Necropsy
4 Euthanasia No Necropsy

AGE (25)
0 0 to 2 wks
1 – 2 wks to 2 mos
2 – 2 to 6 mos
3 6 to 12 mos
4 1 to 2 yrs
5 2 to 4 yrs
6 4 to 7 yrs
7 7 to 10 yrs
8 10 to 15 yrs
9 15 yrs and older

WEIGHT (POUNDS) (26)
Large Animal
0 0 to 3
1 3 to 15
2 15 to 50
3 50 to 150
4 150 to 300
5 – 300 to 600
6 – 600 to 1000
7 1000 to 1300
8 1300 and over

Small Animal
0 – 0 to 1
1 – 1 to 5
2 – 5 to 15
3 15 to 30
4 30 to 50
5 50 to 75
6 75 to 100
7 100 and over

FIRST DIAGNOSIS
27 Initial / Recheck (✓) — 28 29 30 31 32 33 34 35 36

SECOND DIAGNOSIS
37 Initial / Recheck (✓) — 38 39 40 41 42 43 44 45 46

THIRD DIAGNOSIS
47 Initial / Recheck (✓) — 48 49 50 51 52 53 54 55 56

FIRST OPERATION — 57 58 59 60 61

SECOND OPERATION — 62 63 64 65 66

NON-DIAGNOSTIC (67)
0 – Not applicable
1 – Total exam – normal
2 – Bone & joint exam – normal
3 – Sensory organs exam – normal
4 – Reproductive exam – normal
5 – Cardio vascular exam – normal
6 – Integumentary exam normal
7 – Other exam – normal
8 – Biologic donor
9 – Other (boarder, etc.)

DIAGNOSTIC PROCEDURES ("X" Appropriate Boxes)
68 Clinical Diagnosis **ONLY**
69 Gross Pathology
70 Histopathology
71 Serology
72 Microbiology
73 Radiology
74 Electrophysiology
75 Hematology
76 Urinalysis
77 Chemistry
78 Parasitology
79 Other not specified

Notes Comments

NIH 1457 1
Rev. 8-73

VETERINARY MEDICAL CASE ABSTRACT

FORM APPROVED
O.M.B. No. 68-R1119

Fig. 14–1. Case abstract form used for Veterinary Medical Data Program in veterinary colleges in United States and Canada (U.S. National Cancer Institute).

DIAGNOSTIC LABORATORY RECORDS OF MORBIDITY AND MORTALITY. It is vital that government field services in veterinary medicine be provided with adequate laboratory backup. This backup is required for seroepidemiologic surveys as well as for most special investigations, or intensive follow-ups, of cases or outbreaks of disease. All these types of laboratory data should feed into surveillance programs.

The same or other government, as well as private, veterinary laboratories may also provide an essentially unorganized on-demand type of diagnostic service to private veterinary practitioners and, sometimes, directly to farmers. These diagnostic data also constitute potentially useful epidemiologic surveillance information, particularly by suggesting onsets of outbreaks and by being a source of information of unusual or otherwise interesting case reports for intensive follow-up. However, rarely is there now fully adequate liaison in this regard between veterinary diagnostic laboratory services and veterinary epidemiologic services in government. To these ends, it obviously is highly desirable that veterinary laboratory services employ records based upon systems for disease nomenclature and classification fully compatible with those in epidemiologic use.

For such laboratory data to have epidemiologic value to private herd health-type veterinary practitioners as well, it is essential that practitioners employ suitable sampling techniques for selecting the animals from their study population that are to undergo necropsy, biopsy, or culture. The animals chosen determine whether the data yielded are representative of the ill animals and the existing pattern of diseases in the herd. Only if the sampling technique is suitable can these laboratory results be analyzed or interpreted in terms of epidemiologically interesting factors such as age, sex, breed, or management variables. This epidemiological aspect of clinical studies is generally neglected, with the result that diagnostic laboratory results often provide only a small portion of their potential value and sometimes even obscure completely possible determinants of disease frequency. *In a herd-based veterinary practice, laboratory specimens should yield much more diagnostic information than merely an organism isolated, a toxin detected, or a pathologic change noted.*

When laboratory specimens are selected properly and described so as to give a private practitioner their maximal immediate diagnostic value, they at the same time yield a type of laboratory record that serves as a valuable intelligence source for wider scale government disease surveillance programs.

SPECIAL PROGRAMS FOR INCIDENCE DATA. Sometimes special registers exist for particular classes of diseases, or there are other special programs that have intelligence usefulness. Two examples are mentioned.

Alameda and Contra Costa counties animal tumor registry.[8] This registry was established to obtain epidemiologic information on neoplasms in cats and dogs, with the idea that such data might provide clues about environmental or other determinants of human cancer. At the time this registry was established in the early 1960s, the large increase in the number of veterinarians specializing in small animal medicine and the increasing willingness of pet owners to seek veterinary services suggested that epidemiologic studies of neoplasm incidence based on such a registry would be profitable.

Alameda and Contra Costa counties in California were selected as the study area. These counties form a contiguous geographic and demographic unit bounded by water on the west and north and sparsely populated on their eastern and southern borders. The human population in the two counties was approximately 1.5 million when the registry began in 1963, and the pet populations in Alameda County were approximately 92,000 dogs and 73,000 cats. By 1970 the human population had increased to 1.6 million, and the pet population in the two counties was 225,000 dogs and 150,000 cats.[9]

This particular study area was chosen mainly because of its large human and pet populations and because of the availability of complementary information. Specifically, the California Tumor Registry collects data on human cancer, and the Human Population Laboratory of the California State Department of Public Health conducts surveys in the area (This laboratory was used, for example, to identify numbers of veterinary-using households and the animal population base.) A preliminary study was carried out in 1962 to determine the characteristics of veterinary practices in the area and their volume of animal admissions. All practices were visited; veterinarians were asked about the number of neoplasms they diagnosed, their use of pathology laboratories, and methods of specimen submission. At that time very few neoplasms clinically diagnosed in the practices were confirmed by histopathologic examination.

A sample of eight practices was chosen for a pilot study in which veterinarians were asked to complete a report form for all suspected neoplasm cases observed in their practices during a four-week period in 1963. They were also asked to submit specimens for histopathologic confirmation. This pilot study was expanded to include all practices, and formal reporting began in 1963. The practitioners submit case reports and specimens from all cases in which a neoplasm is suspected and receive free of charge a histopathologic diagnosis from the registry. One hundred six practitioners (>98% of the total number) participate in this study, and it is believed that 75% of the cat population and 90% of the dog population are included in the study. By 1975 the registry had been in operation for 12 years, and a number of research findings had been published.[10] These articles have included results of interesting demographic studies of the cat and dog populations at risk.

Some other less conventional animal morbidity data sources also exist or could be developed. One attractive mechanism is animal health insurance schemes, such as those used in Israel, Greece, the Canadian province of Quebec, and other areas. Where these insurance programs exist, they may provide a particularly valuable source of morbidity data. The example given next is from Quebec.

Quebec Animal Health Insurance Program.[11] The Quebec insurance program was introduced by the provincial Ministry of Agriculture in 1971. It was designed as a financial aid to Quebec's farmers, not as a disease monitoring tool. Essentially it subsidizes veterinary services for farm animals by: (1) reducing the initial charge to the farmer to a uniform fee per visit whatever the distance, (2) reducing previous consultation fees paid by farmers by 50%, (3) standardizing fees for treatment throughout the province, and (4) reducing to a minimum the farmers' charge for veterinary drugs through their centralized distribution by a governmentally administered agency.

One way for this animal health insurance program to be used as a tool for disease surveillance is through the invoice provided by the veterinarian to the

Ministry of Finance for payment of his fees. This invoice contains the following information: (1) identification of the owner and his address; (2) identification of the animal(s) by species and in some cases by breed, age, and sex; and (3) diagnosis and treatment and its cost (divided into the farmer's share and the government's share).

The only information that the provincial veterinary services retain from these invoices is the number of diagnoses. During the fiscal year 1974-75, approximately 450,000 diagnoses were submitted. These reports were entered on computer by species and by county (there are 78 counties in Quebec). The following diagnostic categories were represented for that year: nutritional and metabolic diseases 27%, infections 33%, reproductive disorders 31%, and miscellaneous diseases 9%. A standard printout, which lists the number of diagnoses by species and by county, is produced every month.

As an example of the surveillance potential of this system, monthly rates for reported diagnoses of bovine arthritis derived from these printouts are shown in Figure 14–2 for a period of almost 2½ years. The sizes of the populations at risk were obtained from semiannual censuses of livestock in Quebec. When plotted on a graph, these rates suggest the possibility of a seasonal pattern and slight upward trend in frequency of this diagnosis. The latter could be explained by the fact that the number of reporting veterinarians increased from 116 in August, 1971, to 190 in March, 1974. The seasonal pattern, however, repeats itself over the recording period, with a low in September, a first peak in November-December, and a second peak in April-May. This first peak coincides with the beginning of the period of confinement of cattle in barns in Quebec, and the second with calving time and the end of their confinement. Further study of this observed pattern over a period of time, with appropriate data analyses, might lead to a better understanding of the determinants of bovine arthritis.

Some information for such analyses could be obtained by retrieval of the individual records or from specially requested computer printouts. Programming the computer to produce special request printouts (in addition to standard monthly summaries) could extend the surveillance value of the Quebec Animal Health Insurance Program in several ways. For example, data generated by the system could be cross-linked with other computerized programs, such as the metabolic profile testing programs and the Canadian Dairy Herd Improvement Analysis System (D.H.I.A.S.), to yield local surveillance data useful to private practitioners conducting herd health-type practices. Practitioners, or regional practitioners' associations, also could use pooled data from farms of particular types in given geographic areas to obtain average area data values useful in identifying special disease-related factors or disease occurrences on individual farms.

Full surveillance value is being derived now from few, if any, such ongoing disease incidence reporting systems in veterinary medicine. Indications for their

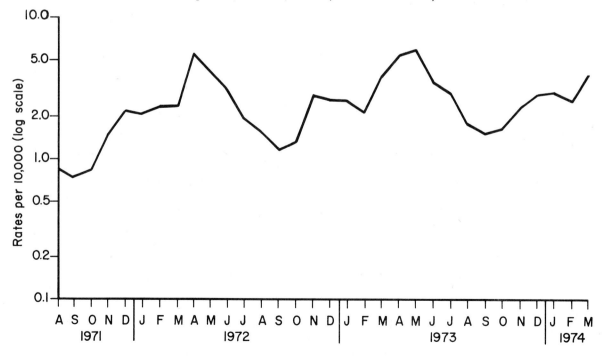

Fig. 14–2. Reported diagnoses of bovine arthritis from August, 1971, to March, 1974, in the province of Quebec. Incidence rates per 10,000 cattle per month.

expanded usefulness are clear, however, particularly for detecting newly occurring diseases, the onset of disease outbreaks, and the spread of diseases in an area. Veterinary medicine has made much greater past use of prevalence surveys.

MORBIDITY PREVALENCE MONITORING OR SURVEY. To date, prevalence surveys have provided the most useful data base for development of the overall surveillance process in veterinary medicine; but, like available incidence reporting mechanisms, they have rarely been utilized to full advantage. Unquestionably, periodic mass field-surveys of entire animal populations by immunodiagnostic testing methods or, less often, by other mass diagnostic tests have been the backbone of livestock disease control programs. Their use has been almost exclusively as a case and herd-finding procedure, however, rather than as part of an overall disease surveillance system.

Virtually all past uses of this powerful intelligence technique have been focused upon individual diseases and on-going programs for their control. Oddly, little extended *general* surveillance use has been made of continuing seroepidemiological programs of this type, and there have been few attempts to substitute sampling procedures for complete population coverage in such programs. With rare exceptions, large numbers of serum samples collected from animal populations at great effort and cost in programs of this type have been discarded following a *single* specific use, such as for *Brucella* testing.

Another even more valuable general morbidity prevalence monitoring opportunity is provided in veterinary medicine by the availability of almost *all* animals of some species for necropsy examination and diagnosis in the abattoir. Blood and other tissue specimens are readily obtainable from such animals. This situation provides a potentially ideal system for many aspects of disease surveillance and is, in fact, the backbone for bovine tuberculosis eradication efforts in the United States.

One problem in extending the surveillance use of this unique data resource is the fact that most long-established veterinary programs in abattoirs were designed for consumer protection *only*. For many of them, this pattern of responsibilities has not been very amenable to change. These veterinary programs have served their human health function reasonably well. It is unfortunate that their epidemiological potential for case-finding and infected herd-finding, for disease prevalence estimation, and for general animal disease surveillance has been so often neglected. Their overall surveillance use has been particularly thwarted in some countries by the government's administrative separation of veterinary food protection services from those for animal disease control. This clearly unnecessary administrative liability should be remedied in the interest of efficient and effective veterinary services. Part of the remedy is

to provide epidemiological training to more veterinary food protection officers.

Extended usage of sera obtained in seroepidemiologic surveys. Potential epidemiological uses of sera and blood clots now collected in mass testing efforts in veterinary medicine include (1) one-time, periodic, or routine surveys for *any infections* of the animal species surveyed if appropriate serological tests exist; (2) prevalence estimate surveys (and case-finding or early detection) for anemias, nutritional deficiency diseases, metabolic diseases, and toxicities detectable by serum or blood cell examination; (3) mapping of distributions and frequencies of genetic markers, such as blood groups and abnormal hemoglobins; (4) use of animal populations for the *biological monitoring of the environment* generally for radiation, pesticides, and other pollutants; and (5) banking of highly selected specimens for future studies. Such obviously valuable extensions of on-going serum collection programs may require nothing more than an increase in sample size, if even that. The following example of an extended pilot use of the existing Market Cattle Identification (M.C.I.) Program in the United States is concerned with surveillance of anaplasmosis.

In 1968-69 a pilot project was undertaken by a U.S. Department of Agriculture veterinarian in California[12] to determine the suitability of the M.C.I. Program (initiated as a brucellosis beef herd-finding procedure) for more general epidemiological surveillance of cattle diseases. In California, the M.C.I. system principally samples beef breeding animals two years of age or older. Dairy cattle, feedlot cattle (steers), and calves are among the classes of cattle generally excluded. During the spring of 1968, an effort was made to obtain all M.C.I. blood samples that had been tested previously for brucellosis in three California State Veterinary Diagnostic Laboratories (Sacramento, Fresno, Petaluma), which tested samples collected at slaughterhouses in the northern two-thirds of California. Clotted samples from two of these laboratories were received by courier, while the third laboratory forwarded by mail unrefrigerated samples from which the clots had been removed. The immediate practical focus of this pilot project was to estimate the prevalence and distribution of bovine anaplasmosis in northern California.

Upon receipt by the investigator, the samples were centrifuged, the separated sera transferred to clean tubes, and a preservative added. These sera samples, with all available M.C.I. identification for each, were then sent to a central U.S. Department of Agriculture laboratory to be tested by the complement fixation test for anaplasmosis. The samples as received originally from the state laboratories were identified by a backtag number (see Fig. 3-2) and/or the herd owner's name and address and sometimes also by other identifying number or brand, age, breed, and sex, as well as by the identifying number of the slaughtering establishment and date of sample collection. For backtagged cattle, the owner's name and address were supplied by the State Animal Health Division office in Sacramento. Test result, sample condition, and the identifying data for each sample then were transferred in coded form to computer data cards and analyzed. Some of the resulting data are shown in Table 14-1 and Figure 14-3.

Although this study indicated a need for drastic improvements in the M.C.I. system, particularly with respect to care in fully identifying animals and in handling samples, the system was suitable for yielding useful anaplasmosis prevalence estimate data for northern California. Identification of some of the biases of M.C.I.-type data in general was indicated on page 80. Newer techniques of particular value for such seroepidemiologic purposes include collection, shipment, and storage of antibody samples as blood dried on filter paper, availability of simple field centrifuges, various blood drop and microtests, automated serological techniques, and immunofluorescence slide methods for large-scale applications. In addition to the preceding, a variety of other useful sources of surveillance data is sometimes available or could be made available with sufficient effort. A few possibilities are considered next.

SURVEILLANCE DATA FROM LESS CONVENTIONAL SOURCES. For the United States, other livestock morbidity data are available from several sources. An important problem that arises in use of veterinary practitioners as sole or principal sources of disease intelligence is that, at least in some animal industries, practicing veterinarians see or are interested in only a portion of the spectrum of diseases present—and often only a very small proportion of the total of all animal diseases. This source of underestimation and bias is suggested by Figure 14-4 for the sheep industry of California.

Disease intelligence by the interview approach. A novel approach to the acquisition of certain types of surveillance data by interviews has been proposed recently.[13] Using the sheep industry of California for a pilot study of the uses and limitations of this approach, an epidemiologist showed that veterinarians, other animal scientists, animal producers, animal buyers, meat packers, farm advisors, and agricultural economists all are potential sources of useful intelligence data about animal morbidity and mortality and associated economic parameters, but that each source tends to recognize and emphasize the role of specific and rarely overlapping categories of disease from their quite different perspectives (Fig. 14-4).

Table 14-1.   Number of Herds with Range of Prevalence of Positive Reactors to Complement Fixation Test for Bovine Anaplasmosis in 15 Northern California Counties, 1968-69[12]

County	No. herds	Range of prevalence (%) observed within a herd*	Avg. observed prevalence for the county*
Alameda	44	85.2–96.5	65.4
Amador	61	30.6–56.0	47.1
Calaveras	47	92.7–100.0	78.8
Fresno	95	0.0–82.4	27.6
Humboldt	119	22.2–80.0	55.1
Merced	268	1.6–46.7	20.0
Monterey	136	17.6–100.0	61.6
Placer	183	6.3–62.5	38.4
Sacramento	202	4.5–76.7	29.8
San Joaquin	162	1.9–78.3	31.4
Shasta	296	18.4–97.5	56.9
Siskiyou	144	35.3–38.7	37.4
Sonoma	136	36.8–55.5	33.2
Stanislaus	89	0.0–100.0	32.9
Tehama	192	34.2–54.7	40.1
Total	2174	0.0–100.0	41.9

*Only herds represented by 30 or more animals tested were used to obtain these prevalences. If herds with 30 or more results were not available, the two largest samples from the county were used for these figures. All prevalence figures are given as percentages.

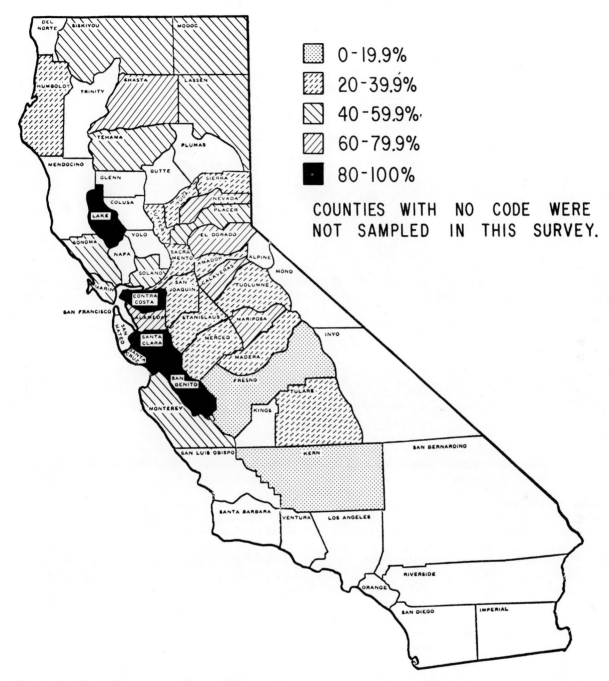

Fig. 14-3. Distribution of positive complement fixation tests for bovine anaplasmosis in beef breeding animals, by county, California, 1969-1970.[12]

In contrast to usual levels of cooperation in the reporting and return of written questionnaires, there was 100% cooperation in this study from interviewees in the several categories mentioned. These interviews were conducted by one veterinarian as a part-time activity over a six-month period. Interviews, following a standard protocol, were carried out in the field, and each lasted from one to several hours. Suitable outline maps were available for direct re-

cording of certain data during interview sessions. These interviews, following the standard protocol given next but allowing for relevant digressions, sought information concerning: (1) general description of the local sheep industry or parts thereof; (2) numbers and distribution of sheep in areas of interviewee's familiarity; (3) descriptions of management and husbandry practices; (4) assessment of productivity in different sectors and areas, e.g.,

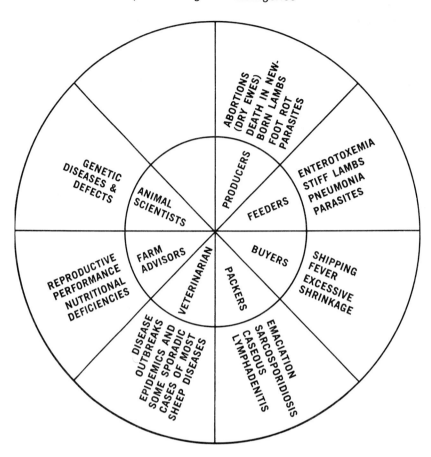

Fig. 14-4. Diagram showing diseases of interest to different persons associated with sheep industry in California (from Ruppanner, R.[13])

relative proportions of feeder lambs versus finished lambs produced; (5) diseases in terms of major problems seen or understood; (6) quantitative morbidity and mortality data in terms of numbers and rates; (7) prevention and treatment of diseases; and (8) costs of disease treatments.

This pilot study yielded a variety of types of useful surveillance information such as relative importance of various diseases in different areas, losses experienced from some diseases, costs of prevention and control, the extent to which recommended preventive procedures actually were followed, information about current outbreaks, neonatal mortality estimates, and data about possible disease determinants. Such an interviewing program was considered a good means to yield worthwhile surveillance information that could be either used in the form collected or applied to the design of surveys or intensive follow-ups. This type of surveillance could be one important function of epidemiologically qualified extension veterinarians.

Other "diagnostic" statistics are derived, for example, from more or less cursory antemortem examination of animals for slaughter, examinations of animals passing through sales yards, and checking of animals intended for shipment interstate. The diag-

nosticians in such instances often are lay livestock inspectors; in any event, such diagnoses usually are purely clinical and are most often made without close examination of the animal.

Despite the relative unreliability of diagnoses of these types on an *individual* animal basis, with the proper evaluation of diagnostic criteria and their accuracy, epidemiologically useful information on unusual levels of disease or unusual diseases sometimes can be obtained from such sources and used when more reliable data are unavailable, or when there is a need to supplement more reliable data. Successful application of new research techniques, such as the ability to obtain not only animal identification information, but also accurate body temperature information, from animals remotely with inexpensive transponder implants, heightens such data collection possibilities immeasurably.

Useful surveillance information other than diagnostic data. Sometimes it is also possible to obtain usable disease frequency data in less direct ways, particularly for diseases often diagnosed and treated by the animal owner himself. One source is a monitoring of drug sales to animal owners; such drugs might include mastitis preparations, ophthalmic preparations, or therapeutic agents specific for one disease or a limited number of diseases. In the case of easy-to-diagnose conditions, fairly accurate incidence data might be obtained in this way. Unusual drug purchases, or unexpectedly large purchases of a drug by one or more farmers, might suggest an intensive follow-up study.

Development and improvement in organization of data sources

On the level of national or other large-scale programs in veterinary medicine, the conclusion is that data collection for the purposes of epidemiological surveillance is not being carried out today except on a piecemeal basis. What is still required generally is the development of multifaceted intelligence programs staffed by qualified epidemiologists, statisticians, and disease economists and well tied-in to facilities for diagnostic laboratory backup and to veterinary food protection and extension services. This need has been recognized recently in the United States in the report of a committee of the National Academy of Sciences.[14] Despite the common absence of comprehensive data collection machinery, the collection aspects of existing veterinary mortality and morbidity data programs probably are more adequate than are their analysis, interpretation, and dissemination aspects.

COLLATION AND ANALYSIS OF DATA

Surveillance data must be collated, reduced, and presented in usable forms or there is no point to their collection. Generally they also must be subjected to some degree of immediate analysis. Beyond such initial treatment, they provide a data bank for more detailed future analyses on an "as needed" basis, especially for studies to identify determinants of disease and studies in animal health economics.

While a variety of government and non-government agencies may be responsible for collection of the types of disease data indicated previously, the surveillance agency *per se* is responsible for pulling all these materials together *promptly* and collating and analyzing them. These aspects of surveillance are some of the most important responsibilities of epidemiologists concerned with animal disease control. There is no simple formula for undertaking these tasks, and many of the techniques and approaches outlined in this book will be employed in the process.

EXPRESSION, INTERPRETATION, AND PROMPT DISSEMINATION OF DATA

Essential to the success of surveillance is the prompt dissemination of the collated and analyzed data, together with appropriately interpreted evaluations of current problems, to (1) those who sub-

mitted the basic data, (2) those others who have a need to know or are in a position to participate in some directed action, and (3) within limits, the public.

This need for *prompt* dissemination cannot be satisfied by annual, semiannual, or quarterly reports, although periodic summaries and more in-depth analyses of certain types of surveillance data at such intervals may be appropriate. What is required is a general disease surveillance document issued frequently and regularly, preferably on a weekly or biweekly or, at the very least, a monthly basis. Appropriate to such a document are such things as (1) current, cumulative, and comparative tabular data of reported occurrences of a variety of diseases subject to continuous surveillance; (2) periodic, more in-depth data on selected diseases; (3) on-going reports of progress in specific control efforts; (4) alerts warning of existing or potential problems; (5) notice of relevant changes in legislation; (6) informative synopses of specific intensive follow-ups of cases or outbreaks; (7) predictions of future disease patterns or events; (8) official or other authoritative procedural recommendations; as well as (9) significant literature abstracts or other types of disease intelligence information. Figures 14–5 and 14–6 show some of these types of material from the Weekly Morbidity and Mortality Report, the basic weekly surveillance report issued by the U.S. Public Health Service.

Summary reports published less frequently often focus upon a single disease or related group of diseases and provide the greatest degree of in-depth analysis that the available data will sustain. The summarized partial contents of one such report of the U.S. Center for Disease Control are shown for illustrative purposes in Figure 14–7.

Various forms of data expression appropriate to surveillance reports, including but certainly not limited to tabular, graphic, statistical, and cartographic techniques, have been introduced in Chapters 5, 6, and 7. Different types of surveillance reports may be appropriate to different intended audiences. For example, those reports seeking to alert, educate, or generally inform the public might take the form of press releases and audio- or television tapes. Extension veterinarians with epidemiological training are in an ideal situation not only to feed important data into disease surveillance systems, but also to assure its prompt verbal and written dissemination to private veterinary practitioners and livestock owners.

Surveillance should never become routine. It should always be looked upon as a "pilot project" amenable to change and adaptation. For this reason, and also to make the best use of surveillance data, there should be on-going programs and research using these data. In veterinary medicine, some of the more important of these uses include (1) attempts to identify disease

CENTER FOR DISEASE CONTROL

Morbidity and Mortality

Vol. 24, No. 34

For
Week Ending
August 23, 1975

U.S. DEPARTMENT OF HEALTH, EDUCATION, AND WELFARE PUBLIC HEALTH SERVICE
DATE OF RELEASE: JULY 4, 1975 — ATLANTA, GEORGIA 30333

EPIDEMIOLOGIC NOTES AND REPORTS
TOXOPLASMOSIS - Pennsylvania

(Reported by: William G Lord, DVM, Public Health Veterinarian; Frank Boni, MD, Alvin Bodek, MD, Robert W Hilberg, MD, Rita Rosini, MD, private physicians; Frank B Clack, DVM, Director, Allegheny County Health Department; and the Parasitic Diseases Branch, Bureau of Epidemiology, CDC.)

On September 2, 1974, 2 male members of a wedding party became ill with low-grade fever, chills, generalized aches, fatigue, and swollen cervical lymph nodes. On September 4, another male member became similarly ill. On September 30, a female member also became ill with identical symptoms but did not have swollen cervical lymph nodes. The fever, chills, and generalized aches in these 4 persons subsided unevenly over a period of weeks; the fatigue and swollen lymph nodes persisted for months.

The patients were at first treated symptomatically and with antibiotics by their respective physicians. When the illness persisted, however, toxoplasmosis was suspected, and sera were drawn in November and December from 3 of the 4

CONTENTS

Epidemiologic Notes and Reports
   Toxoplasmosis - Pennsylvania 285
Current Trends
   Regulations for Importation of Nonhuman Primates –
      United States 286
   Primary and Secondary Syphilis – United States,
      June 1975 291
   Follow Up on St. Louis Encephalitis – Mississippi,
      United States 291

ill persons. Results by indirect fluorescent antibody (IFA) test were positive in all 3 persons for toxoplasmosis (Table I).

These results indicated a possible common source outbreak, and epidemiologic investigation revealed that on August 23, 1974, the 4 ill persons were among a group of 19 people attending a wedding rehearsal supper at a Syrian restaurant. Food histories were obtained from 15 of the 19

TABLE I. CASES OF SPECIFIED NOTIFIABLE DISEASES: UNITED STATES
(Cumulative totals include revised and delayed reports through previous weeks)

DISEASE	34th WEEK ENDING August 23, 1975	34th WEEK ENDING August 24, 1974	MEDIAN 1970-1974	CUMULATIVE, FIRST 34 WEEKS August 23, 1975	CUMULATIVE, FIRST 34 WEEKS August 24, 1974	MEDIAN 1970-1974
Aseptic meningitis	124	129	230	1,832	1,746	2,498
Brucellosis	6	1	3	151	104	120
Chickenpox	358	253		116,285	98,925	
Diphtheria	4	3	3	205	165	119
Encephalitis {Primary	58	41	38	573	593	852
Encephalitis {Post-Infectious	6	10	6	226	184	204
Hepatitis, Viral {Type B	273	192	167	7,511	6,190	5,534
Hepatitis, Viral {Type A	653	860	1,119	22,856	27,695	36,021
Hepatitis, Viral {Type unspecified	162	158		5,268	5,479	
Malaria	17	10	13	268	133	665
Measles (rubeola)	93	107	185	21,079	19,580	26,651
Meningococcal infections, total	23	17	17	1,031	931	1,012
Civilian	23	17	17	1,009	906	987
Military	–	–	–	22	25	38
Mumps	259	350	350	46,137	43,881	55,991
Pertussis	52	64		969	1,046	
Rubella (German measles)	51	140	149	14,651	9,565	25,773
Tetanus	6	2	2	58	60	68
Tuberculosis	679	611		21,907	20,064	
Tularemia	–	1	4	80	92	
Typhoid fever	6	6	10	200	245	224
Typhus, tick-borne (Rky. Mt. spotted fever)	32	34	23	611	606	376
Venereal Diseases:						
Gonorrhea {Civilian	20,751	18,067		635,420	571,104	
Gonorrhea {Military	576	626		19,719	19,216	
Syphilis, primary and secondary {Civilian	466	508		16,708	16,446	
Syphilis, primary and secondary {Military	1	9		234	303	
Rabies in animals	36	59	63	1,621	1,929	2,441

TABLE II. NOTIFIABLE DISEASES OF LOW FREQUENCY

	Cum.		Cum.
Anthrax: Ohio 1	1	Poliomyelitis, total	3
Botulism	14	Paralytic	3
Congenital rubella syndrome	17	Psittacosis: Ore. 1, Calif. 1	30
Leprosy: N.Y.C. 2	112	Rabies in man	1
Leptospirosis: Ark. 2	29	Trichinosis: * Conn. 2, Upstate N.Y. 1, N.J. 1, Alaska 1	62
Plague	'9	Typhus, murine: Texas 1	24

Fig. 14-5. Sample page from weekly disease surveillance report of U.S. Public Health Service, Center for Disease Control. Page shows types of tabular data presented and an example of a narrative report of the intensive follow-up investigation of an epidemic of a zoonotic infection.

determinants; (2) prophylactic, therapeutic, and other disease control trials; (3) predictions of future disease incidence; (4) inputs into decision-making models; and (5) evaluations of animal health economics. The predictive use of surveillance is illustrated next, and some of these other uses are considered in the next two chapters.

EPIDEMIOLOGICAL SURVEILLANCE AS A PREDICTIVE TOOL

One of the more important aspects of a surveillance system may be the ability to predict the occurrence or severity of disease problems, and to take appropriate actions. An example of such a usage is shown

Morbidity and Mortality Weekly Report

FIFTH DISEASE – Pennsylvania

From January through April 1975 an outbreak of rash illness occurred in 64 of 162 pupils (40%) in grades 1-6 at an elementary school in Clearville, Pennsylvania (Table 1). The illness was described as primarily a rash seen first on the face, then on the arms, and less frequently on the legs. Basically an erythema, the face rash gave a "slapped-cheek" appearance. The rash on the extremities was maculopapular and occasionally became reticulated. Usually no fever was noted, and the patient did not feel ill. In some individuals the rash recurred.

Table 1
Occurrence of Rash Illness in Elementary Students, Clearville, Pennsylvania, January-April 15, 1975

Month	Cases
January	2
February	3
March	18
April	40
Unknown	1
Total	64

Investigation of absenteeism records showed that from January 6 through February 28 mean daily absenteeism was 9.6, while from March 3 through April 14 it was 15.2, 59% higher. Plotting onsets by 3-day intervals, a gradual increase in cases occurred through March and peaked in early April (Figure 1).

FIGURE 1
ONSET OF RASH ILLNESS AT AN ELEMENTARY SCHOOL, BY 3-DAY INTERVALS, CLEARVILLE, PENNSYLVANIA, MARCH 1-APRIL 15, 1975

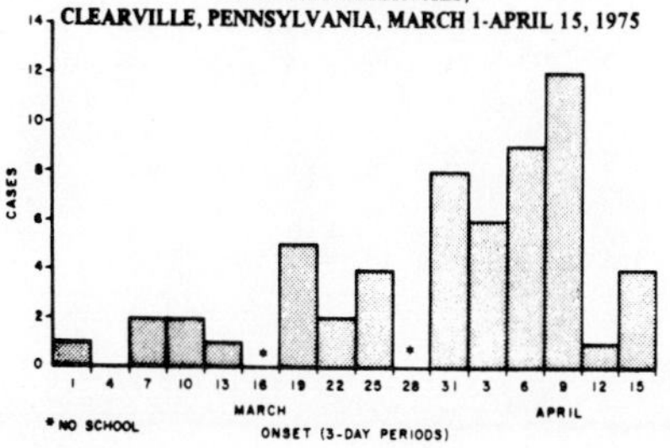

Analyzing the occurrence of rash by grade, the initial cases occurred in grades 1-3, with 52% of the ill children having their onset in March and a preponderance of cases occurring among second graders (Table 2). In addition, 92% of the cases in grades 4-6 had onset in April.

As of April 15, no cases of this type of rash had been recognized in any of the other elementary schools in this district. Two cases in students at the junior-senior high school had been reported, but no further cases were noted. Apparently some younger siblings of the ill elementary school children subsequently had the same rash at home.

Editorial Note

Based upon examinations of ill children, descriptions of the illness, and epidemiologic information, a diagnosis of epidemic erythema infectiosum, or Fifth disease, was made in this outbreak. Fifth disease is a benign illness of presumed viral etiology. It predominantly affects children ages 4-15, although adults can occasionally contract the disease. The mode of transmission is unknown, but assumed to be spread person-to-person by droplet infection. The incubation period is estimated at 4-15 days. The rash classically begins as an intense malar erythema ("slapped-cheek appearance"), spreads in maculopapular fashion to the extremities and trunk, becomes reticulated, and disappears in a few days to 5 weeks. The rash may be evanescent with recurrences related to changes in temperature, exercise, stress, or emotion. Associated fever is rare, and systemic illness is unusual except in adults, who can develop arthralgias or actual arthritis. The diagnosis of Fifth disease is based solely on clinical findings; there are no confirmatory laboratory tests. Authorities agree that since the

Table 2
Occurrence of Rash Illness by Grade at an Elementary School, Clearville, Pennsylvania, March 1-April 15, 1975

Grade	Students	No. with Rash	% with Rash	Onset March	Onset April	% March Onset
1	29	8	28	6	2	75
2	22	16	73	6	10	38
3	25	7	28	4	3	57
4	27	10	37	0	10	0
5	33	10	30	1	9	10
6	26	7	27	1	6	14
Total	162	58	36	18	40	31

illness is so benign and has no known complications, children need not be excluded from school if they otherwise feel well. *(Reported by Ruth Foor, RN, Everett Area School District; William E Parkin, DVM, Chief, Epidemiology Section, Division of Communicable Diseases, Pennsylvania Department of Health; and an EIS Officer.)*

Fig. 14-6. Sample page from weekly disease surveillance report of U.S. Public Health Service, Center for Disease Control. Example shows a narrative report, including an epidemic curve and tabular data, for an outbreak of an unusual disease of unknown etiology.

in the following paragraphs, which discuss the control of western equine encephalomyelitis.

Western equine encephalomyelitis

Some of the epidemiological complexities of western equine encephalomyelitis (WE) virus infection and the temporal sequence of events preceding summer epidemics of the disease in horses and man are reviewed in Chapters 4 and 6. The extensive epidemic of WE that occurred in Colorado in the summer of 1965 was predicted accurately[15] as the result of an on-going surveillance effort. The first indicators of that epidemic were the spring weather conditions (Fig. 14–8). Excess rainfall was noted beginning in early June and continuing into July. Major flooding resulted. In addition, "day-degrees above 70°F." did not begin to accumulate until

unusually late and 10 day-degrees above 70°F. were not reached until June 30. WE virus amplification in Colorado was known from past surveillance records to be partially dependent upon unusually cool and wet weather conditions in the spring. This prediction was confirmed by the end of June when *Culex tarsalis* populations had reached several times their expected levels, and their infection rates with WE virus also were well above the usual.

As a consequence of these observations, a special weekly surveillance newsletter was begun to alert veterinarians and health officers. Emergency aerial spraying for mosquitoes was initiated in late June, and a public education effort was begun. Continued surveillance (Figs. 14–8 and 14–9) showed seroconversion of sentinel chickens to have begun about mid-July, rather than as expected in normal years in

CENTER FOR DISEASE CONTROL

BRUCELLOSIS

| ANNUAL SUMMARY |
| BRUCELLOSIS — 1973 |

SURVEILLANCE

Center for Disease Control . . . . David J. Sencer, M.D., Director

Bureau of Epidemiology . . . . Philip S. Brachman, M.D., Director

Bacterial Diseases Division. . . . . John V. Bennett, M.D., Chief

Bacterial Zoonoses Branch . . . . Arnold K. Kaufmann, D.V.M., Chief
Marshall D. Fox, D.V.M.

Table 3   Brucellosis Cases* by Most Probable Source of Infection, United
States, 1968-1973

| Most Probable Source | Year | | | | | |
of Infection	1968	1969	1970	1971	1972	1973
Contact with Swine	90	114	85	88	88	51
Contact with Cattle	26	20	21	16	33	43
Contact with Cattle or Swine	21	16	31	16	15	15
Ingestion of Unpasteurized Dairy Products	29	5	6	26	13	33
Laboratory or Vaccine Accident	10	5	8	5	6	5
Other	3	4	4	2	7	6
Unknown	28	31	47	18	17	13
Totals	207	195	202	171	179	166

*Includes only cases for which case reports were received.

III. REPORTS FROM THE STATES

A. Human Brucella canis Infection - Tennessee: Reported by A. E. Horne, M.D., private practitioner, Memphis; Wilton A. Rightsel, Ph.D., Technical Director, Microbiology, Baptist Memorial Hospital, Memphis; George S. Lovejoy, M.D., Director, Memphis-Shelby County Health Department; Luther E. Fredrickson, D.V.M., Director, Veterinary Medicine, and Robert H. Hutcheson, Jr., M.D., State Epidemiologist, Tennessee Department of Public Health; and an EIS Officer.
An 18-year-old man was hospitalized in Memphis, on April 11, 1973, with a history of headache, nonproductive cough, low back pain, nausea, vomiting, and weight loss, over a 2-week period. He developed fever and chills on the day prior to admission. Blood cultures obtained on April 15 and 16 were positive for a gram-negative rod subsequently identified as Brucella canis.
Following hospital discharge on April 17, the patient was treated with ampicillin 250 mg 4 times daily for 8 days. Ampicillin treatment was discontinued when a generalized macular rash developed. Because of headache, sore throat, and low back pain, the

Fig. 14-7. Composite sample page from annual surveillance summary for brucellosis, U.S. Public Health Service, Center for Disease Control. Such summaries contain detailed tabular and graphic data as well as narrative reports of descriptive studies and intensive follow-up investigations.

early August. The conversion rate increased rapidly to unprecedented levels.

Reporting of clinical cases of encephalitis in horses began in the first week in July, and these were soon serologically confirmed as WE. The human index case had its onset on July 12, and the human epidemic peaked in mid-August. The declining epidemic curve for human infections beginning in late August followed a decline in the mosquito population, which started in early August.

ACTIVE DISEASE MONITORING OF INDIVIDUAL HERDS

Most of the examples given in this chapter are of surveillance-type epidemiological intelligence in large populations as aids to planning and carrying out government disease control programs. However, organized surveillance in individual herds is becoming more and more important. Animal agriculture is evolving generally, and quite rapidly, toward large

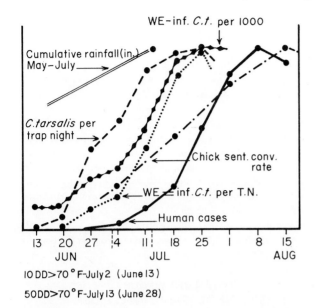

Fig. 14–8. Sequential relationships between selected indices and human epidemic curve during western equine encephalitis (WE) outbreak in eastern Colorado during 1965. All data except weather data are plotted as moving averages (redrawn from Hess, A.D., and Hayes, R.O. 1967. Seasonal dynamics of western encephalitis virus. Am. J. Med. Sci. 253:333).

integrated or coordinated operations in both the fattening-type and breeding-type industries. This process and its epidemiological significance are discussed in Chapter 17. These changes demand new types of veterinary practice input including, in particular, a continuous surveillance capability as a basis for epidemiological predictions and for epidemiologic and economic decision-making. An example to illustrate this use of herd surveillance in a beef feedlot practice is given in Chapter 16.

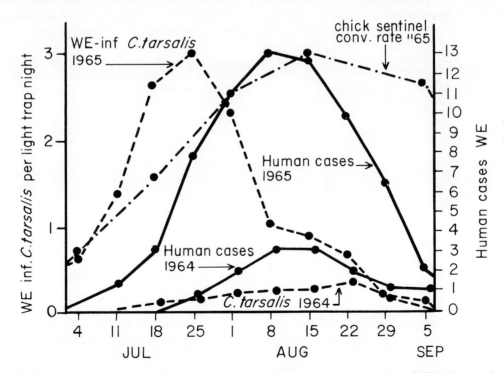

Fig. 14–9. Relationships between population levels of western equine encephalitis (WE)-infected *C. tarsalis* and human cases of WE encephalitis in eastern Colorado during epidemic year, 1965, and nonepidemic year, 1964. The relationship between WE antibody (HAI) conversion rates in sentinel chickens and human cases of WE is also shown for the epidemic year, 1965. All data are plotted as moving averages (redrawn from Hess, A.D., and Hayes, R.O. 1967. Seasonal dynamics of western encephalitis virus. Am. J. Med. Sci. 253:333).

INTENSIVE FOLLOW-UP

In addition to an on-going surveillance program, organizations concerned with livestock disease investigation and control, as well as individuals and groups in other aspects of veterinary practice, often require a more flexible and adaptable intelligence mechanism that can be quickly responsive to unanticipated disease events or unusual intelligence opportunities. Responses to such situations generally must be in-depth and often of relatively short duration. Common situations for intensive follow-up include suspected introductions of exotic infections, other epidemic occurrences of diseases, "problem herds" encountered during on-going disease control programs and other "unusual" disease events, as well as more frequent needs for contact, traceback, or case-finding efforts. Intensive follow-up efforts may be undertaken, of course, by the individual private practitioner or members of a group practice.

However, the capacity of a government veterinary organization for intensive epidemiological follow-up on a continuing "as needed" basis requires the availability (for such *ad hoc* assignments) of a mobile force of *trained* field investigators bulwarked by good facilities for the prompt laboratory examination of field specimens. The Epidemic Intelligence Service of the U.S. Center for Disease Control is an excellent example of such a field-based organization. This service consists of relatively few senior epidemiologists plus a highly mobile cadre of selected young physicians and veterinarians, frequently recruited and trained for limited assignment periods of about two years. A somewhat more specialized field force, the Emergency Disease Program, in the Animal and Plant Health Inspection Service of the U.S. Department of Agriculture, is specifically oriented to the intensive follow-up of suspected instances of the introduction of exotic livestock pathogens into the United States.[16]

Intensive follow-up efforts are varied in format and may call upon, in different combinations, virtually all of the methods in the epidemiologist's armamentarium. Several examples of intelligence efforts of this type have been given, with respect to epidemic or outbreak investigations and for case-finding and traceback efforts, in other sections of this book. A requisite of every such intensive effort is a written report of the event and follow-up, including appropriate analyses of data and a statement of conclusions, with *prompt* feed-in to the overall surveillance system of interim reports as required, and, wherever appropriate, fuller final reporting in the scientific literature.

FUTURE NEEDS IN EPIDEMIOLOGICAL INTELLIGENCE

Unquestionably, one of the greatest needs in veterinary medicine throughout the world today is the perfection of comprehensive epidemiological intelligence systems. This will probably become the single most important area of government veterinary services *per se*, and will provide accurate documentation of the importance of animal diseases, the sole basis for rational priority determinations with respect to research and possible actions against animal diseases, an accurate measure of progress in campaigns against diseases, a mechanism for program evaluation, the basis for an effective liaison between different veterinary services in government, and, finally, a rational basis for development of future cooperative efforts between the public and private sectors of veterinary medicine.

Chapter 15

ECONOMIC PARAMETERS IN EPIDEMIOLOGY

THE economic losses caused by livestock diseases are undoubtedly high but, with few exceptions, they are not known with any precision. General estimates for the United States are between 3 and 6 billion dollars annually.[1] The generally low reliability of published figures on overall losses or on those from specific diseases is attributable to the fact that most of them have been based upon crude estimates. Important sources of error result not only from inadequate surveillance data on animal morbidity and on difficulties of even crudely estimating indirect social costs of animal diseases, but also from a tendency to discuss disease losses as if they represent values that could be totally recaptured if the disease were brought under control.[2] Since it costs money to prevent or control diseases, the net gain resulting will not be the avoided disease losses *per se*, but the avoided disease losses minus the cost of controlling the disease.

Even so, measurement of gross disease losses alone is an important first step in helping to establish relative priorities in veterinary medicine and to indicate the potential of control and eradication approaches. Were two diseases shown to be of equal gross dollar value and technical control feasibility, then consideration would have to be given to such factors as costs of alternative control possibilities and social costs. (For example, one of the diseases might occur totally unpredictably and with often disastrous consequences to individual farmers.)

Economic aspects of veterinary medicine have received increasing attention in recent years and no doubt will receive even more attention in the future. This chapter considers costs from the standpoint of: (1) traditional food-animal practice, (2) preventive herd health-type practice, and (3) public practice carried out by state or federal veterinary agencies for control or eradication of defined diseases in large areas. There is no discussion of the more complex problem of trying to put dollar and cents values on urban companion-animal veterinary practices. The problem in that practice area of veterinary medicine resembles the problem of an economic evaluation of the impact of human diseases and human medical practice. Until more substantial progress is made in the human field, any attempt to assess similar questions in veterinary medicine would be premature.[3]

TRADITIONAL FOOD-ANIMAL PRACTICE

Veterinary service in the food-animal practice sector must be considered in an economic sense as a resource in animal production. In other words, it is an *input* factor in the production of meat, milk, eggs, and other animal products, and must be evaluated economically in the same way as are other inputs such as feed, pesticides, labor, housing, and managerial variables. A farmer acting rationally would utilize a veterinary service until the marginal value of its productivity equals the marginal value of productivity of some other input; that is, veterinary services would be used until the last dollar spent on them gives the farmer the same return as the last dollar spent, for example, on feed. The optimal amount of veterinary service used would depend on the degree of substitutability of feed and other input factors for veterinary service and on their relative prices. Because of the complexity of this type of situation, it is not surprising that few farmers attempt to have such economic evaluations carried out. However, it is likely that many successful and experienced farmers instinctively use veterinary service at a level that is close to the economic optimum.

This instinctive use concept was illustrated in a published study[4] designed to measure the contribution of the veterinary service expense component to dairy enterprise income in Minnesota, assuming that veterinary service like other resources is subject to the law of diminishing returns. Data were obtained on the value of milk produced plus changes in animal inventory, less the cost of feed consumed by dairy animals. A production function was estimated, with income as a function of cow numbers, veterinary services expense, drug expense, calves that died, and cows that were culled. Cow numbers were used as a proxy for land, labor, and capital devoted to the dairy enterprise. Calves that died and cows culled were used as a proxy for the general health conditions in the herds. Veterinary services expense was considered to be the total of veterinary bills, including drugs used or prescribed by the veterinarian. Drug expences *per se* represented the farmers' own purchases of drugs.

The estimated marginal product value of veterinary services (i.e., the return on the last dollar spent on veterinary services) varied from $8.03 for farms that used $0 to $6 of veterinary service per cow per year to $1.82 for farms that used more than $12 of veterinary services. The average value of $2.96 is similar to the value of the marginal product for other inputs such as pesticides. The farmers who used veterinary services most seemed to be closest to the optimal level of use, assuming unconstrained production budgets.

The value of marginal product for the farmers' own use of drugs was $6.28, which is higher than expected and seems to contradict the belief that farmers frequently buy drugs of low marginal productivity. However, the high value in this study may reflect in large part the inclusion of iodine teat dip purchases. It is possible, too, that certain unmeasured aspects of management improvements are associated with drug use.

Rigorous cow culling appeared to result in a high payoff. This economic return again might partially have resulted from association of culling with other aspects of management; that is, culling *per se* may not have been independent of such other factors.

Interpretation of this type of study, in which the effects of veterinary services are treated as an economic production function, may be difficult because veterinary service also may not be independent of certain management factors that are not measured but may have a strong economic impact. However, it may be possible to correct for such interdependences, and analyses of this type should be encouraged because they do provide insight into the economic value of veterinary inputs in terms of food-animal production.

HERD HEALTH PROGRAMS

In evaluation of the economic effect of herd health programs, more direct measurements of change in disease losses have been attempted than those in the production-type equation illustrated previously. In the final analysis, it is the total income of the farm that is important, and costing of animal diseases and herd health programs must be considered in that context. This "whole farm" point of view has been discussed by Morris and several other investigators.[5] Use of linear programming has been one technique advocated to determine such things as optimum herd size, calving distribution, and level of control for various diseases, all of which can be achieved within the limitations of resource restrictions in available land, labor, capital, veterinary services, and other areas. One published proposal[6] has outlined methods for analysis of the components of a dairy preventive medicine program that is divided into these four components: improvement of reproductive efficiency, improved mastitis control, reduced calf losses, and control of other diseases. It was proposed to integrate these four disease components to produce plans for whole-farm health programs.

In that example, the economic value of preventive actions taken within each section of the program was measured by gross margin analysis in which the extra *cost* incurred by some directed action (i.e., a therapeutic or preventive measure) was subtracted from the economic value of the response (benefit *or* cost). If more than one method had been available for prevention or cure of a particular syndrome, the method with the highest gross margin would be chosen, other things being equal.

For such analyses, it is important to be able to anticipate the types of response elicited in order to estimate such gross margins correctly. For instance, treatment and prevention of a phosphorus deficiency in cows may result in improved reproduction and improved milk yield. Both of these factors should be included in the response realized. Conversely, restricting intake of estrogenic clover may improve fertility but at the same time reduce production. In another case, diminishing response in fertility improvement resulting from a relative energy deficiency might be anticipated if feed supplementation continued to be increased. Production functions can be used to determine the economically optimal levels of inputs in such situations.

In the evaluation of the economic impact of diseases that temporarily reduce growth rate, attention should be paid to a possible compensatory gain that may occur following control of the disease. This rebound effect will influence the economically optimal level of disease control measures. This factor seems to be especially evident in parasite control. Also, there is some indication that a moderate depression of growth rate during rearing of calves does not affect their subsequent production.

Few published descriptions of a whole-farm approach in disease control have yet appeared, and generally these have not benefitted from detailed analyses. A number of publications do, however, consider economic aspects of therapeutic and prophylactic intervention against specific diseases.[7] Such studies are valuable and may help in determining economically optimal interventions for a whole-farm program.

Benefits from changes in disease control and breeding regimens

A published example concerning control of bovine mastitis, and including an investment appraisal, is illustrated next.[8] In this analysis, a representative dairy farm that milks 100 cows converts from a mastitis control program consisting of udder washing, teat-cup dipping in an antiseptic solution, and treatment of clinical mastitis to a control program consisting of udder washing with running water, teat dipping, backflushing of teat-cups, and dry period treatment of diagnosed infected quarters. With this program change, the prevalence of subclinical mastitis is reduced from 30% of quarters to 5%. Because of the time delay between the change in program and realization of a reduction in the infection level, the costs and the gains in this analysis should have been *discounted* back to the time of the program change. For simplicity of illustration, this discounting was not done. (Discounting is discussed under the subject of cost-benefit analysis.)

The analysis in the illustration was as follows, with all the monetary values given in Australian dollars:

(1) Additional returns

Cows have longer herd life since the number sold because of low production caused by mastitis is reduced from 35% to almost zero. As a result, some heifers that would otherwise have entered the herd can be sold.

Sale per year of 5.2 animals at two years of age and 19.8 at 5.05 lactations	$2725
Increased genetic gains — Higher milk production from older cows	Not counted

(2) Returns no longer obtained

Sale of 25 cows after four lactations	$2575

(3) Extra cost

Diagnostic testing	$70
Antibiotic for dry treatment of 10% of quarters annually	$36
Teat dip	$60
Depreciation of backflushing system	$10
Annual maintenance of milking machine	$15

(4) Costs no longer incurred

Reduced loss of production because of mastitis	$1500
Sanitizers for udder and teat-cup dipping	$50
Reduced treatment of clinical mastitis	$117
Change in income (1+4−2−3) =	$1626

One problem with this type of approach is that it treats the situation as a static one, and it raises the question of when it would be reasonable to change the program. In fact, farmers are strongly tempted to discontinue such successful programs after a number of years. This problem can be alleviated partially by

developing a predictive model to forecast the situation that will exist after application for a given number of years of a defined replacement/culling program combined with mastitis control. Epidemiological modeling is considered in the following chapter.

In another instance, a published control program based upon chemotherapy for fascioliasis in cattle included determination of production losses but not an investment appraisal.[9] Two hundred fifteen milking cows were examined for the presence of fluke eggs, and 65 were found to be positive. The infected cows were divided randomly into groups (I and II); the uninfected cows constituted group III. The milk yield of each cow was recorded prior to and after anthelmintic treatment. The results showed that milk yield of cows in group I (after treatment) was 8% better than yields in group II and that group III had a 6% higher yield than group I. The conclusion was that low levels of liver fluke infections caused at least an 8% reduction in milk yield, corresponding to loss of 0.5 pounds sterling per cow per month. The costs of alternatives for control (e.g., chemotherapy, use of molluscicides, drainage, and fencing) were not discussed. In a further example of an improved estrus detection program, the author reported a gross margin of 13.5 pounds sterling per cow per year.[10] Although information about economic returns on herd health programs is still limited, it seems certain that such programs at their initiation have the potential to yield higher values of marginal product than do more traditional veterinary services.

Need for research

As has been suggested at other points in this book, successful conduct of herd health programs in veterinary medicine requires generation of types of knowledge uncommonly produced today by veterinary research. A basic epidemiological approach to describing and analyzing overall herd problems has not been developed for any animal industry. Generally, little research has been carried out on transformation of biological and epidemiological information into economically and managerially sound guidelines for field veterinarians and farmers.[11] In a herd health-type situation, field *research* should be virtually indistinguishable from *practice*.

As indicated at several points by example, it often is not essential to define precisely the etiology of a disease before being able to control it. Epidemiology is concerned *often* with quite indirect but valid determinants of diseases. Similarly, Morris[5] has suggested that the carrying out of an economic analysis may not be dependent upon precise etiological data. For example, it may be possible from the records of a dairy herd to make hypotheses about some of the likely causes of reproductive inefficiency, such as nutritional deficiency, vibriosis, or less direct factors;

to examine these retrospectively (Chapters 11 and 13); and then to determine quickly through prospective corrective trials (Chapter 12) the most expedient and economic way of tackling the problem even without waiting for a precise laboratory-confirmed diagnosis. Laboratory diagnoses take precious time and often are less than satisfactory, particularly when multiple agents may be involved. Ultimately, the study of etiology may suggest better control methods. The previous approach is economically sound not only in disastrous outbreak situations such as the parathion poisoning epidemic in a cattle feedlot, but also in endemic situations.[5]

Many so-called herd health programs attempt to omit the steps just discussed and empirically prescribe prophylactic or therapeutic action without first carrying out proper retrospective analyses and prospective corrective pilot trials. This uncontrolled, unscientific approach is understandable perhaps when purely routine cases are being dealt with—but it hardly recommends itself as a general approach if for no other reason than that it does not yield convincing information for future use.

The field research procedure outlined does not necessarily cause a delay in the treatment that a herd may need. With a reasonable series of hypotheses in hand, trials yielding unbiased responses can be achieved in some situations through an evolutionary operation system (EVOP) in which trials are conducted in a continuous fashion within the herd in order to evolve optimal health control conditions. In such a system, the variables in the trials are changed to a degree that is small enough to avoid major economic losses or increased health hazards in the operation, yet large enough to be measured.

What is generally overlooked, even when the value of such a stepwise system of prospective trials is appreciated, is that the type of information needed to design trials is sometimes available in farm records and can be evaluated through retrospective epidemiological studies. Useful techniques for this purpose are discussed throughout this book. In particular, multivariate retrospective field studies may make it possible rather quickly to obtain more precise information about meaningful disease determinants than would be gained by a succession of expensive laboratory searches for *a* specific agent. This approach is illustrated in the example on dairy calf mortality in Chapter 13. These observations do not discount at all the great value of laboratory support—quite the contrary—but merely warn against an exclusive dependence on laboratory diagnosis (often a biased sample of sick or dead animals).

PUBLIC PROGRAMS IN DISEASE CONTROL AND PREVENTION

The economic evaluation of public veterinary practice, the third sector for emphasis, is carried out through cost-benefit analyses, which apply a technique that attempts to evaluate the social costs and social benefits of investment projects. Their purpose is to help the veterinarian decide whether a particular project should be undertaken, and, if it should, what program alternatives recommend themselves. The essential difference between cost-benefit analysis and ordinary investment appraisal methods used for individual farms is the stress in cost-benefit analysis on *social* costs and benefits.

The aim is to identify and measure the losses and gains in economic welfare that are incurred by *society as a whole* if the particular project is undertaken. In calculating the benefits of constructing a new public transport system, not only the revenue from ticket sales would be taken into consideration but also the value of reductions in travelling time to users, congestion cost to motorists, and comparable aspects. Similarly, in calculating costs of a new airport, the costs of land acquisition, construction, and subsequent operation, plus losses, for such matters as aircraft noise and spoilage of scenic beauty, would all be included. There are many difficulties in cost-benefit analysis—the main one being the placement of dollar values on costs and benefits that have no market price. Cost-benefit analysis nevertheless is an important method of making the best possible information available to government decision makers. Items that cannot be given monetary value, so-called intangibles, are at least listed in such an analysis.

The original rationale of cost-benefit criteria is that of a Pareto improvement, defined as a change in economic organization that makes one or more members of society better off without making anybody worse off. However, some public projects clearly make some people worse off (those exposed to airport noise) and some people better off (those who benefit from the airport but are not bothered by the noise). Therefore, the rationale of cost-benefit criteria usually is considered in terms of a *potential* Pareto improvement, which is defined as a change that—if costless transfers of goods and/or money among members of a society are assumed—*can* make everyone better off in the aggregate. In other words, a project with positive benefits is one which produces *total* gains that *exceed* total losses.[12]

In 1950 general principles and rules for cost-benefit analysis were established by an interagency government committee in the United States. These rules were developed into a planning-programming-budgeting (P.P.B.) system introduced by presidential order in 1965 to apply to all federal departments and agencies. Thus, since 1965 the veterinary services of the U.S. Department of Agriculture have been obliged to carry out cost-benefit analyses of their animal disease control and eradication programs. The value of cost-benefit analysis is not solely that it helps to insure that proposed disease control projects have a positive effect, and permits the choice of the economically best approach to control among alternatives, but also that it provides a valuable insight into the behavior of diseases in populations and helps define the need for additional knowledge.

The following examples illustrate some of the components that go into cost-benefit analysis of animal disease control programs. General principles of cost-benefit analysis are discussed in more detail by Mishan.[13]

Principles of project evaluation

In a disease control project, as in most other projects, benefits and costs occur in different quantities at different times.[12,13] Typically most of the costs occur first while the benefits show up later. A profile for an engineering project, such as building a dam that will generate hydroelectric power and provide for irrigation, may resemble that shown in Figure 15–1. In disease control or eradication programs, one can generally expect a different profile because continued vigilance is required to prevent reintroduction of the disease, and this action incurs continued cost. The cost-benefit profile of brucellosis eradication in a country may resemble Figure 15–2.

Irrespective of the shape of the cost-benefit profile, the general approach to comparison between costs and benefits is to discount the costs and benefits incurred each year of the project back to a present value using a predetermined interest rate. The general discount/compound formula is: $(1+r)^n$, where r is the interest rate and n equals the number of years. In compounding, PV (present value) in n years is worth $PV(1+r)^n = FV$ (future value). In discounting, $\frac{FV}{(1+r)^n} = PV$.

If the following are streams of cost and benefits in a project,

Year	0	1	2	3	4
Costs ($)	1000	0	0	0	0
Benefits ($)	0	200	300	400	400

and the interest rate is 8%, the present value of the benefits is:

$$\frac{200}{(1+0.08)^1} + \frac{300}{(1+0.08)^2} + \frac{400}{(1+0.08)^3} + \frac{400}{(1+0.08)^4} = \$1054,$$

while the present value of the cost is $1000. The net benefit becomes $1054 - $1000 = $54, and the benefit-cost ratio is $\frac{1054}{1000}$ = 1.054. Thus, discounting also takes into consideration interest yield on the money for the program if it were invested in an alternative fashion.

It is clear that the outcome of this type of calculation depends on the pattern in which benefits and costs occur over the years, the interest rate that is used, and the duration of the project (the number of years for which benefits and costs are calculated). Mishan[13] offers a detailed discussion of investment criteria, including the use of internal rate of return calculations. These considerations are important, but the project analyst often does not have a choice with respect to investment criteria. In fact, the use of present value calculations with a fixed discount rate has been established by authorities in some countries. In 1975 it was 10% in the United States and 8% in the United Kingdom. With respect to the duration of projects, it is difficult to give fixed rules because projects are very different. However, in disease control programs it would rarely be advisable to project for more than 20 years.

Hypothetical example of control of a tick-borne disease[14]

This example is purely hypothetical and given for illustrative purposes only. Suppose that a region is stocked with 10,000 breeding head of cattle at a stocking rate of 5 acres per breeding head. Annual value of production (net of variable cost) equals $250 per breeding head. The annual crude death rate of cattle is closely related to the density of a tick population that serves as vectors for a disease agent.

The annual crude death rate (%) is $\alpha + \beta x^2$, where α = 2, β = 0.008, and x = tick population per acre divided by 10,000.

Before the control program, the tick population is 150,000 per acre; and this ecological equilibrium

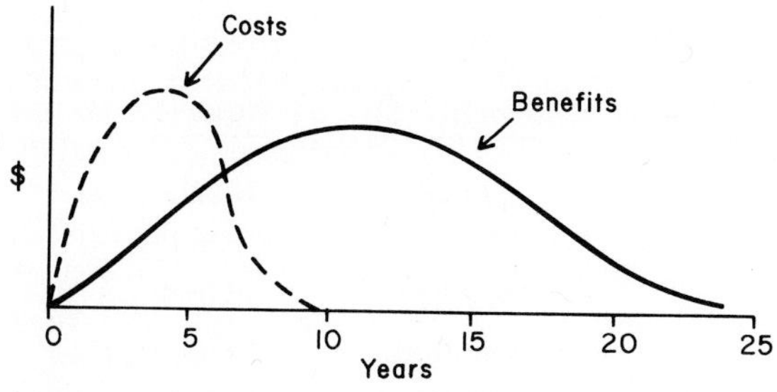

Fig. 15–1. Hypothetical cost-benefit profile for public engineering project.

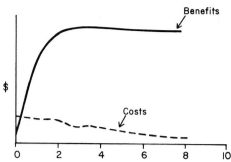

Fig. 15-2. Hypothetical cost-benefit profile for animal disease eradication program.

(climax) population is affected by spraying and rainfall. The tick population has ability to recover because of the presence of wildlife hosts. The spraying technology is known, and spraying costs 20 cents per acre per year. The degree of kill is dependent on rainfall, according to the following function:

$$\frac{\text{No. killed/year/acre}}{100} = 240 - 4R,$$

where R, the annual rainfall, is a random variable with a mean of 35 inches and standard deviation of 25 inches.

From these data the effect of spray can be calculated. Using an average rainfall of 35 inches, x is the number of ticks expected to be killed:

$$\frac{x}{100} = 240 - (4 \times 35)$$
$$x = 10,000.$$

Remaining numbers of ticks = 150,000 – 10,000 = 140,000.

The expected percent of cattle dying annually when no spraying is applied is:

$$2 + 0.08(\frac{150,000}{10,000})^2 = 20.$$

Expected annual percent mortality when spraying is applied is:

$$2 + 0.08(\frac{140,000}{10,000})^2 = 17.68.$$

The benefit of spraying equals 20% – 17.68% = 2.32% decrease in annual mortality. In money value this figure is equal to:

$$\frac{10,000 \times 2.32 \times \$250}{100} = \$58,000 \text{ per year.}$$

The cost of spraying equals 50,000 x 0.2 = $10,000 per year.

The expected streams of costs and benefits remain constant as long as the program lasts, with a net benefit of $48,000 per year. Running the program for four years (10% interest) results in net benefits of $167,000 and a benefit-cost ratio of 5.8. Extension of the program will increase the net benefit but not change the benefit-cost ratio. A decrease of the discount rate to 8% will increase present value of four years' net benefit to $179,000 but leave the benefit-cost ratio unchanged.

Several suggestions can be made with respect to the program just described. It might be that the rate of spraying is not optimal; i.e., that $1 of extra input of spray will result in more than $1 saved by reduced annual mortality. This amount can be determined by field studies and development of a production function. However, one would have to consider additional costs or benefits caused by the effect of higher pesticide levels on fauna and on animal and human health. Furthermore, the program might be improved by elimination of the wildlife reservoir for the tick, with the result that the tick population does not recover after spraying.

Elimination of the wildlife reservoir might bring in $100,000 in benefit from sales of meat in the first year but incur a loss of $20,000 per year because of elimination of tourism.

Keeping the rate of spraying constant, the calculations now become:

Year	No. ticks surviving/acre	Cattle killed (%)	Value of cattle saved ($)
0	150,000	20	0
1	140,000	17.68	58,000
2	130,000	15.52	112,000
3	120,000	13.52	162,000
4	110,000	11.68	208,000
5	100,000	10	250,000

Year	Benefits ($)	Costs ($)
0	100,000	20,000
1	58,000	30,000
2	112,000	30,000
3	162,000	30,000
4	208,000	30,000
5	250,000	30,000

With a 10% interest rate, present value of benefits is $314,000 and of cost $85,000, giving a net benefit of $229,000 and a benefit-cost ratio of 3.32. If the interest rate is 8%, the values become $397,000, $102,000, $295,000, and 3.9. This example illustrates that a difference in benefits (or costs) from year to year also influences the benefit-cost ratio when the interest rate is changed.

If the analysis were continued over additional years, it would be found that, after a certain number of years, the cost of spraying would equal the value of additional cattle lives saved. At this time, the program should be reevaluated; e.g., the economic consequences of completely eradicating ticks and barring wildlife hosts of the tick from reentering the region should be analyzed.

A number of other areas should be considered. The assumption of average rainfall is arbitrary. One could carry out a so-called sensitivity test by repeating the cost-benefit analysis using average rainfall plus one standard deviation. If net benefits are still positive, it can be assumed with higher assurance that this project meets the required criteria.

Another consideration that must enter the cost-benefit analysis is the opportunity cost of the land, i.e., the value of the land in its best alternative use. The value of the land as a tourist area has already been included in the analysis, but, if its best alternative value is as cropland, the value of this use should be entered as a cost. Another consideration is that cattle and/or crop production may create income for small livestock holders who would otherwise remain unemployed. The principles in dealing with these items are discussed by Mishan.[12,13] Also, the possible damaging effect of pesticides and the fact that wildlife may be permanently eliminated should be listed as losses although it might be difficult to put dollar values on these—apart from the lost tourist income, which has already been mentioned.

Finally, it should be pointed out that the way benefits were calculated in the preceding example is not entirely correct. The social benefit is not simply estimated as the reduced economic losses of beef production, but is also determined as an increase in consumers' surplus resulting from the improved cattle production economy. The increase in consumers' surplus can be estimated on the bases of the demand curve for beef, the price elasticity of beef, and the increase in supply. These principles also are discussed by Mishan[12,13] and appear in an analysis of tsetse fly control in Uganda.[15]

It must be emphasized that the validity of the cost-benefit analysis of disease control programs depends on reliable data obtained through epidemiological studies. Thus, epidemiological studies and economic studies go hand in glove. Unfortunately, data of the necessary quality often are lacking today.

Cost-benefit evaluation of alternative control policies for foot-and-mouth disease in Great Britain

Following the 1967-68 foot-and-mouth disease epidemic in England, it was suggested that vaccination be substituted for the traditional slaughter policy as a method to control this disease.[16]

(1) Slaughter policy

All susceptible animals on a farm where the disease has been detected are slaughtered, and exposed animals are traced and slaughtered. A 10-mile quarantine zone is established around the affected farm, and a larger controlled area is established if exposed animals that have been moved cannot be traced and slaughtered.

(2) Vaccination policy

All cattle, sheep, and goats (not pigs) three months old would be vaccinated with a trivalent inactivated vaccine. Two vaccinations would be given the first year, and after that there would be one vaccination per year. When outbreaks occurred, the approach described under the slaughter policy would apply, and there would be area vaccination with monovalent vaccine.

(3) Benefits

The benefits accrued to society were measured as the costs avoided in the absence of the disease. The net benefit to society of each of the alternative control policies was estimated as the difference between cost of an endemic situation and cost of controlling the disease by alternative methods. It was assumed that, if foot-and-mouth disease went uncontrolled in Great Britain, there would be a 25% yearly incidence rate, and livestock production would decrease as follows:

(a) Decrease of 25% in milk production during the first four years, then a 12.5% decrease for the following years.

(b) Reduction of 15% in output of beef, mutton, and lamb during the first two years and then a reduction of 12.5% during the following years (reduced fertility 6%; increased mortality 2% in young, 0.5% in adult; loss of weight gain 2%; delayed calving 2%).

(c) Reduction of 20% in pork production.

These data were only estimates. However, as shown in the following paragraphs, even if they were grossly overestimated, a net benefit would accrue from both control policies.

(1) Slaughter cost

A probability analysis based on number of outbreaks in previous years gave an expected annual number of outbreaks (number of affected farms) of 175. Cost of slaughter and compensation to farmers was evaluated as 51 pounds sterling per animal (1968 prices), and the consequential cost to the community was set at the same level.

Marketing inefficiencies and higher distribution costs because of quarantine restrictions caused an approximately 5% increase in meat prices during the 1967-68 epidemic. To this figure must be added certain nonquantified costs, such as distress of farmers having their livestock slaughtered, genetic loss due to slaughter of pedigree herds, and upset of breeding programs due to interruption of artificial insemination service. Other interests affected are food wholesalers, industries and organizations supplying goods and services to agriculture, public works (e.g., road construction), sport, and tourism. Losses that are not costs to society but merely transfer payments could be identified; e.g., agricultural workers lost some overtime earnings, which were offset by reduced labor cost to the farmers.

(2) Vaccination cost

It was assumed that the general vaccination would reduce primary outbreaks by 50% and secondary outbreaks by 90% (all herds within a 5-mile radius of a primary outbreak would be revaccinated with monovalent vaccine); and it was assumed that consequential losses would be reduced to 25% of the direct costs of slaughtering. The main expense is the vaccine.

For 1969 the cost of a vaccine dose for cattle would be 12.5p and 4.2p per sheep. The prices were expected to drop 15% by 1970 with a further drop of 25% by 1972. Allowance of 10% was made for vaccine wastage, and corrections were made for increasing numbers of animals to be vaccinated over the years (because of expected increase in livestock populations). Vaccination fees were set at 10p per head for cattle and 5p per head for sheep.

The net present value (benefits minus costs discounted at 8% for a 16-year period) was 1414 million pounds sterling for the slaughter policy and 1389 for vaccination. These figures are so close that ranking was based on relative costs (Table 15–1). Based on the total costs the slaughter policy was recommended. These calculations of benefit have some wide error margins because of lack of reliable figures for disease losses and spread of disease. Also the projected future number of livestock may be in error.

The estimated cost differences between the two policies depend on three sets of assumptions: vaccine cost, veterinary fees, and outbreak numbers. Outbreak numbers could decline considerably because of improvement in foot-and-mouth disease situations in countries that export meat to Great Britain. This change would favor the slaughter policy. The authors carried out a sensitivity analysis with increased consequential costs and increased vaccination cost, respectively. This cost increase did not change the ranking of policies. This summary does not do justice to an interesting study, which is one of the first published cost-benefit analyses related to veterinary medicine. It should be read in its entirety.

Problem 20. Calculation of economic losses associated with calf mortality on a dairy farm

The economic problems of calf mortality could be encountered by veterinarians in private herd health or public practice.[17] The herd setting and circumstances for this problem are as described in Problem 18 in Chapter 12. Now you will make use of the life table calculated for that problem. It should resemble the one shown in Table 15–2 (although the notation

Table 15–1.   Estimated Costs of Alternative Foot-and-Mouth Disease Control Programs for Great Britain[16]

	Millions £ Sterling	
	Slaughter policy	Vaccination policy
Direct costs	6	48
Slaughtering	6	1
Vaccination	0	47
Consequential costs	29	12
Miscellaneous costs in distribution sector	6	0.4
Compensating payments for slaughtering	22	2.5
Allowance for risk	1	0.1
Costs involved in assembling stock for vaccination	0	9
Total	35	60

Table 15–2.   Life Table of Survivorship for Heifer Dairy Calves on Standard Farm (Problem 20)[17]*

Time (in weeks) after birth	No. calves alive at least i weeks after birth	No. calves dying between the ith and the ith + 1 week	Probability of dying during the ith to the ith + 1 week for calves alive at time i	Probability of those calves alive at time i surviving until the ith + 1 week ($p_i = 1 - q_i$)	Proportion of calves surviving i weeks
i	0_i	d_i	q_i	p_i	P_i
0	100	8	0.080	0.920	100.0
1	92	7	0.076	0.924	92.0
2	85	3	0.035	0.965	85.0
3	82	1	0.012	0.988	82.0
4	81	1	0.012	0.988	81.1
5	80	—	—	—	80.1

*See text.

used is slightly different from that described in Chapter 12).

Assume that if calf deaths do not occur, the per-item costs to raise each heifer calf are as shown in Table 15–3.

Calculate the cumulative costs by week to raise a heifer calf to five weeks of age.

Assume the average value of a heifer calf at birth to be $70 ($V_0$), and assume that it increases in value by $10 each week (i.e., $V_1 = \$80$, $V_2 = \$90$).

You can now make use of the stochastic model illustrated in Chapter 16. Assume that heifer calves are not sold until they reach the end of the fourth week of life (i.e., five weeks of age). The probability of selling a calf before that time, therefore, is zero.

Substituting the appropriate data in the model equation, calculate the total expected return per calf if surviving calves are all sold at five weeks of age.

What would the farmer's profit have been per calf at five weeks of age if no calf mortality had occurred?

What was the profit margin loss per calf because of this experienced 20% mortality rate?

Figure 15–3 plots the effects of different levels of calf mortality on expected net return per animal given the circumstances of this problem.

DEVELOPING MORE ADEQUATE DATA

This chapter concludes by pointing to the possibilities suggested in a few published studies, which recommend providing more complete input data to economic studies considering the costs of animal diseases.

Cost of fever

In an energy-based theoretical approach to the more accurate estimation of costs of animal diseases,

Table 15–3.   Cost to Raise Heifer Dairy Calves to Five Weeks of Age (Problem 20)[17]*

Item	Cost
Building[†] costs per calf	$3.50
Labor[†] costs per calf	$5.00
Feed costs per calf	
Whole milk	$2.50/week (week 0–3)
Powdered milk	$1.00/week (week 3–5)
Concentrate	$0.25/week (week 3–5)
Hay	$0.15/week (week 2–5)
Veterinary services and drug costs per calf	$0.40/week

*See text.
†The figures in this example are considered fixed costs.

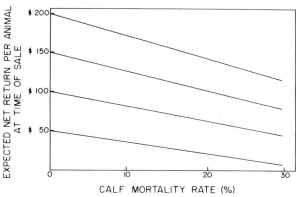

Fig. 15–3. Effect of calf mortality on expected net return per calf at time of sale (Problem 20).[17]

the added feed cost of fever in accelerating protein and caloric energy metabolism was estimated for one year in the cattle population of Canada.[18] Published data on frequency of the four most common diagnoses in cattle in 12 major North American veterinary clinics (all four diseases usually accompanied by fever) were used in a conservative hypothesis that 25% of Canadian cattle experience in any one year a febrile episode of 3°F. rise in temperature of an average 3 days' duration. Thus, a total of 27 million "degree-days" per year were calculated for the 12 million cattle population of Canada.

Assuming that an average digestible energy requirement is 20,000 kcal per day per animal and also assuming, from published estimates, that each degree of fever requires 7% of this daily value, then each degree-day would utilize 1400 kcal. From the calculated estimate of total degree-days per year for Canada, 37.8 billion kcal would have to be expended annually to maintain bovine fevers. Converting to wheat or barley grain, 11,812 tons of grain would be required per year merely to maintain fever, or enough grain to supply the full energy requirements of 250,000 cattle for one week. Certainly, a considerable refinement of such estimates could be made using real data, and these numbers could be converted to economic terms.

Costs of subclinical parasitism

In another example the biomass of parasites was interestingly computed in the case of human ascariasis in China before World War II.[19] Extrapolations of prevalence data on *Ascaris lumbricoides* infections in Chinese indicated a total of 335×10^6 infected people in 1937. Considering the mean infection level as 18 worms per infected individual, the total ascarids harbored by the population was calculated as 6×10^9. That worm biomass equalled that of 442,000 men. It had an annual reproductive capacity of 22×10^{16} eggs, that is, 18,000 tons of ascarid eggs. The author of this estimate could have carried this analysis further by calculating dollars required per year just to nourish this particular parasite population and to sustain its reproductive capacity. Similar calculations would be apt in attempting to estimate the true costs of a number of parasitic diseases or complexes of livestock.

Because of wide interest in this subject and a highly scattered literature, further references on economic studies of animal diseases are included with the notes.[20] Like some other types of population studies of disease, those designed to yield economic data may lend themselves to construction of epidemiological or decision-making models. One example is included in this chapter, and the general subject of epidemiological modelling is discussed in Chapter 16.

Chapter 16

EPIDEMIOLOGICAL MODELS

THE purpose of modelling in epidemiology is (1) to make predictions of disease incidence or prevalence, (2) to better understand the underlying biomedical mechanism, or (3) to test hypotheses about the mechanism. One should be cautioned, however, that the predictive capacity of a model depends upon the determinants that influence the disease behaving in the same way in the future. For this reason predictive epidemiological models should be updated frequently and based on the latest observational information.

The important requirements of a model are that (1) it should behave in a biologically and mathematically reasonable way; (2) it must be sensitive to important factors and insensitive to unimportant factors; (3) its mechanisms should be intuitively acceptable; and (4) it should mimic real life situations.

Models can be constructed inductively, deductively, or in a combination of ways. They can be categorized in several ways, e.g., as predictive or explanatory models, or as iconic, analogic, or analytic models.[1] Models also may be deterministic or stochastic. Deterministic models are concerned with the *average* circumstance or individual, and the mathematical solution of the model equation is always the same, subject to the restrictions imposed by the initial conditions specified in the model. A stochastic model, on the other hand, includes an element of *randomness*, and the model equation can produce several outcomes depending upon the laws of chance. Stochastic models often are more realistic than corresponding deterministic models, but they are also more complex.

In mathematical modelling of a biomedical phenomenon, a chief aim may be to characterize that phenomenon, reducing it to its essential elements, so that the relationships among its components can be studied mathematically. The cost of reducing a phenomenon to its essential elements can be great, particularly when a great deal of interesting detail must be ignored. Also, medical and other biological phenomena are usually so complex that only a few factors can be chosen for model building; thus, there

may be some question as to whether the so-called essential elements included in the model are the truly essential or relevant elements. In spite of these limitations, there are several definite advantages to studying reduced numbers of factors. In particular, it may be possible to study the effects of single elements mathematically in a model even when such elements do not occur alone in nature.

Possibly the greatest advantage of a well-conceived mathematical model is the fact that it contains a detailed and precisely described structure. In other words, model building in epidemiology forces us to decide which elements are useful to include, as well as which elements of the phenomenon are not essential. Methods described in Chapter 13 may aid in selection of factors chosen for the model. Thus, this detailed scrutiny of the phenomenon, irrespective of whether it ultimately leads to model building, does improve one's understanding of nature. Another advantage of mathematical modelling lies in the fact that mathematical frontiers also may be expanded in seeking solutions to the equations that are developed as parts of mathematical models.

Another advantage of modelling lies in the fact that a model's greatest *analytical* power is a direct consequence of the mathematical formulation. Unfortunately, the equations that are the basis for the model may be analytically intractable. However, with the use of computers, epidemiologists can often resort to various numerical techniques to obtain solutions. Although such computer-based procedures can be troublesome, difficult, and sometimes fallacious, if veterinarians interested in such procedures consult and use the advice of experts, computed solutions to model equations can supply usable information.

Additional computational difficulties also may occur. For example, one may be able to formulate the mathematical equations for the system or phenomenon, yet be unable to solve the equations analytically or numerically. *Simulation studies* then may be profitable investigative strategies. Although simulation studies do not provide algebraic solutions

255

to the problem inherent in the model, they are usually relatively simple to perform, relying on sufficiently large numbers of repetitions to describe the solution statistically. Perhaps the major advantage of simulation studies lies in the fact that parameters can be altered at any stage, thereby arriving at some optimal solution. Such optimality naturally depends on the model having been sufficiently elaborate to be realistic in the phenomenological sense.

As indicated in earlier chapters, testing hypotheses is an essential part of the scientific method, and any worthwhile scientific hypothesis has at least some quantitative aspects. In fact, whenever data are collected in order to test a statistical hypothesis, testing involves whether the data are compatible with the *model* described in the hypothesis. Thus, the statistical hypotheses tested are, in effect, partial accounts of certain aspects of reality. Modelling in this sense is certainly a far-reaching activity. Also, many mathematical biologists and epidemiologists would concur with the notion that mathematical models have the same logical status as other scientific and statistical hypotheses, and therefore require justification and manipulation according to standard scientific methodological criteria.

The formulation of a mathematical, statistical, or epidemiological model has several advantages as well as disadvantages. Curiously, the advantages and disadvantages are often the same features of the model. In particular, such models often have great clarity, yet this clarity makes the difficulties, oversimplifications, and unrealities readily perceivable. On the one hand, formulation of a model requires verification by suitable practical experiments or surveys; on the other hand, mathematical analysis usually augments our theoretical knowledge about the model's structure *per se*.

EARLY RINDERPEST MODEL

Modern mathematical representations of the behavior and course of epidemics can be traced to William Farr's study of several smallpox outbreaks in the late 1830s in England and Wales. Farr, recognizing that a certain orderliness existed in the epidemic patterns of several diseases, essentially fit a normal frequency curve to smoothed smallpox death frequencies.

Significantly, Farr also modelled empirically a rinderpest outbreak in cattle that began late in 1865 in England. His mathematical approach to this epidemic of cattle plague was based on an assumption that the third ratios of successive pairs of frequencies of reported cases during four-week periods were constant, whereas in epidemics of human smallpox he had used only second ratios. As shown in Table 16–1, Farr forecast the peak of the epidemic earlier than it really occurred, and also predicted a rapid decline. Although his predictions of the outcome of the rinderpest outbreak were not overly accurate, they, and his earlier formulations with data from smallpox epidemics, were adequate demonstrations of Farr's views on the essentially regular pattern in infectious disease outbreaks.

Chapters 5 and 13 discuss some mathematical approaches for solving epidemiological problems. This chapter has moved to another level of abstraction, examining some mathematical models of veterinary medical phenomena.

The literature on mathematical models in epidemiology is extensive.[2] Thus, this textbook cannot, and

Table 16–1. Rinderpest Outbreak in Cattle in England, 1865-66: Cases Reported, and Cases Forecast by William Farr*

Year	4-week period	Reported cases	Farr's calculated cases	Cases finally reported
1865	Oct. 7–Nov. 4	9597	9597	9597
	Nov. 5–Dec. 2	18,817	18,817	18,817
	Dec. 3–Dec. 30	33,835	33,835	33,835
1866	Dec. 31–Jan. 27	47,191	47,191	47,287
			Farr's predictions	
	Jan. 28–Feb. 24		43,182	57,004
	Feb. 25–Mar. 24		21,927	27,958
	Mar. 25–Apr. 21		5226	15,856
	Apr. 22–May 19		494	14,734
	May 20–June 16		16	Approx. 5000

*After R. E. Serfling. 1952. Historical review of epidemic theory. Human Biology 24:145-166.

should not, attempt to produce a mathematical treatise. On the other hand, some mathematical terminology and manipulation of symbols are necessary. The remainder of this chapter outlines selected examples of epidemiological models.

CONSTRUCTION OF A SIMPLE EPIDEMIOLOGIC MODEL

Before considering the mathematical details of building a model, it will be useful to review some general biological and clinical ideas and limitations underlying epidemic model building. For purposes of illustration, a model of a simple epidemic has been selected.

Epidemic models can be formulated at various levels of sophistication and complexity, but this one is concerned with an epidemic infection spreading in a population of individuals, say, cattle. Within this population are one or more individuals *susceptible* to infection who acquire the infection as a result of the presence of some other *infectious* individual (infective). The disease transmission may occur directly or indirectly, depending upon the particular disease under consideration. Following exposure of the susceptible animal to the infective, there may be a prepatent period during which the newly exposed animal develops the infection internally to the point that transmission from this individual to others is possible. Following this period, the individual is infectious, and liable to transmit the infection to other susceptible animals. If the infectious animal develops signs and symptoms of the disease, chances are that it will be removed from circulation among the population until it recovers or dies.

Not uncommonly, it is assumed that all individuals in the population being modelled are mixing continually and randomly. However, it is well known that social distance among individual animals is not necessarily equal; to wit, the pecking order among avian species and other evidence of social stratification among species can and does affect disease transmission. Nevertheless, although the assumption of continuous random mixing is an oversimplification, it is usually adequate as a first approximation.

A model of an epidemic can be formulated for large groups or for small groups of individuals. Models constructed for large groups or populations provide general insight into the epidemic and may be useful for public health, livestock disease control, or other government health agencies. Models of small groups, such as litters or families, provide more detailed results, and can provide information about specific clinical features such as length of incubation period or length of infectious period. Situations exist where both types of models may be useful, as in modelling trypanosomiasis in cattle in the north central state of

Nigeria (large group), while also looking at the behavior of trypanosomes in specific types of husbandry (large subgroup) situations, and in specific herds (small group). It should be clear that the study of large groups and of small groups is complementary, yet each kind of study can be instructive in itself.

Specifically, this example concerns a simple epidemic spreading among a herd of susceptible cattle in which there is no removal from the population as a result of death, isolation, or recovery. Whether such a formulation is realistic is, at this stage, irrelevant. Two types of model formulation are being demonstrated, and arguments concerning realism should be raised later. Let the number of susceptibles be n, and suppose a single infectious animal (the primary case) is introduced to the population at the beginning of the period of observation (say, at time t=0). A deterministic model and a stochastic model will be formulated to enable comparison and contrast of the two formulations.

Deterministic model

This model formulation assumes the n+1 individuals mix homogeneously. Furthermore, at some time t>0, there will be s susceptibles and f infectives ($s + f$ = n+1). It is assumed further that the average number of new infections in a time interval Δt is proportional to the number of infectives as well as the number of susceptibles. If it is assumed further that the contact rate between members of this population is C, then the *average* number of new cases in the time interval Δt will be $Csf\Delta t$.[3] If Δs designates the change in the number of susceptibles, all the foregoing can be summarized as

$$(\Delta s) = -Csf(\Delta t), \qquad (16.1)$$

where the coefficient is negative because the number of susceptibles decreases or remains the same, but never increases. Using a little calculus, and replacing Ct by τ as the time scale, the model can be written as

$$\frac{ds}{d\tau} = -s\,(n-s+1), \qquad (16.2)$$

where τ=0 and s=n at time t=0.

Several points should be clear in the preceding model: (1) the period between infection and ability to infect is zero; (2) the deterministic model is concerned only with averages; and (3) s has not yet been determined.

Solving for s, subject to assumptions restated in (16.2), produces

$$s = \frac{n(n+1)}{n + \exp[(n+1)\tau]}.$$

In practice, epidemics are generally recorded as numbers of new cases appearing each month, week, or day, so that it may be more appropriate to consider the rate at which new cases accrue. This rate, $-ds/d\tau$, represents the epidemic curve, given by

$$\frac{-ds}{d\tau} = s(n-s+1) = \frac{n(n+1)^2 \exp[(n+1)\tau]}{\{n + \exp[(n+1)\tau]\}^2}$$

The epidemic curve is symmetric, unimodal, and has its maximum at

$$\tau = \frac{\log n}{n+1} .$$

Curiously, this epidemic curve has the characteristic property of epidemics; namely, the rate at which new cases appear increases rapidly at first, reaches a maximum, and then decreases to zero. However, being symmetric, the epidemic curve may not be a realistic characterization in many circumstances. It is also worth noting that the rapid rate of spread of infection at the height of the epidemic (in this model) is a simple mathematical consequence of the assumption that the average number of new infectives is proportional to the number of infectives already in the population as well as to the number of susceptibles. This interesting note serves to reiterate that the underlying assumptions have far-reaching consequences in the solution of the model.

The deterministic model has been concerned with the behavior of an *average* individual. Introducing the notions of chance and probability offers a little more in the way of realism.

Stochastic model

Reconsider the same epidemic model in its stochastic framework, with $s(t)$ = number of susceptibles at time t. In a manner analogous to what was done for the average individual in the deterministic model, in the stochastic model one assumes that the probability of a *single* new case is proportional to both the number of infectives and the number of susceptibles. Using the notation defined earlier, the transition probability associated with a time change Δt can be written as $Cs(n-s+1)\Delta t$. If the time scale is changed to $\tau = Ct$ as before, and calculus is applied, the result is the partial differential equation

$$\frac{\partial P}{\partial \tau} = (1-s) \left(n\frac{\partial P}{\partial s} - s\frac{\partial^2 P}{\partial s^2} \right)$$

for the probability generating function. As before, the assumption is that the period from infection to ability to transmit is zero, and $P(s,o) = s^n$.

After applying calculus and elementary algebra, one obtains the stochastic solution

$$P_r(\tau) = \sum_{k=1}^{n-r+1} c_{rk} \exp[-k(n-k+1)\tau]$$

where

$$c_{rk} = \frac{(-1)^{k-1} (n-2k+1)n! (n-r)! (r-k-1)!}{r! (k-1)! (n-k)! (n-r-k+1)!}$$

(In the preceding equation, r refers to the number of susceptibles, $r > \frac{1}{2}n$, and n is even).

This solution is of little interest to most epidemiologists or veterinarians. However, it does serve to illustrate the complexity that one encounters in calculating exact probabilities for even the simplest stochastic models.[4]

The simple epidemic model has been extended and improved by various refinements, for example, by including the possibility of recovery from the disease and removal from the population. Furthermore, several diseases *per se* have been modelled with relatively simple mathematical structures, the most noteworthy being deterministic models of endemic malaria produced by MacDonald and Armitage,[5] extending the notions of Ross. These latter extensions of simple epidemics naturally have included a generalization to the host and vector situation. Stochastic modelling of animal diseases has been discussed by Morris.[5]

Another class of epidemic models permits a more detailed look at the pattern of epidemics in small groups such as families, litters, and small herds of susceptible animals. Of these, chain binomial models are, perhaps, the best known.

Chain binomial models

L.J. Reed and W.H. Frost developed a model for classroom work at Johns Hopkins University. This model, described in detail and extended by Abbey, was a modification of a model proposed by Soper.[6] The Reed-Frost model is based on the assumptions:

The infection is spread directly from infected individuals to others by a certain kind of contact (adequate contact) and in no other way.

Any non-immune individual in the group, after such contact with an infectious individual in a given period, will develop the infection and will be infectious to others only within the following time period, after which he is wholly immune.

Each individual has a fixed probability of coming into adequate contact with any other specified individual in the group within one time interval, and this probability is the same for every member of the group.

The individuals are wholly segregated from others outside the group.

These conditions remain constant during the epidemic.

The time interval chosen was a length equal to the average period during which a new case was infectious.

Consider a small backyard flock of chickens. Let p denote the probability of adequate contact between any two members of this flock so as to transmit the infection if one bird is susceptible and the other infectious. Let C_t be the number of cases produced during time interval t in this flock. Then q^{C_t} is the probability that a specified chicken avoids contact with all C_t cases during the time interval, and $1-q^{C_t}$ is the probability that the specified individual has adequate contact with at least one of the infected birds. Furthermore, let S_t denote the number of susceptible individuals at time t. The average number of cases produced at time t+1 is the product of S_t and the probability of adequate contact with an infectious bird,

$$C_{t+1} = S_t(1-q^{C_t}).$$

With this deterministic formulation, it is possible to calculate the numbers of cases at successive periods of time; hence, a chain model results.

Suppose that one infected bird is introduced into a group of 100 susceptible chickens, and, for illustration, assume p = 0.04. The epidemic, as detailed in Table 16–2, terminates after six time periods, with 99 immune birds and two susceptible birds.

The preceding deterministic model can be modified by introducing a chance element: Replace the equation $C_{t+1} = S_t(1-q^{C_t})$ by saying that the probability of C_{t+1} cases at time t+1 is

$$P(C_{t+1}|S_t,C_t) = \binom{S_t}{C_{t+1}}(1-q^{C_t})^{C_{t+1}}(q^{C_t})^{S_{t+1}},$$

recalling that there were S_t susceptibles and C_t cases at time t. This expression is clearly an ordinary binomial probability with $(1-q^{C_t})$ being the probability that a susceptible individual becomes a case at time t+1.

The infectious process proceeds by steps through time; at each point in time there is such a binomial probability statement, hence the name *chain binomial*.

With the binomial probability just described, it is possible to write down the probabilities for any chain of cases. For example, suppose that, in a large number of litters of kittens, each litter has four kittens, and one from each litter is infected initially by a certain virus. Within each of these litters, several epidemic chains are possible; e.g., the infection may

Table 16–2.   Calculation of Theoretical Epidemic from Reed-Frost Chain Model (p = 0.04)

Time interval t	No. susceptibles S_t	No. cases C_t	No. immunes I_t	Calculations for C_{t+1} and S_{t+1}
0	100	1	—	$C_1 = 100(1-.96) = 4$ $S_1 = 100-4 = 96$
1	96	4	1	$C_2 = 96(1-.96^4) = 14$ $S_2 = 96-14 = 82$
2	82	14	5	$C_3 = 82(1-.96^{14}) = 36$ $S_3 = 82-36 = 46$
3	46	36	19	$C_4 = 46(1-.96^{36}) = 35$ $S_4 = 46-35 = 11$
4	11	35	55	$C_5 = 11(1-.96^{35}) = 8$ $S_5 = 11-8 = 3$
5	3	8	90	$C_6 = 3(1-.96^8) = 1$ $S_6 = 3-1 = 2$
6	2	1	98	$C_7 = 2(1-.96^1) = 0$ $S_7 = 2-0 = 2$
7	2	0	99	— —

be transmitted to none of the other kittens (chain 1), or it may be transmitted to only one other kitten (1,1), or it may be transmitted to only one, who in turn infects a third kitten (1,1,1), etc. For litters of four with one initial case, the possible chains are (1), (1,1), (1,1,1), (1,2), (1,1,1,1), (1,1,2), (1,2,1), and (1,3), which can be represented conveniently as (1), (1^2), (1^3), (12), (1^4), $(1^2 2)$, (121), and (13). If the conditions specified under the assumptions for the Reed-Frost model prevail, the following distribution of types of chains would be expected in n epidemics in four-kitten litters having one initial case:

Type of chain	Expected no. litters
1	nq^3
1^2	$3npq^4$
1^3	$6np^2 q^4$
12	$3np^2 q^3$
1^4	$6np^3 q^3$
$1^2 2$	$3np^3 q^2$
121	$3np^3 q(1+q)$
13	np^3
	n

It is now possible to examine the proportions of such epidemics leading to 1,2,3, or 4 cases:

No. cases	Types of chains	Expected proportion of epidemics
1	1	q^3
2	1^2	$3pq^4$
3	1^3,12	$6p^2 q^4 + 3p^2 q^3 = 3p^2 q^3 (2q+1)$
4	1^4,$1^2 2$,121,13	$p^3 (6q^3 + 6q^2 + 3q + 1)$

Thus, the Reed-Frost formulation would anticipate q^3 as the proportion of these epidemics that would abort; i.e., q^3 is the relative frequency of four-kitten litters in which no infections would occur other than the initial case. This property could be used to estimate q, and therefore p=(1−q).

Unfortunately, it is unlikely that the probability p, assumed to be constant within any epidemic, remains the same across all epidemics. That is, the kitten-kitten contacts in four-kitten litters are unlikely to be the same among all such litters. Therefore, more sophisticated models have been developed, but they are outside the scope of the present discussion.

Many models such as those just described can be designed for a number of practical population problems in veterinary medicine. For example, one stochastic model that has been published is useful to help visualize and quantify the economic costs associated with dairy calf mortality.

STOCHASTIC MODEL OF ECONOMIC COSTS OF DAIRY CALF MORTALITY[7]

This model of dairy calf raising is concerned with the successive weekly probabilities of two events, death (D) of a calf or its sale (S), the latter event being conditional upon its survival $(\overline{D})$. As the discrete time intervals of one week, used for calculating these successive risks, are short compared to the average life span of dairy calves, and there is no interval between successive trials, such a model reasonably approximates a calf-raising operation that takes place in continuous time. In constructing a tree diagram to illustrate the various pathways that each calf might take during any week i following its birth, for its first t weeks of life (Fig. 16–1), the following additional notations were used:

q_i = probability of dying during the ith week of age.

$1-q_i$ = probability of surviving through the ith week to the beginning of the ith + 1 week of age.

s_i = conditional probability of being sold during the ith week of age, given that the calf survives through the ith-1 week.

$1-s_i$ = conditional probability of calf not being sold during the ith week of age, given survival through the ith-1 week.

T = completed lifetime in weeks after birth.

t = variable time index taking integer values from 0 to T.

Considering the second week of life from t=1 to t=2 as an example (see Fig. 16–1), the following events are possible in the life of a calf surviving the previous week (t=0 to t=1) and not sold:

(1) The calf dies (D) during the week.

(2) The calf survives the week and is sold at the end of the week $(S/\overline{D})$.

(3) The calf survives the week, is not sold, and remains in the population to again be at risk of these three events in the next week $(\overline{S}|\overline{D})$.

The probabilities of these three events in week 2 (i.e., after surviving one week) are:

$$P(D) = (1-q_0)(1-s_0)q_1$$
$$P(S|\overline{D}) = (1-q_0)(1-s_0)(1-q_1)s_1$$
$$P(\overline{S}|\overline{D}) = (1-q_0)(1-s_0)(1-q_1)(1-s_1)$$

For the second part of the model, a second tree diagram is constructed (Fig. 16–2) indicating the monetary returns associated with the events shown in Figure 16–1.

For constructing this diagram, use the following additional notations:

V_t = sale price of calf at week t

B_i = portion of building depreciation attributable to the care of a given calf during the ith week of age

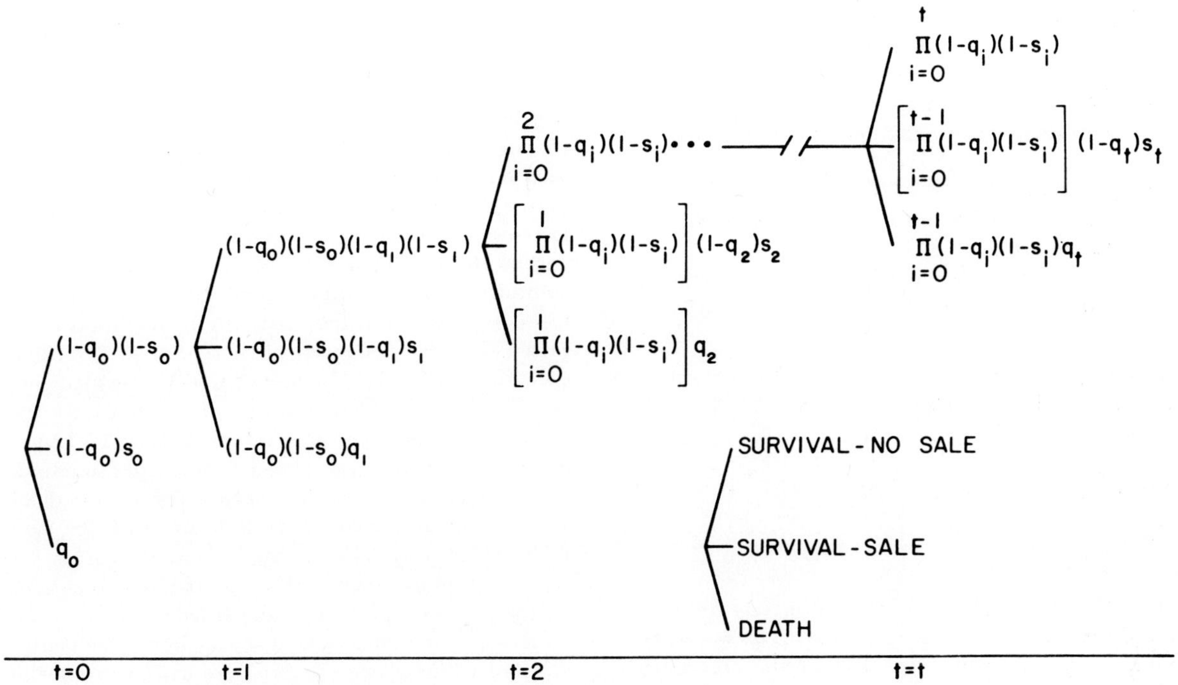

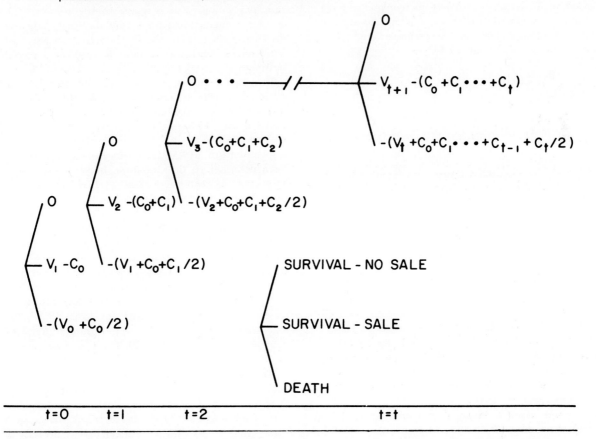

Fig. 16-1. Tree diagram representing various possible fates of calf during first t weeks of life, together with probabilities of those fates (see text for notations).[7]

Fig. 16-2. Tree diagram representing various possible fates of calf during first t weeks of life, together with monetary return to dairyman associated with those fates (see text for notations).[7]

L_i = portion of the cost of labor attributable to the care of a given calf during the ith week of age

F_i = portion of the cost of feed attributable to the care of a given calf during the ith week of age

M_i = portion of the cost of veterinary medical care attributable to the care of a given calf during the ith week of age

C_i = total cost $(B_i+L_i+F_i+M_i)$ attributable to the care of a given calf during the ith week of age

Taking again as an example the second week of life following birth (see Figs. 16–1 and 16–2), the monetary returns, respectively, are:

$$\text{Returns (D)} = -(V_1 + C_0 + \frac{C_1}{2})$$
$$\text{Returns (S|}\overline{D}) = V_2 - (C_0 + C_1)$$
$$\text{Returns (}\overline{S}|\overline{D}) = 0$$

Then the expected or average monetary returns realized for that week in association with these events would be the respective products of the preceding probabilities and monetary returns for D, S|$\overline{D}$, and $\overline{S}$|$\overline{D}$, respectively (see Fig. 16–2).

To obtain the total expected monetary return for a period of T weeks, the weekly incremental average returns are summed; that is, the expected or average return to the dairyman (in T weeks) associated solely with the death of the calf $(E(R_D))$ is

$$E(R_D) = -q_0 \left(V_0 + \frac{C_0}{2} \right) -$$

$$\sum_{t=1}^{T} \left[\prod_{i=0}^{t-1} (1-q_i)(1-s_i) \right] q_t \left[V_t + \sum_{i=0}^{t-1} C_i + \frac{C_t}{2} \right]$$

Similarly, the expected return associated with calf survival and subsequent sale $(E(R_{S|\overline{D}}))$ is

$$E(R_{S|\overline{D}}) = (1-q_0)\, s_0\, (V_1 - C_0) +$$

$$\sum_{t=1}^{T} \left[\prod_{i=0}^{t-1} (1-q_i)(1-s_i) \right] (1-q_t)\, s_t (V_{t+1} - \sum_{i=0}^{t} C_i)$$

The total expected return to the dairyman is the sum of $E(R_D)$ and $E(R_{S|\overline{D}})$. This latter equation constitutes the stochastic model. An economic problem based upon this model is given in Chapter 15. Another type of stochastic model useful for epidemiological decision-making by a veterinarian is outlined next. It involves an immunodiagnostic screening program.

TESTING FOR CYSTICERCOSIS IN A CATTLE FEEDLOT[8]

In this example, the person conducting the program is a beef feedlot consultant. One of his clients plans to purchase 1000 750-lb. yearling Corriente steers. The intention is to feed them to 1075 lbs. weight over a 130-day period. These steers cost $240 each ($32 per hundredweight) in Mexico. Their delivered cost to the feedlot is $247.50 each, including buying commission and transportation. Their value for immediate slaughter as they arrive in the feedlot is $225 each ($30 per hundredweight). The cost of feeding each steer to 1075 lbs. is $195.84, including medicine and vaccination ($6 per head), death loss at 1.0% ($2.54 per head), and interest at 12.0% ($14.32 per head). The cost of the ration is $5.53 per hundredweight, including overhead charges. The average daily weight gain and feed conversion are 2.51 lbs. and 8.79, respectively. The amount paid by the packer for each good grade steer is $451.50 ($42 per hundredweight). Average profit per animal fed is $8.16.

Carcasses of animals found at slaughter to be lightly infected with *Cysticercus bovis* are frozen to kill the parasite and then marketed. The price paid the feedlot in such cases is discounted so much per pound carcass weight, and a freezing charge of an additional sum per pound also is made to the feedlot. The average monetary loss for a 1000-lb. lightly infected fattened steer is $70. Heavily infected carcasses are condemned, and the feedlot is paid or charged nothing.

Three serological tests for bovine cysticercosis are assumed to be available. In local field trials, an indirect hemagglutination test (IHT) showed a sensitivity of only 45%, but a specificity of 90%. A latex agglutination test (LAT) had a sensitivity of 90% but a specificity of 50%. (Tests with these qualities have been described in the literature, but few have been subjected to extensive field evaluation.) A new hypothetical test (X) is assumed to be available; it is both 90% sensitive and 90% specific. The cost of testing is considered to be $1 per animal.

At the present time, feedlot operators can, and do, take out insurance against cysticercosis losses at a premium of approximately $0.10 per head per month. For 1000 steers fattened for four months, this premium would be $400. In fact, such insurance is often a bank requirement for loans to feedlot operations. For the future, some insurers intend to increase insurance rates to $0.40 per head per month or discontinue coverage.

The average prevalence rate for cysticercosis in slaughter cattle originating in Mexico is taken to be 2.0%. Prevalence rates per lot of cattle are assumed to vary from 0 to 20%. Marketing arrangements are such that the losses from cysticercosis detected at slaughter are passed on from the slaughterhouse to the feedlot operator and must be absorbed by him.

Consideration is being given to the possibility of testing these 1000 feeder steers for cysticercosis (1) before purchase and with purchase subject to test results, or (2) after purchase, with no recourse to seller. In both cases, the consultant wants to make certain epidemiologic and economic decisions concerning the disposition of these steers. A stochastic model for this purpose has been designed, and several decision-making possibilities are illustrated.

He begins by elucidating two classes of events, which will serve to distinguish the various possible strategies available to a veterinarian who is interested in maximizing the economic return (or minimizing the losses) from a feedlot's operations. The first class is a class of nonrandom events and can be thought of largely as equivalent to the making of policy decisions. He decides that the four events constituting this first class of events are:

(1) The feedlot owner elects to carry or not to carry insurance.

(2) The veterinarian elects to perform or not to perform diagnostic testing of the feeder calves.

(3) If he performs diagnostic testing, he can choose to test either before or after purchase.

(4) Finally, if he tests, then he can elect either to be guided by the test results or to ignore the test results.

A second class of events consists of those that are random in character, hence governed by probability laws.

He decides that these latter events are as follows:

(1) A given animal is either infected or uninfected.

(2) If infected, a given animal is either lightly or heavily infected.

(3) The outcome of a diagnostic test on a given animal is either positive or negative, with probabilities depending upon the infection status of the animal and upon the particular diagnostic test used.

He now proceeds to a detailed examination of the various possible strategies available, together with probabilities, monetary returns, and expected monetary returns associated with each strategy.

Case 1

(1) The feedlot owner is uninsured against losses due to cysticercosis.

(2) The consultant decides to conduct serologic testing at, say, $1 per head.

(3) He tests before purchase, with the option of buying or refusing to buy any given animal.

(4) He decides to follow, or be guided by, the results of the test.

Associated with Case 1 is the tree diagram of Figure 16–3. Each branch is labelled with a random event connected with the occurrence or nonoccurrence of *Cysticercus bovis*, together with the probabilities of these events. At the terminus of each path through the tree diagram are numbers arranged in three columns. The first of these numbers, in the column labelled *P*, *gives the probability associated with each path*, or joint event in the tree diagram. For example, if he follows, in order, the path labelled "Infected Lightly–T+", he names the event consisting of a positive serologic test of a lightly infected animal. The event consisting of infection is assumed, for the purposes of this model, to occur with probability of 0.02. Given that an animal is infected, the conditional probability that it is lightly infected is taken to be 1-h, where, for the present, h is an unspecified positive number between 0 and 1. Finally the conditional event T+, a serologically positive test of a lightly infected animal, is assumed to occur with conditional probability s, which is the same as the sensitivity of the test used. As with h, the number s is a positive number lying between 0 and 1. Thus, the path, or event, "Infected Lightly–T+," is seen to have probability P = 0.02(1-h)s.

The second column, labelled *R*, *gives the return to the feedlot owner associated with a given joint event.* Thus, if the feedlot owner decides to adopt the strategy of Case 1, his return for the joint event "Infected Lightly T+" is negative $1. In other words, since the serologic test is positive, the owner elects not to purchase the animal; hence his out-of-pocket cost is just the cost of conducting the test. Notice that in Case 1 the return is negative $1 for each serologically positive animal. If the animal is serologically negative, then the consultant assumes that the feedlot owner is willing to buy the animal for fattening, and in fact does so. If the animal is uninfected and serologically negative, the feedlot owner, after purchase and fattening, makes a profit of $8.16, minus the $1 for testing, for a net profit of $7.16 per animal. If the animal is lightly infected but serologically negative, it is purchased for fattening and the light infection is not discovered until slaughter time. The return to the owner (actually a loss) is $76.25. Finally, if the animal is heavily infected but serologically negative, again it is purchased for fattening and, as before, the infection is not discovered until slaughter time. In this case the entire carcass is condemned, and the return to the owner is –$444.34.

The third column, labelled $E(R)$, *is the expected, or average, return to the feedlot owner* associated with a given joint event. It is the product of the entries in the first two columns. Adding all the entries in the third column, the consultant obtains the expected return to the feedlot owner summed over all possible joint events. For Case 1, this equation $E(R) = 7.9968\sigma + 1.5050s - 7.3618h(1-s) - 2.505$ constitutes the stochastic model. This expected overall return is generally found to depend on s and σ, the sensitivity

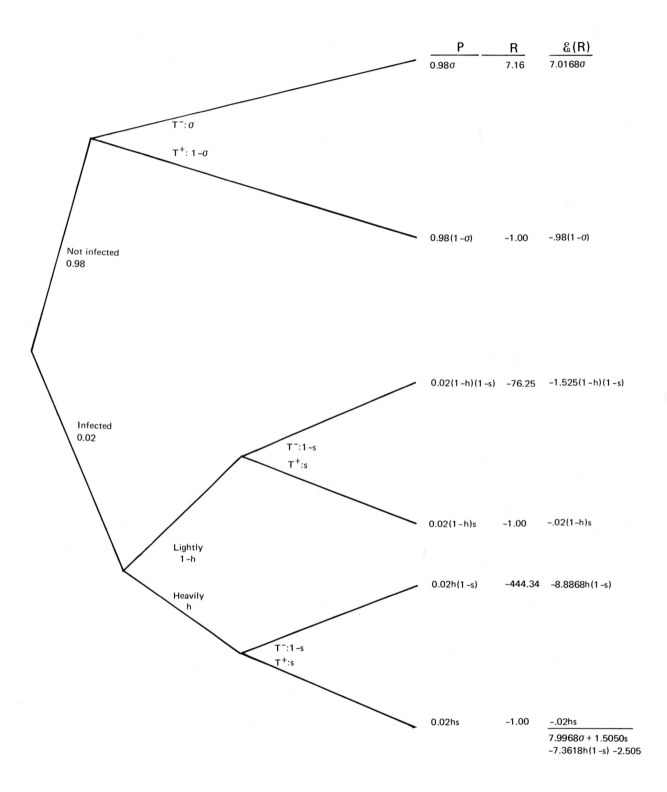

Fig. 16–3. Tree diagram for Case 1 (animals uninsured, tested before purchase at $1/head and test results followed) in economic decision-making model concerning cysticercosis in beef feedlot (see text for notations).

and specificity, respectively, of the serologic test used; and upon h, the conditional probability that if an animal is infected, it is infected heavily.

The present problem considers the indirect hemagglutination test (IHT) with s = 0.45 and σ = 0.90, the latex agglutination test (LAT) with s = 0.90 and σ = 0.50, and a hypothetical X–test (XT) with s = 0.90 and σ = 0.90. Under a choice of one of these three serologic tests, s and σ become known; hence the expected overall return depends linearly on h, the proportion of heavily infected animals among all infected animals. For Case 1 and for each of the three tests, IH, LA and XT, the expected return is plotted as a linear function of h in Figure 16–4. Note that the X-test dominates both the IH test and the LA test over the whole range of h; that is to say, no matter what the proportion of heavily infected animals, it is always more profitable to use the X-test. However, if only the IH-test and the LA-test are available, it is more profitable to use the IH-test up to h = 0.77 and to use the LA-test for 0.77 < h ⩽ 1.

Problem 21. Use of stochastic economic decision-making model

Referring to the preceding material, list all of the other possible combinations of decision choices available to the veterinarian other than the combination considered in Case 1.

Using Case 1 as an example, construct the probability tree diagrams necessary for one of these other cases and carry out the appropriate calculations. Write the equation for your stochastic model.

Calculate the expected average monetary return E(R) for each test as a linear function of h, and plot these data.

Another example of modelling combines an experimental study with computer simulation of the experimental results.

EPIDEMIC SIMULATION OF DISTEMPER

An epidemic of distemper was induced experimentally in a colony of ferrets at Washington State University.[9] A 29×5 grid of pens had been constructed; but with every third row empty, the occupied pens actually constituted a 20×5 grid. The empty row was a walkway providing access to all pens for husbandry purposes. The epidemic was initiated by placing a single infected ferret in the center of the first row, a susceptible ferret having been placed in each of the remaining 99 pens. The epidemic lasted 85 days, at which time 97 of the susceptible animals had died, and the two survivors were found to be immune.

It was known that an exposed ferret becomes infectious six days after infection and remains infectious until death at about day 15. It was also known that distemper among ferrets spreads by air-borne transmission as well as by direct contact between animals. Using a six-day prepatent period followed by an eight-day infectious period, the experimental epidemic was simulated on a computer. The simulation studies indicated that the pattern of spread of the experimental epidemic was influenced by pen structure as well as by the draftiness of the building in which the experiment was conducted.

One additional model will be considered. It, like the chain binomial formulation, is based on a "chain" approach. In this instance, however, a matrix algebra method will be used.

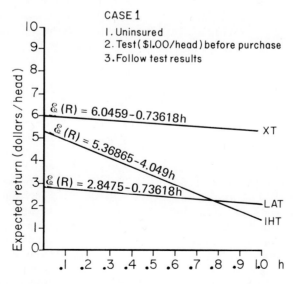

Fig. 16–4. Monetary returns in Case 1 (see Fig. 16–3) of economic decision-making model concerning cysticercosis in beef feedlot (see text for notations).

MODEL OF BOVINE MASTITIS—MARKOV CHAIN APPROACH

The following is a deterministic model of bovine mastitis based on eight years' laboratory diagnostic data from a herd in Minnesota.[10] The data consisted of results from laboratory testing of milk samples from individual cows for pathogenic bacteria two to three times per year. Included was information about culling and replacement rates. For the sake of simplicity, the culling rate in the present example is assumed to be constant. The data did not provide record linkage for individual cows; e.g., it is not possible to find *which* of the cows with *Streptococcus agalactiae* infection were culled.

The situation in a herd can be described by the following graphic model, which contains all possible changes of state that can occur with respect to mastitis. The length of the time interval may vary depending, among other things, on how detailed the data are. In the present situation, the length was chosen to be approximately a calving interval (a year) because the data available did not permit the use of shorter intervals. During a period of this length, in reality there may be several changes for an individual cow between the states: clean $\rightleftarrows$ mastitis. This possibility, however, is of minor importance because only a persistent state of mastitis has serious economic consequences. The present model assumes that all animal replacements are free of mastitis.

TIME INTERVAL

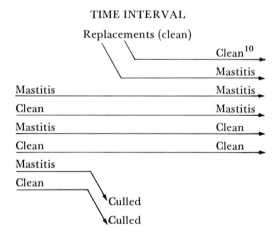

A Markov process is a mathematical model that makes it possible to study complex systems. Its basic concepts are those of the "state" of a system and "transitions" between (or among) states. In the present model, states are "mastitis," "clean," and "culled." The state of mastitis means a laboratory diagnosed infection. It is subdivided into infections with *Streptococcus agalactiae*, other streptococci, *Staphylococcus* spp., and other infections (coliforms or yeast in at least one quarter of the udder). The probability of transition from the present state to a new state is a function only of the present state and not of the history of the system before its arrival in the present state. The probabilities of transition can be represented conveniently in a transition matrix. If there are two possible states in the system, the transition matrix is

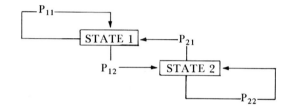

where P_{ij} is the probability that an individual in state i moves to state j during the time interval, $P_{11} + P_{12} = 1$, and $P_{21} + P_{22} = 1$.

The probabilities of transition from one state to another can be illustrated schematically as follows:

If $\underset{\sim}{F}_0$ is an initial distribution vector (in this case describing the fractions F_i of a herd in the different states described previously), then

$$\underset{\sim}{F}_1 = \underset{\sim}{F}_0 \times \underset{\sim}{T}, \text{ and in general}$$

$$\underset{\sim}{F}_{n+1} = \underset{\sim}{F}_n \times \underset{\sim}{T}$$

These multiplications are carried out according to the rules for matrix multiplication as shown in the following example.

The transition matrix for the mastitis model considered here has the form shown in Table 16–3. The elements represent the transition from one state to another. The sum of probabilities in each row is one. The meanings of the elements are as shown in the following examples:

$P_{C \to C}$ = the probability of a cow remaining noninfected (clean).

$P_{C \to SA}$ = the probability of a clean cow becoming infected with *Streptococcus agalactiae*.

$P_{C \to OS}$ = the probability of a clean cow becoming infected with other streptococci.

$P_{C \to ST}$ = the probability of a clean cow becoming infected with staphylococci.

$P_{C \to OI}$ = the probability of a clean cow getting other infections (usually coliforms or yeast).

$P_{C \to CU}$ = the probability of a clean cow being culled.

Table 16–3.   Transition Matrix for Mastitis Model (see text)

	Clean	*S. agalactiae*	Other streptococci	Staphylococci	Other infections	Culled
Clean	C→C	C→SA	C→OS	C→ST	C→OI	C→CU
Streptococcus agalactiae	SA→C	SA→SA	SA→OS	SA→ST	SA→OI	SA→CU
Other streptococci	OS→C	OS→SA	OS→OS	OS→ST	OS→OI	OS→CU
Staphylococci	ST→C	ST→SA	ST→OS	ST→ST	ST→OI	ST→CU
Other infections	OI→C	OI→SA	OI→OS	OI→ST	OI→OI	OI→CU
Culled	/	/	/	/	/	CU→CU

/ = No culled animal is returned to the herd; no culled animal can be culled a second time.

$P_{SA \to C}$ = the probability of a cow infected with *S. agalactiae* becoming cured.

$P_{SA \to SA}$ = the probability of a cow infected with *S. agalactiae* remaining infected.

$P_{SA \to OS}$ = the probability of a *S. agalactiae*-infected cow becoming infected with other streptococci instead.

$P_{SA \to ST}$ = the probability that a cow recovered from *S. agalactiae* infection became infected with staphylococci.

It should be noted that "double" or "mixed" infections are not considered in this model although they do occur occasionally. Also there is no distinction between infection in one and more than one quarter.

The meanings of the remaining elements in Table 16–3 are evident from what has already been explained. In the bottom row of Table 16–3, culled cows remain culled and cannot become infected or go from an infected to a clean state. $P_{CU \to CU}$ is therefore equal to one.

Data from a dairy herd that had a mastitis program consisting of treatment of clinical mastitis and treatment of infected cows with penicillin during the dry period indicated the approximate probabilities of transition shown in the following matrix (Table 16–4). The aims of the management were to cull per year 29% of cows that had the lowest (actual or potential) yields irrespective of their mastitis status, with the exception that 50% of the cows with staphylococcal infection were culled.

There are 1000 cows in the herd, and laboratory examinations show the following distribution of cattle in the herd at the beginning of the year when *Staphylococcus* infections became a serious problem.

Table 16–4.   Transition Matrix for Markov Model for Dairy Herd with Mastitis Program Consisting of Treatment of Infected Quarters with Penicillin and Extensive Culling of Cows Infected with Staphylococci (see text)

	Clean	*S. agalactiae*	Other streptococci	Staphylococci	Other infections	Culled	Sum
Clean	0.52	0.03	0.02	0.12	0.02	0.29	1.00
Streptococcus agalactiae	0.70	0.01				0.29	1.00
Other streptococci	0.70		0.01			0.29	1.00
Staphylococci	0.10			0.40		0.50	1.00
Other infections	0.71					0.29	1.00
Culled						1.00	1.00

Number of Cows by Infection Status			
Beginning of year	Clean	S. agalactiae	Other streptococci
0	803	52	52

	Staphylococcus	Other infections	Culled
	79	14	0

This breakdown is the initial distribution vector (803, 52, 52, 79, 14, 0), and the state of the herd at the end of the year is determined by finding the matrix product of the distribution vector with the transition matrix

Clean cows: $803 \times 0.52 + 52 \times 0.70 + 52 \times 0.70 + 79 \times 0.1 + 14 \times 0.71 = 508.2$

Cows infected with S. agalactiae: $803 \times 0.03 + 52 \times 0.01 = 24.61$

Cows infected with other streptococci: $803 \times 0.02 + 52 \times 0.01 = 16.58$

Cows infected with Staphylococcus: $803 \times 0.12 + 79 \times 0.4 = 127.96$

Cows with other infections: $803 \times 0.02 = 16.06$

Culled cows: $803 \times 0.29 + 52 \times 0.29 + 52 \times 0.29 + 79 \times 0.5 + 14 \times 0.29 = 306.59$

The distribution of animals in each state at the end of the period is thus described as follows.

Number of Cows		
Clean	S. agalactiae	Other streptococci
508.20	24.61	16.58

Staphylococci	Other infections	Culled
127.96	16.06	306.59

In this model, the culled cows are now replaced with clean cows, and the animals in each state at the beginning of the next period are distributed as follows.

Number of Cows by Status, by beginning of period 2		
Clean	S. agalactiae	Other streptococci
814.79	24.61	16.58

Staphylococci	Other infections	Culled
127.96	16.06	0

To find the status at the end of this period, multiply the new vector with the transition matrix, for example,

Clean cows: $814.79 \times 0.52 + 24.61 \times 0.70 + 16.58 \times 0.70 + 127.96 \times 0.10 + 16.06 \times 0.71 = 476.72$.

Table 16–5.   Changes in Mastitis Prevalence in Herd of 1000 Cows (see text)

Year	Clean	S. agalactiae	Other streptococci	Staphylococci	Other infections	Culled
1	815	25	17	128	16	
	477	25	16	149	16	317
2	794	25	16	149	16	
	468	24	16	155	16	321
3	789	24	16	155	16	
	465	24	16	156	16	323
4	788	24	16	157	16	
	464	24	16	157	16	323
5	787	24	16	157	16	
	464	24	16	157	16	323

The purpose of calculating with fractions of cows is to attain higher precision. After completion of the calculations for all periods, the numbers should be rounded.

Table 16–5 shows the changes, with integer values, over a five-year period.

The results of applying the Markov chain model indicate that the mastitis program has not been very efficient; the streptococcal and "other" infections have remained fairly low, but the prevalence of staphylococcal infection first increased and then leveled off at 15.7%. This result was obtained with a transition matrix based on previous experience. In a real life situation, the matrix should be updated every year.

Because of the inefficiency of the mastitis program, the following changes were made: teat dipping in a disinfectant was initiated, *all* dry cows were treated, and less extensive culling was done among staphylococcal infected cows (Table 16–6). The predicted change in efficiency achieved by the new program is considerable during the first couple of years; then an almost static situation is reached, with about 1% prevalence of the streptococcal infections and 3.6%

prevalence of staphylococcal infection (Table 16–7).

The data obtained with the Markov model can be used for economic evaluation of a control program, and the model can be made as detailed as desired if sufficient data are available. An advantage of the Markov chain model is that it is simple and flexible. Such a model can be constructed on a rather limited number of data, and it is easily updated and changed into a more detailed form. The model, as already mentioned, can also be changed to take account of infections spreading from animal to animal.

In the present model—and also in the classic Markov process—the elements of the transition matrix are constant through each iteration, the assumption here being that mastitis is an infectious but not readily communicable disease; i.e., the probability of infection is not highly dependent on the number of cows already infected. In other infectious diseases, this assumption may not be true; and the transition probability changes accordingly with respect to the duration of the outbreak, or with respect to the number of individuals already infected. A Markov model has been constructed under such circumstances for foot-and-mouth disease.[11]

Table 16–6.   Transition Matrix After Change in Mastitis Program (see text)

	Clean	*S. agalactiae*	Other streptococci	Staphylococci	Other infections	Culled	Sum
Clean	0.65	0.01	0.01	0.03	0.01	0.29	1.00
Streptococcus agalactiae	0.70	0.01				0.29	1.00
Other streptococci	0.70		0.01			0.29	1.00
Staphylococci	0.50			0.21		0.29	1.00
Other infections	0.50			0.21		0.29	1.00
Culled						1.00	1.00

Table 16–7.   Changes in Mastitis Prevalence After Introduction of New Mastitis Control Policy (see text)

Year	Clean	*S. agalactiae*	Other streptococci	Staphylococci	Other infections	Culled
6	787	24	16	157	16	
	626	8	8	60	8	290
7	916	8	8	60	8	
	641	9	9	42	9	290
8	931	9	9	42	9	
	643	9	9	39	9	290
9	933	9	9	39	9	
	644	9	9	39	9	290
10	933	9	9	39	9	
	644	9	9	38	9	290

Part 5

AREAS OF APPLICATION

*"A veterinary practitioner
with an ideal can alter the
economic and health aspect
of a rural community . . ."*
K. F. Meyer

Chapter 17

EPIDEMIOLOGY'S ROLES IN VETERINARY PRACTICE

IT is clear to most veterinarians that veterinary medicine is called upon today to contribute to the solution of an increasing variety of important social problems. Though few professions are engaged in so wide a range of activities as individual veterinarians now are, the veterinary input is far too thin in many of them. The increasing urgency in meeting a number of mankind's most basic needs demands a more substantial overall contribution by veterinarians in the immediate future. Some of the problems for which they can help obtain solutions are familiar to veterinarians from long experience. One such is food production. The profession is much less familiar though with other major problem areas, like population limitation, to which it is also able to provide important inputs. Two main avenues are open for these overall efforts by veterinarians; one is through a variety of activities in fairly basic research, including epidemiological research. The other avenue is through various types of public and private veterinary practice. A characteristic of most problems approachable by this latter avenue is that they are population-related and, therefore, susceptible to epidemiological attack.

SOCIAL PROBLEMS REQUIRING VETERINARY INPUT

Unquestionably, most past expenditures of the veterinary profession's energies and talents have been directed toward creating viable food-animal industries in the countries now considered "economically developed." The rather phenomenal successes of these efforts are resulting in major changes in animal production systems in most of these countries. With these changes, important new challenges to the profession's ingenuity have arisen in recent years. Since the world protein problem is unlikely to be solved by the development of unconventional sources of protein, it is clear that renewed creativity in epidemiology is called for in response to new disease challenges posed by intensified animal production, in achieving the optimal balance between animal and plant agriculture, as well as in meeting familiar and unfamiliar problems in the economically developing and economically underdeveloped worlds. Fresh epidemiological inputs are urgently required throughout this whole most vital area of veterinary practice. This area for future action has been addressed repeatedly throughout the book.[1]

Through the past century, veterinary medicine also has assumed ever more important functions in the protection of human health.[2] As the branch of general allopathic medicine directly concerned with health and disease in all animals other than man, veterinary medicine plays a significant human health role through basic and comparative medical research. Experimental medicine still is mostly animal medicine and is likely to remain so in the future. It is not surprising therefore that, despite their relatively small numbers, veterinarians have been the second most productive of the several health professions from the standpoint of research. One of the more important areas for their past contribution to man's health was methodological research in epidemiology, which led to many of the first techniques for approaching and controlling diseases at a population level. This contribution has been mentioned in Chapters 3 and 4.

Tremendous opportunities exist today, not only for new methodological progress by veterinarians in epidemiology, which would have multiple repercussions, including direct ones to human health; but also for an expansion of comparative epidemiological research on spontaneously occurring diseases of unknown etiology, for example, cancer as well as cardiovascular and other degenerative diseases. This broad health science function of veterinary medicine also manifests itself in facing the many new and intriguing medical ecology problems that emerge each year as men intrude into new ecosystems or interact with lower animals in new ways. Still needed too are heightened efforts to reduce the overall risks to man of many comparatively well-known infections that he acquires from other members of the animal kingdom. In this connection, an expanded role for food protection services is needed. Food hygiene veterinarians must cooperate in the evolution of active and more widely conceived epidemiological surveillance efforts. This need has been discussed in some detail in Chapter 14.

Overdue attention also is beginning to be directed toward the long-term threats to plant, animal, and human life resulting from the accumulation of chemical and physical pollutants in the environment. At the present time, the veterinary profession contributes to solutions to these problems through comparative medical research on the pathogenic effects of air, water, and soil pollutants and through help in determining safety standards for foods and drugs. One other area for a potentially important veterinary impact is the use of animal populations for continuous monitoring of the environment for biologically significant levels of pollution as well as for identification of specific untoward biological effects of continuing pollution. Tools for such monitoring efforts partially exist; and this area could well become a very important one for public service in veterinary medicine. A recently published report of the World Health Organization on *The Veterinary Contribution to Public Health Practice* discusses several important aspects of veterinary activities in this overall environmental sphere.[3]

Limitation of human population growth is a further imperative for the future. Veterinarians have long been concerned with problems of mammalian reproduction. Most of this past effort has taken the form of basic research aimed at *increased* fertility and fecundity and accelerated population growth in domestic animal species important to man as sources of food and other valuable products. Pioneering work on the physiology of reproduction—artificial insemination, sperm and ovum physiology, ovum- and embryo-transplantation, and other aspects of the subject—has been part of this effort. Today these long-term veterinary interests and experiences are beginning to be redirected toward problems related to *control* of human population growth. A veterinarian now heads Great Britain's national laboratory for research on human reproduction, and 11 veterinarians hold current positions in this field in American medical schools. This immense problem area is in need of much expanded efforts, to many of which veterinarians can bring unusual skills and experience.

An ideal experimental arena for epidemiological input to aspects of population biology and control is through trials of various approaches to population control among excess populations of owned and ownerless dogs and cats in many of our cities. Both private and public veterinary practitioners can contribute to this effort. Recent development—by a veterinary scientist and his group—of an implantable and biodegradable long-term birth control capsule is an example of a research step that might receive large-scale epidemiological field evaluation through trials among excess populations of dogs and cats.

A last area of social need that can be approached through population studies undertaken by veterinarians is the role of the veterinary profession itself as an agent for social good.[4] Despite the fact that veterinary medicine's origins predate man's historical records, no profession so widely contributing to solutions to important human problems is so little known and understood as is the veterinary profession. Much of veterinary medicine's future effectiveness and role depends upon fuller documentation of its present and past efforts over its broad area of service.

Documentation requires acquisition of *specific data* that can be obtained only through surveys of the veterinary population as an agent influencing human problems and events. This need to document veterinary medicine's record is apropos to the several areas mentioned for veterinary service, but it is especially required to indicate the veterinary profession's role as an instrument for promotion of humane values in society. The fact that many men and women have chosen to apply their high levels of medical skills and knowledge not to heal people directly but to alleviate suffering in dumb animals has a moral content and value easily understood by children the world over but poorly recognized generally for *its* social value. The veterinary profession as an agent for demonstration and promotion in a community of such badly needed humane values as compassion, kindness, empathy, and love in an often inhumane world is an area highly worthy of serious study. The design, conduct, and reporting of results of such studies make use of methods common to epidemiological research.

The remainder of this chapter enlarges upon the two most prominent of the problem areas that need substantial epidemiological inputs from veterinary medicine. Possibly the most critical area for heightened activity is food-animal production. To visualize what can be done about current problems in this area of veterinary practice in economically developing and economically developed countries requires some historical perspective. Though the examples chosen reflect the experience of the United States, similar changes also are occurring in other countries.

EVOLUTION OF PRACTICE IN FOOD-ANIMAL MEDICINE IN UNITED STATES

In the mid-1800s, the newly developing animal industries of the United States were not only satisfying our domestic needs but were also major exporters of products and important earners of foreign exchange. The agricultural economy of much of this country was becoming geared to a European market to dispose of its excess swine and cattle. In this respect the United States closely resembled many Third World countries today. At that time veterinary education was virtually nonexistent in the United States, and government veterinary services were completely lacking. Then several things happened.

In the midst of the nascent swine industry of Ohio and Indiana, a new and highly fatal disease appeared for the first time in 1833. It was named hog cholera; and before long it was estimated to have destroyed up to 60% of the total swine population in large areas of the American Midwest. By 1870 its yearly toll was at least $20 million; and farmers threatened by disaster clamored loudly for something to be done about this untreatable disease of unknown cause.

During this same period the development of the soon-to-be-great southwestern cattle industry was beginning to take place on the vast lands seized from Mexico in the Mexican War. However, as these cattle began to be driven by tens of thousands to the markets of St. Louis, Omaha, and Chicago, the native cattle of the northern states through which they passed fell ill in large numbers and died from another "new" disease. The association of this disastrous disease— "Spanish staggers" or Texas fever— with southern cattle drives was clear to northern farmers. To meet this threat, they imposed the "Winchester quarantine," a barrier of armed men across the cattle trails, desperately seeking in this way to protect their own animals and livelihood. Their anguished cries to the government for help were soon joined to those of the swine raisers of the Middle West.

In the meantime, two further animal disease tragedies were unfolding. In the 1870s, European investigators developed techniques to detect *Trichinella spiralis* in swine carcasses, and they designed programs to combat high levels of this serious infection in much of the European human population. As part of this effort, veterinarians discovered that swine imported from America were infected with trichinosis at a *higher* rate than that for their own animals. As a consequence, Italy banned the import of all American swine in 1879; and that country's lead was soon followed by most of the other European states. Thus, America's developing agricultural economy began to face serious challenge abroad as well as at home. Animal disease was becoming a serious restraint to America's trade—and to the country's future.

Furthermore, as if all of those situations were not concern enough, contagious bovine pleuropneumonia by then had spread throughout most of the eastern third of the United States. This highly fatal disease was introduced into New York in 1843 by a cow purchased from a British ship. By 1880, it was a problem of such magnitude that several eastern states appointed veterinary officials for the first time in efforts to combat its rapid spread, but they achieved only spotty successes. The affected eastern farmers, like the swine raisers and cattlemen, could do little more than complain. Finally, however, their complaints reached a crescendo when reports of "rampant bovine pleuropneumonia" in American cattle appeared in the British press in 1881, and that country placed an embargo on import of all cattle from the United States.

Creation of a government veterinary service

Faced with these combined onslaughts of hog cholera, Texas fever, pleuropneumonia, trichinosis, and other only slightly less important animal diseases—threatening as they did loss of much overseas commerce and destruction of the most important domestic animal industries—the U.S. Congress finally acted. Roughly 100 years after Europe's example, Daniel Elmer Salmon was appointed by the U.S. federal government in 1883 to establish a government veterinary service for the United States. In 1884 this service became the Bureau of Animal Industry (B.A.I.). That Salmon's choice was a wise one was soon clear, for the enabling legislation that he drafted for the Congress indicated at the onset the boldness of the approach he planned to follow. Partially by employing methods recently demonstrated in Europe—on a comparatively smaller scale—as effective against rinderpest, Salmon set out to "extirpate" the major epidemic livestock diseases from the entire United States. Heading a completely new organization, Salmon had an advantage. He was not bound by a hundred years of tradition as was Europe, but was free to strike out in new directions if the methods of Europe appeared inadequate.

With his small force of recruits, Salmon first tackled contagious bovine pleuropneumonia. His techniques were mass diagnostic survey (an immense effort covering every farm), quarantine, and selective slaughter, with the result that, just eight years after Salmon's appointment, Secretary of Agriculture J.M. Rusk was able to officially declare "that the United States is free from the disease known as contagious pleuropneumonia." This single accomplishment took place six years before the etiologic agent of pleuropneumonia was identified! Other eradication successes followed in the battle against Texas fever, dourine, and glanders; and hog cholera soon was brought under a reasonable level of control through mass vaccination campaigns. In this great overall effort, a number of new methods for combating diseases *en masse* were developed, tested, and proven.

It is necessary to recount something of these historical events not only to understand the threat that livestock diseases posed to the developing American economy in the late 1800s, but also to understand the fundamental advances in epidemiology and disease control realized through these early efforts of the B.A.I. For some years, the B.A.I. was the preeminent *medical* research organization in the United States.[5] Such lessons should be particularly instructive to veterinarians working in economically developing countries today.

Accomplishments of the B.A.I. included the following:

(1) Demonstration of the high level of methodological innovation possible when field research is built into efforts toward disease control and is a significant

activity of many of the individuals involved in control. Salmon and his immediate successors showed nothing if they did not demonstrate that *disease control depends upon field research, that is, upon epidemiology.*

(2) Identification of the *group* of most highly disruptive livestock diseases, and animal diseases of great public health importance, that could be effectively controlled or eradicated by a combination of these, for the most part novel, methods.

(3) Establishment of a federal veterinary infrastructure reaching throughout the United States and early recognition of the necessity in such ambitious programs for cooperation not only between veterinary forces at different levels of government, but also between government and the industries concerned plus the veterinary profession at large. One result was formation of a highly effective and influential sanctioning, coordinating, and standard-setting body known now as the United States Animal Health Association. Another important result was the early establishment of an effective pattern of cooperation in the United States between the privately practicing and publicly practicing veterinary profession. Without the aid of the 50% or more private American veterinarians who, over the years, have worked on a part-time fee basis on public programs, the phenomenal successes of the B.A.I. would not have been achieved.

The population units of concern in these early animal disease control efforts were those of whole states or other large geographical areas; this situation was possible because the epidemiologies of most of the diseases chosen for attack were quite straightforward and ecologically simple. Since their determinants showed little apparent variation from farm to farm, the control efforts could be highly centralized with relatively little decision-making in the field.

As a consequence, it was possible to focus these proven tools (mass diagnostic survey, quarantine, mass treatment, mass immunization, and selective slaughter) upon one formidable disease problem after another. Over a period of 90 years, the initial programs were completed; and tuberculosis, brucellosis, glanders, scabies, foot-and-mouth disease, fowl plague, scrapie, vesicular exanthema, screwworms, Venezuelan equine encephalomyelitis, and Asian Newcastle disease have been added to the list of animal diseases faced successfully in the United States.

Rarely during this entire period of minor setbacks and major successes were the basic methods developed in the late 1800s and early 1900s found wanting. An undesirable but understandable consequence, therefore, was that *ongoing epidemiological research, including methodological research, ceased to be part of the job of officials responsible for*

disease control. Basic bench-type research on animal diseases was delegated to other branches of government, including the universities; and population-based field research tended to "fall between the chairs."

At the same time, other diseases such as anthrax, blackleg, and other clostridial infections, including a number of poultry infections, were brought under reasonable control through less organized efforts. Where veterinary research yielded effective vaccines, as it did in many such instances, routine immunization by private practitioners and owners generally prevented or aborted major disruptive occurrences of these types of infections. By their nature, however, these approaches represented continuing and undiminished efforts, and potential problems remain.

Intensification of animal production

The lasting consequence of this total veterinary effort in the United States was that the major epidemic diseases of livestock, which would have continually disrupted our agriculture and prevented the development of viable animal industries, were beaten back one by one. The not well-appreciated result of all this great effort was the possibility for the first time in human history of the development of intensive systems of animal husbandry. Such changes began to take place first in the poultry meat industry in the 1930s; and a veritable revolution, comparable to the more recent "Green Revolution" with wheat and rice, occurred. With production of healthy animals possible, rapid refinements in nutrition and breeding also were possible; and enormous populations of birds then could be managed in what are best described as "broiler cities." This process now has been repeated in a number of countries, and chicken meat produced quickly at low cost with a high rate of feed conversion has become available to a significant portion of the world's population for which chicken or other meat was a rare luxury not many years ago.

Similar changes are occurring today in mammoth feedlot operations for fattening beef cattle, in intensified systems of swine production, in the turkey and egg industries, and in the evolution of dairies of 1000 and more milking animals. Real nutritional progress and crossbreeding progress now are possible in these industries, too, although innovative breeding efforts for some species are still partially in a "lag phase."

These benefits of successful disease control in the economically developed countries of the world have made possible the more economical production of animal protein. They indicate clearly some of the things that can be done in the economically developing countries. At the same time they present *new* and exciting, but formidable, challenges to veterinary medicine.

NEW EPIDEMIOLOGICAL PROBLEMS AND NEW APPROACHES.   Despite the considerable successes that have been realized in veterinary medicine in the so-called economically developed countries in the past century, it is conservatively estimated for the United States that the annual toll for livestock diseases, principally of food animals, is at least $4 billion. What kinds of disease problems do such losses represent?

In general the veterinary problems of this and similar countries of Western Europe, Japan, and Australasia are of five types:

(1) Those actually or potentially disruptive national or regional infections of food-producing animals which are still uncontrolled. For the United States, these diseases include anaplasmosis, infectious bovine rhinotracheitis, bovine virus diarrhea, and avian mycoplasma infections.

(2) Some inadequately controlled livestock infections, such as trichinosis, bovine cysticercosis, hydatid disease, and salmonellosis, which are of considerable public health importance in a number of well-developed countries.

(3) Low-level residua of infections that have been reduced from previously high levels by ongoing large-scale programs, such as those against tuberculosis and brucellosis.

(4) Continuing dangers from many important highly disruptive infections now absent and excluded from a country. Experiences in the United States with Asian Newcastle disease and Venezuelan equine encephalomyelitis in recent years clearly indicate this ever-present risk.

(5) Most important of all, the many less dramatic and epidemiologically complicated diseases or disease complexes that insidiously affect food production efficiency by raising the unit cost of producing food. When they are not at unusually high levels, problems like these tend to be overlooked by farmers or regarded as fixed costs of operation.[6] Some of the most important problems of this type are neonatal death losses and reproductive inefficiencies in all species, mixed parasitisms, stress-related or similar syndromes in which various opportunistic microorganisms may play a role, bovine mastitis, and various metabolic diseases.

Conventional problems remaining. It is likely that some of the disease problems in these first two categories can and should be combatted successfully by using the proven methods of the past century. Certainly trichinosis falls into this category, although plans for trichinosis eradication from swine also include improved features of surveillance and intensive follow-up that have been little used to date.

The keys to the reduction or elimination of other diseases in these categories are the development of sufficient interest, enthusiasm, and demand on the part of the industries and the public; initiative by the veterinary services; and increased research support.

Diseases such as salmonellosis clearly merit such interest, initiative, and support now. For some such diseases, decisions are also required as to whether directed eradication possibilities exist in place of ongoing and largely undirected control through mass vaccination or mass chemotherapy programs on individual farms. Many programs of these types represent undiminishing efforts or permanent fixed costs of disease prevention, hence of food production. Deciding the possibilities and priorities with respect to these two groups of problems must be the function of an organized program of overall disease surveillance, with the capacity of field trials of alternative control approaches, including, ultimately, the development of well-conceived pilot projects.

Residua of successfully combatted infections. The residua of previously prevalent infections, such as those of hog cholera, brucellosis, and tuberculosis, are being attacked through intensive epidemiological follow-up investigations of problem herd situations and, in specific instances, by total depopulation of such herds. Where apparently unexplainable sporadic occurrences of these infections persist, possibilities such as those suggested on page 13 must be considered. It is clearly recognized that the costs of locating and combatting residual infections in the terminal stages of eradication campaigns are high but essential. In the instance of tuberculosis in the United States, federal veterinary authorities have estimated the timetables and benefit-cost ratios of several alternatives for facing this type of situation.

Exclusion of exotic diseases. The problem of excluding or rapidly stamping out foreign disease invaders will remain with the developed countries until the whole world has realized their standards of animal health. This situation has two aspects. One, efforts in international veterinary medicine require highest priorities and support not only because they relate directly to the increasing global problem of inadequate animal protein—a problem of protein starvation in some countries—but also because they directly protect our own animal populations and assure our own domestic food supply. Two, during this probably lengthy period, there must always be maintained a sufficiently well-prepared, responsive, and mobile government veterinary force able to meet all such emergencies.

In this connection, it must be clear to U.S. politicians and the public that present highly intensive systems of animal production, in which very large populations of animals are maintained in close proximity to one another, are *highly vulnerable* to potentially devastating attacks by many animal diseases not now present. While a national disaster was averted a few years ago by destroying an Asian Newcastle disease foothold in southern California, an obvious lesson from that recent experience, as well as from the experience with Venezuelan equine encephalomyelitis in the Southwest, was that most of our government veterinary reserves had to be used to accomplish these results. Scarce manpower was temporarily diverted from other high-priority programs, including recruitment of veterinarians from other government services such as the military; and private practitioners were co-opted. Less than adequate support of a government's veterinary forces poses a continuing threat to that country's future.

While the ongoing intensification of animal production—with concentration of production in fewer but larger enterprises—poses new disease risks to a nation's agriculture, it also heightens prospects for new and more scientific approaches to public and private preventive food animal medicine. Some of these prospects are considered in the following paragraphs.

EMERGENCE OF EPIDEMIOLOGICALLY BASED PRACTICES. The population, preventive, and economic bases of veterinary practice have always been prominent. In private food-animal practice in the past, however, economic considerations tended to thwart the development of optimal preventive herd programs of disease management because animal populations tended to be too small and too numerous and veterinarians too few. Harassed practitioners commonly found themselves with too little time even to meet fully an endless series of medical treatment emergencies, often for individual animals, on many widely scattered farms. They frequently spent more time in their cars than with their patients; and the economics and logistics of the situation were such that rarely could they be adequately recompensed in money, or sometimes even in satisfaction, for their high level of skills and knowledge. This situation was aptly called "fire engine" practice; and, for many veterinarians, continually putting out such "fires," often at night after the farmer himself and his neighbors had given up, did not fully call upon their abilities to practice veterinary medicine.

Now, the situation has completely changed. Larger, integrated or coordinated production units for fattening market poultry, hogs, and beef cattle present opportunities for a more enlightened and rational practitioner effort. Dairy farms, breeder operations, and egg production units also present such prospects, but of a somewhat different nature. The result is that several new types of private practice patterns are emerging.

Specialty group and herd health plan practices. The need for veterinary specialists in the intensified food-animal industries is clear, and this pattern of education in veterinary medicine is becoming more and more evident today. For a group practice involved in operations producing fattened stock for market (e.g., feedlots, broiler and turkey farms), such specialties might include epidemiology, clinical medicine, pathology, clinical pathology, nutrition, and microbiology. For breeder-type operations (e.g., cow-calf ranches, egg ranches, dairy farms), specialists in reproduction and genetics also would be highly desirable. Such group practices sometimes have been set up to offer a contract-type service in which the producer-owner arranges with the veterinary group for an overall herd health program or for specified types of services on a routine basis, as well as for provision of required emergency services.

For fattening operations, with rapid turnover of animal populations, often on an "all in—all out" basis, this type of practice relationship is easily visualized on a continuing basis. In some situations with breeder-type operations, however, there is much less turnover of the population, and individual animals tend to be kept as long as they seem to be highly productive of offspring, eggs, or milk. In these instances, there has sometimes been a tendency for owners to value routine herd health plans less once the really critical or acute loss problems, such as in dairy cattle with mastitis, neonatal mortality, or gross reproductive failures, are under reasonable control. Part of this question would be resolved if such practices had ongoing epidemiological (including cost-benefit) inputs that were more frequent and more sophisticated.

Consultant practices. A slightly different emerging practice pattern is that offered by individual veterinary consultants or consultant groups. The principal difference in this approach from the preceding one is that the consultant sells to the owner-manager diagnoses and analyses of problems, the design of solutions and programs, assessments of programs and other recommendations only. The consultant is not responsible for direct clinical or laboratory services, or sometimes even with ongoing epidemiological surveillance efforts, which must otherwise be provided for by the management.

Single enterprise practices. For very large animal production enterprises, often the most rational approach is for the management to employ one or more full-time veterinarians on a salaried basis. This pattern has been common in the poultry industry for some time. In that industry, most of the full-time veterinarians have been pathologists or microbiologists, with far fewer veterinary specialists from other fields. Fairly commonly, however, these individual poultry veterinarians have broadened their initial interests and area of scientific management concern; in the largest organizations, some of them now direct the activities of the other veterinary and animal science specialists and exercise overall scientific management responsibilities.

Because of this management role, it has been suggested that new graduate programs be set up to train veterinarians (including disciplinary specialists) more broadly with respect to the overall problems of a particular animal industry. These programs would offer subjects such as epidemiology, computer science, statistics, economics, nutrition, and genetics, in addition to clinical medicine and pathology. One or two poultry practice graduate programs of this general type have been established in the United States and could provide a pattern for similar practice in other industries.

Because it is uniquely holistic in outlook, and is population-and-prevention-based, epidemiology best serves as the integrating discipline for educational programs of this type. In general the specialist in epidemiology is particularly well suited for overall scientific manager positions with large animal production enterprises.

NEW POPULATION UNITS FOR PRACTICE. Each of these newer private practice patterns in food-animal medicine focuses attention upon the whole herd or farm unit as the "patient." This new focus represents a departure from the most prevalent private practice pattern of the immediate past; in the earlier pattern, most of the veterinarian's training tended to be directed toward intensive treatment of the individual sick animal. As indicated, additional skills are required for newer forms of practice.

On the other hand, the government veterinary services could concentrate most of their past efforts upon *very large* population units—for example, all the animals of a species in a particular country or state—with expectation of little epidemiological variability in the disease they were controlling from one farm unit to the next. Recently, however, with more attention needed in ongoing programs for "problem herds," for quickly facing possible introductions of exotic pathogens and for designing control programs for more variable diseases, such as mastitis and trichinosis, the *whole farm-herd unit* of concern figures ever more prominently in more and more public practitioners' activities. In recognition of this need for more intensive attention to more epidemiologically complex problems in the field, government veterinary services, such as those of the United States, are providing opportunities for specialized training in epidemiology for more and more of their field personnel. This trend will unquestionably continue.

What can be said is that, in the past, neither the public nor private sector of veterinary medicine focused as much attention on the farm or herd unit as is being called for today in the economically developed countries. Moreover, even when they did, it was often in undirected or uncoordinated efforts in which different veterinarians might give different and even conflicting advice to the same owner-producer, who often also received still different advice from feed and drug company representatives.

Therefore, as more and more attention in both the public and private practice of food animal medicine is directed to the herd or farm unit—and, increasingly, to ever larger farm units—new patterns of cooperation between the two practice sectors and the livestock industries must emerge. Besides the proven methods of disease control of the past, which have been discussed in Chapters 3 and 4, many of the newer epidemiological, statistical, and economic methods of Chapters 5 and 11 to 16 will see greater use, while still newer methods will need to be visualized and tested in the field.

These changing patterns of practice and cooperation will increasingly demand of the public and private food-animal practitioners, not only traditional skills in clinical medicine and pathology, but also important additional skills in epidemiology, including those in areas of related application to population medicine, such as statistics, computer science, economics, and population genetics. Today's food-animal veterinarian must also be equipped to carry out field research and become an expert in the complementary epidemiological diagnostic methods of intensive follow-up and overall surveillance (as discussed in Chapter 14).

EVOLUTION OF VETERINARY PUBLIC HEALTH PRACTICE IN UNITED STATES

In order to visualize current problems of veterinary practice with respect to human health, it is again necessary to acquire a degree of historical perspective. A relatively large number of veterinarians throughout the world participate in the practice of human herd medicine—or public health. Veterinary medicine's initial input into public health was in the design and execution of programs to protect the consuming public from unsafe meat, milk, and other edible animal products. These efforts commenced in earnest in the middle 1800s and played an important part in the development of the overall field and concepts of public health. Veterinarians such as Robert von Ostertag and Daniel E. Salmon laid the foundation for food protection in general while other public health veterinarians established some of the first public health laboratories for the microbiological examination of milk. By 1900 veterinarians were commonly represented in local public health departments in the United States and other countries, while a number of others served on local and state boards of health.

By the decade of 1920-30, many of the most critical food-related problems in public health were being well controlled in western countries through fairly routine inspection procedures and investigative protocols. Though a few individuals among these veterinary public health pioneers (such as Nathan Sinai) visualized additional veterinary functions in public health,[7] creative new veterinary inputs for public health practice diminished for the next 20 to 25 years.

However, near the end of World War II, it began to be more generally recognized that other veterinary efforts, such as the control of zoonotic diseases in animals and comparative medical research employing animal models, directly affected people's health and that more effective liaison was needed between public health services and veterinary services in government and between research workers in these two branches of allopathic medicine. These ends have been approached by the establishment of small but active veterinary medical units within the World Health Organization and Pan American Health Organization and, in some countries, within their health ministries and health departments at the various levels of government. As a result, large-scale control programs have been undertaken against rabies, brucellosis, tuberculosis, trypanosomiasis, hydatid disease, and other zoonotic infections in a number of countries where such control efforts had not existed previously.[3] These developments are by no means universal, however, and some countries have not yet effectively tapped veterinary skills in the service of human health.

In some countries veterinarians with relevant specialized skills have also begun to participate more commonly in other phases of medical research and human population medicine. This expansion into other areas has been especially evident in epidemi-

ology and medical microbiology—fields in which individual veterinarians such as Edmond Nocard, Gaston Ramon, K.F. Meyer, John Gilruth, Maurice Hall, Willard Wright, Ian Clunies-Ross, and many, many others have contributed actively and importantly.

This overall subject of veterinary medicine and human health has been discussed at length elsewhere.[2] What requires emphasis in this chapter is that, while broad epidemiological and similar generalist roles in public health are being performed increasingly by veterinarians, the continued growth and development of these important avenues for veterinary service demand that creative veterinarians be highly trained in population, preventive, and economic aspects of medical practice and that they also be capable of leadership in new directions in this problem area.

CONCLUSION

This book has been an attempt to introduce the variety of tools and approaches basic to the public or private practice of veterinary medicine on a herd or population basis. These areas of veterinary practice are exciting and rapidly evolving. Skills in the practice of population medicine can help veterinarians seize opportunities for a variety of useful, rewarding careers and at the same time let them contribute to the solutions to some of man's most pressing problems.

CHAPTER
NOTES

Chapter 1

1. Strict etymological considerations may not always be the best guide to word usage. If they were, epidemiology would have to be considered a special branch of epizootiology; and such other generally useful terms as *population* and *demography* would apply only to a single animal species, man. Epidemiology is a more commonly used and understood word than is epizootiology, and there is no need to use different words for the study of diseases in populations of men versus populations of other animals any more than there would be to use two different words for pathology. In summary, epizootiology is not only unwieldy and often mispronounced, but also redundant. As an alternative definition for epidemiology, we believe "the study of the *health status* of populations" to possess considerable merit.

2. This classification is intended in its broadest sense; for example, pathology is considered here as the British use it, to embrace *all* activities (including microbiology and toxicology) generally associated with a diagnostic laboratory.

3. Christopher Graham, V.M.D., M.D., one of the founding partners of the Mayo Clinic and its chief diagnostician, long ago directed attention to this latter feature of veterinary practice in noting that "from the time the historical differentiation between human and veterinary medicine took place, veterinary medicine has been a clearer cut science than human. It is based more on practical experience and investigation, observation of facts, and the truths and principles derived therefrom."

4. The term diagnosis is used in a somewhat broader context (see Table 1–1) in epidemiology than in clinical medicine or pathology. Following such *initial* approaches as intensive follow-up or surveillance, the diagnostic process in epidemiology may well involve a variety of types of planned studies or trials.

5. *The Art of Scientific Investigation* (William Heinemann Ltd., London), written by a well-known veterinarian, W.I.B. Beveridge, is an excellent introduction to use of the scientific method. Its interest to veterinarians is heightened by many medical examples, especially veterinary ones.

6. Detailed keys to use of the veterinary literature are: Kerker, A.E., and Murphy, H.T. 1973. *Comparative and Veterinary Medicine. A Guide to the Resource Literature.* University of Wisconsin Press, Madison, and Schwabe, C.W. 1969. A key to the literature, Chapter 17. *In* Veterinary Medicine and Human Health, 2nd ed. The Williams & Wilkins Co., Baltimore. Also of value for special purposes are Jaboda, G. 1970. *Information Storage and Retrieval Systems for Individual Researchers.* Wiley-Interscience, New York, and Heiner, S., and Vellucci, M.J. 1972. *Selected Federal Computer-Based Information Systems.* Information Resources Press, Washington, D.C. The National Library of

Medicine and American Public Health Association jointly publish *Current Bibliography of Epidemiology.*

7. More detailed discussion of this subject is found in MacMahon, B., and Pugh, T.F. 1970. *Epidemiology. Principles and Methods.* Little, Brown and Co., Boston.

8. Snow's studies on cholera (reprinted in book form as *Snow on Cholera.* Hafner Publishing Co., New York, 1965) are regarded as an epidemiological classic, not solely because he was the first to demonstrate epidemic transmission of a disease through water as a vehicle, but also because he showed clearly the value of a new and most useful research approach to disease, namely, the use of natural experiments that lend themselves to retrospective analysis and interpretation. This account was chosen because there were no comparable early veterinary examples on the use of this now-basic epidemiological technique. The reasons were twofold. First, the veterinarian generally lacked (and still lacks) many of the types of vital statistics data upon which retrospective case-control studies are dependent; second, in contrast to the usual situation in human medicine, the veterinarian has always enjoyed the attractive option of setting up the more direct prospective type of experiment to test hypotheses.

9. Snow ingeniously divided his households (on the same streets) between the water companies supplying them by a simple chemical salinity test that differentiated between brackish (and contaminated) water drawn from the lower Thames and less saline, safe water drawn from further upstream.

10. Webster (see Note 1 for Chapter 9), Topley and Wilson, and others have also used the term *experimental epidemiology* to refer to controlled laboratory studies on the roles of specific epidemiological variables in experimental infections with different pathogens in closed populations of laboratory animals, such as mice. Such an approach is more real than contrived to the veterinarian who is concerned with the health of and the natural occurrence of diseases not only in populations of laboratory animals, but also in similarly closed and manipulatable populations of poultry or (occasionally) other species.

11. Histories of medicine sometimes erroneously credit Theobald Smith with this important discovery of arthropod transmission of microorganisms. In fact, Smith initially opposed conduct of the prospective trials that led to Kilborne's demonstration that ticks transmit the parasite of Texas fever. The source of confusion about this discovery lies in the fact that Kilborne's work on ticks and tick transmission and Smith's on the pathology and microbiology of the disease in cattle appeared in the same Bureau of Animal Industry reports on the disease, with Smith's name listed first. Later, when some physicians also credited Smith with the vector discovery, he failed to reject credit forcefully

enough. The original reports of the Bureau of Animal Industry are clear on this point, however; and a detailed account of the respective roles of Kilborne and Smith, as well as of Cooper Curtice and Daniel Salmon, in Texas fever research has been written by a well-known parasitologist, Maurice Hall (1935. Theobald Smith as a parasitologist. J. Parasitol. 21:231). Briefer accounts are found in J.F. Smithcors (1964. The development of veterinary medical science: some historical aspects and prospects. Adv. Vet. Sci. 9:1) and in C.W. Schwabe (1969. *Veterinary Medicine and Human Health*, 2nd ed. The Williams & Wilkins Co., Baltimore).

Chapter 2

1. Anon. 1874. The effects of the recent fog on the Smithfield Show and London dairies. The Vet. 47:32.

2. You will recall that the appropriate χ^2 statistic is

$$\chi^2 = \sum_{i=1}^{k} \frac{(O_i - E_i)^2}{E_i}$$

or for a fourfold table

$$\chi^2 = \frac{(ad-bc)^2 N}{(a+b)(c+d)(a+c)(b+d)} =$$

$$\frac{[(525)(118,151)-(181,343)(94)]^2 \; 300,113}{(181,868)(118,245)(619)(299,494)} = 152.$$

3. Epidemiology in veterinary practice has come a long way in distinguishing medically significant associations from those that may not be. The quotation that follows is from Orr, S.C. 1889. Cyclops megalostomus archynchus. Am. Vet. Rev. 13:228: "On the morning of the 20th of June I was called to attend a case of difficult parturition in a mare . . . . After a long and tedious operation the head and neck were severed . . . , and the subject of the accompanying cut is what I found . . . . The eyes . . . were both combined in one large eye . . . . There were two pupils . . . . *As the mare has been kept near the railroad it is thought by some that this strange freak of nature was caused by sudden fright at the train after night, as the eye somewhat resembles the head-light of a locomotive.*" (italics ours)

4. Taken literally, *commensalism* means "eating at another's table." It is a symbiotic relationship in which one partner benefits and the other is indifferent. Parasitologists generally differentiate it from other symbiotic relationships, such as *mutualism* where both partners benefit from the relationship, and *parasitism*, where one benefits and the other is harmed.

5. Hall, M.C. 1936. *Control of Animal Parasites*. The North American Veterinarian, Evanston.

6. Dubos, R.J. (Ed.) 1948. *Bacterial and Mycotic Infections of Man*. J.B. Lippincott Co., Philadelphia.

7. In Theobald Smith's words, "Wherever a parasitic microorganism has an opportunity over long periods of time to reach an equilibrium with the host species, the final form taken by the infection will be such as will not seriously interfere with survival of the host species and virulence will be low or moderate." (Smith, T. 1963. *Parasitism and Disease*. Reprint. Hafner Publishing Co., New York).

8. By epidemiological consensus, the term *vector* now is restricted to *invertebrate* animals fulfilling this transmitting role. It is considered loose usage, therefore, to refer to a dog, a fox, or a bat as a vector of rabies.

9. Attack rates: 3/21 = 14.3%, 3/21 = 14.3%; incidence rates: 3/21 = 14.3%, 3/18 = 16.7%. Note that an *average* population for a given time period can be calculated several

ways, e.g., an average of initial and final populations, the midpoint population, or the population on each day divided by the total days. Inspection of the data generally suggests the most suitable procedure. In these two instances, the values obtained by the methods suggested would have been the same.

10. The prevalence rate is 3/18 = 16.7%.

An Answer to a Text Problem: Weather Conditions. The maximum and minimum temperatures were December 1 (75°/42° F), December 2 (72°/42°), December 3 (74°/43°), December 4 (68°/39°), December 5 (65°/39°), December 6 (71°/45°), December 7 (78°/55°), December 8 (78°/55°), December 9 (80°/60°), December 10 (81°/62°), December 11 (79°/60°), and December 12 (75°/49°). There was fog every morning and heavy smog on December 9 and 10. No precipitation.

Chapter 3

1. The highly readable yet factual accounts of episodes in medical detection written by Berton Rouché for the *New Yorker* magazine and also published in book form (*Eleven Blue Men, The Incurable Wound, Annals of Epidemiology*) by Little, Brown and Co., Boston, are "must" reading for epidemiologists. A number of these accounts are about zoonoses and include veterinarians among their disease detectives.

2. This section was contributed by a colleague, Dr. Roger Ruppanner.

3. See Hendricks, S.L. (Chm.) 1966. *Procedure for the Investigation of Foodborne Disease Outbreaks*. Committee on Communicable Diseases Affecting Man. Int. Assoc. Milk, Food and Environment. Sanitar., Shelbyville.

4. This problem was constructed by Dr. Roger Ruppanner.

5. According to Paul, J.R., and White, C. (1973. *Serological Epidemiology*. Academic Press, Inc., New York), it was not until the 1930's that at all comparable large-scale efforts in seroepidemiology had been undertaken in human medicine.

6. Hutton, N.E. (Chm.) 1974. A Nationwide System for Animal Health Surveillance. National Academy of Sciences, Washington, D.C.

7. Of considerable interest are recent isolations of what apparently is vesicular exanthema virus from sea lions and other marine mammals along the Pacific coast of North America.

8. This practice is mentioned by Virgil (1st century B.C.) in his *Georgics*:". . . with quick knife check the mischief, ere it creep with contagion through the unwary herd. Less thick and fast the whirlwind scours the main with tempest in its wake, than swarm the plagues of cattle; nor seize they single lives alone, but sudden clear whole feeding grounds, the flock with all its promise, and extirpate the breed."

9. Hooper, W.D. (Transl.) 1960. *Marcus Porcius Cato on Agriculture, Marcus Terentius Varro on Agriculture*. Harvard University Press, Cambridge. Varro was a contemporary of Heraclides of Tarentum, author of one of the first known veterinary texts. Varro, however, quotes frequently from Mago, a Carthaginian writer on veterinary medicine and agriculture whose works were translated into Latin from Punic by order of the Roman Senate after the fall of Carthage.

10. Forster, E.S., and Heffner, E.H. (Transl.) 1954. *Lucius Junius Moderatus Columella on Agriculture*, vol. 2. Harvard University Press, Cambridge.

11. See Schwabe, C.W. 1969. *Veterinary Medicine and Human Health*, 2nd ed. The Williams & Wilkins Co., Baltimore.

An Answer to a Text Problem: Toxicological Analysis of All Feeds. This request was impractically vague and, if fulfilled, would have required about three weeks.

Chapter 4

1. A notable exception to this generalization was the early discovery by government veterinary practitioners of vector transmission of infections. Later on, a more or less rigid categorization of research and control personnel became evident in many government veterinary services. Research became more exclusively bench research, and methodological and field research suffered as a consequence. In this connection, a major step toward revitalizing public health in the United States in the 1940s was the creation of the Center for Disease Control (C.D.C.) in World War II as a place where epidemiological research with laboratory back-up could be carried out in conjunction with on-going public health programs. Most government veterinary services now lack such an applied field research organization, although, in the United States, a committee of the National Academy of Sciences has recommended a rather similar creation (Hutton, N.E. (Chm.). 1974. *A Nationwide System for Animal Health Surveillance.* National Academy of Sciences, Washington.)

2. The Russian, E.N. Pavlovsky, has been the principal exponent of such concepts. A review of Pavlovsky's ideas about natural foci may be found in an English translation of one of his works (Levine, N.D. (Ed.) 1966. *Natural Nidality of Transmissible Diseases.* University of Illinois Press, Urbana)

3. See Audy, J.R. 1960. Relation of foci of zoonoses to interspersed or mosaic vegetation. Papers of the 2nd W.H.O. Course on Natural Foci of Infections, Moscow U.S.S.R.

4. This case is not the same as the dead-end man represents for some infections acquired from lower animals. Here, the explanation may be a social one, related to disposal of the dead by burial or fire, rather than a biological one. For example, hydatid disease can be transmitted from man to carrion-feeding jackals and dogs among those tribes in East Africa that deliberately expose their dead to these scavengers. The same relationship also exists between the Parsees in India and carrion-feeding birds.

5. This jingle about salmonellae was published in *Lancet:*
"An infection found in beavers
    was transmitted to retrievers
    and carelessly contracted by a 'vet,'
While the organism,
    injected in a toad in Timbuktu,
    was recovered from a tadpole in Tibet."

6. For more detailed information on the zoonoses *per se*, see F.A.O./W.H.O. 1967. *Expert Committee on Zoonoses*, Third Report. W.H.O. Tech. Report Series No. 378; Hubbert, W.T., McCulloch, W.F. and Schnurrenberger, P.R. 1975. *Diseases Transmitted from Animals to Man.* 6th ed. Charles C Thomas, Springfield; Van der Hoeden, J. (Ed.). 1964. *Zoonoses.* Elsevier Publishing Co., New York; Schwabe, C.W. 1969. *Veterinary Medicine and Human Health.* 2nd ed. The Williams & Wilkins Co., Baltimore; Riemann, H. and Bryan, F. (Ed.). 1977. *Food-borne Infections and Intoxications.* 2nd ed. Academic Press, New York.

7. Because of this fact—as well as the fact that attention given to infections in veterinary education today is much greater than that offered in human medical education—more and more veterinarians in American public health departments are being asked to assume responsibility for the epidemiology and prevention of infectious diseases in general.

8. A useful source for this and other currently accepted epidemiological definitions is the American Public Health Association's authoritative manual, *Control of Communicable Diseases in Man.* Formerly, vector was also applied more loosely (and in a purely anthropocentric context) to include, for example, dogs or foxes as vectors of human rabies. The term vector, while epidemiologically useful as currently accepted, is still biased biologically with respect to the general study of diseases in vertebrates and invertebrates.

9. Hanson, R.P. 1957. The natural history of hog cholera. J. Am. Vet. Med. Assoc. 131:211.

10. For a readable account of the effect of plague on life in modern times, read Camus, Albert. 1972. *The Plague.* Random House, New York.

11. See Chapter 7, note 6.

12. Ford, J. 1971. *The Role of the Trypanosomiases in African Ecology.* Clarendon Press, Oxford; Ford, J. 1965. Distribution of *Glossina* and epidemiological patterns in the African trypanosomiases. J. Trop. Med. Hyg. 18:211.

13. See Schwabe, C.W., and Kilejian, A. 1968. Chemical aspects of the ecology of Platyhelminthes. *In* Chemical Zoology, vol. 2. Florkin, M., and Scheer, B.T. (Eds.) Academic Press, New York.

14. The epidemiologist interested in studies of these types should refer to a detailed standard work such as Southwood, T.R.E. 1968. *Ecological Methods.* Methuen and Co., Ltd., London. A manual for techniques in studying rodents and other small mammal populations is Davis, D.E. 1956. *Manual for Analysis of Rodent Populations*, School of Hygiene and Public Health, Johns Hopkins University, Baltimore. For references to wildlife in general, see individual issues of *Wildlife Review*, a key to this literature, published by the Fish and Wildlife Service of the U.S. Department of Interior.

15. Weitz, B. 1956. Identification of blood meals of blood-sucking arthropods. Bull. W.H.O. 15:473.

16. Marcus Vitruvius Pollio, who lived in Augustan Rome and published on architecture and agriculture, advocated placing animals upon a piece of land before selecting it as a townsite and then rejecting or accepting the site depending upon whether, at slaughter, the animals' livers appeared abnormal or normal. Birds have been used similarly in mines as sentinel animals for poisonous gases.

17. Constantine, D. 1962. Rabies transmission by the nonbite route. Public Health Rep. 77:287.

18. The interesting roles of many of the early veterinarians involved in unfolding basic knowledge about this whole group of arthropod-borne viral infections is introduced in Schwabe, C.W. 1969. *Veterinary Medicine and Human Health*, 2nd ed. The Williams & Wilkins Co., Baltimore, p. 49 and in Johnson, H.N. 1960. Public health in relation to birds: arthropod-borne viruses. Wildlife Natl. Res. Conf. Proc., p. 121.

19. Reeves, W.C. 1967. Factors that influence the probability of epidemics of western equine, St. Louis and California encephalitis in California. Vector News 14:13 (data derived, too, from the annual reports of Dr. Reeves' long-term project in this field).

20. A veterinary parasitologist and pathologist, Harry W. Graybill, together with Theobald Smith, first demonstrated in 1920 that helminths may serve as vectors of infectious microorganisms when they showed that the protozoan, *Histomonas meleagridis*, the agent of blackhead in turkeys, was transmitted by the nematode *Heterakis*.

21. The subject is extensively reviewed by Knapp, S.E., and Millemann, R.E. 1970. Salmon poisoning disease, Chapter 36. *In* Infectious Diseases of Wild Mammals. Davis, J.W., Karstad, L.H., and Trainer, D.O. (Eds.). Iowa State University Press, Ames.

22. Diseases like salmon poisoning prove the truth of Jonathan Swift's:
"So, naturalists observe, a flea
  hath smaller fleas that on him prey;
  And these have smaller still to bite 'em.
  and so proceed *ad infinitum*."

23. Madin, S.H. 1973. Pigs, sealions and vesicular exanthema, *In* Proc. Second Int. Conf. Foot-and-Mouth Disease. Pollard, M. (Ed.). The Gustav Stern Foundation, New York. The general account of vesicular exanthema is abridged from Bankowski, R.A. 1965. Vesicular exanthema. Adv. Vet. Sci. 10:23.

24. Because this vector was a tick, itself a parasite, and access to it was gained by dipping cattle in a parasiticidal bath, Curtice's effort was at the same time the first large-scale demonstration of mass chemotherapy.

An Answer to a Text Problem: Movement of Animals. Pens 9, 10, 12, 19, 20, and 56 were empty on December 9 and filled on December 10 with cattle trucked in on that day. Pens 14, 15, 18, 26, 47, 54, and 55 were stocked on December 8 with cattle trucked in on that day. No other animals were added to the complex during the week prior to the outbreak, and no animals were moved from pen to pen.

Chapter 5

1. Much of the terminology of this chapter has been adapted to conform to recommendations of the Subsection on Teaching of Statistics in the Health Sciences, American Statistical Association, at its Annual Meeting, St. Louis, August 26, 1974.

2. Pearson, E.S., and Hartley, H.O. (Eds.) 1958. Biometrika Tables for Statisticians. vol. 1, 2nd ed. Cambridge University Press, Cambridge.

3. Cross-over groups are such that part of the study subjects receive a treatment, say A, at the beginning of the trial, and part receive another, say B. After some specified time, the treatments are switched, or "crossed-over." It should be noted that one of these treatments is in fact a control, i.e., either no treatment or the treatment advocated on the basis of conventional, current veterinary wisdom.

4. Adler, H.E., and Wiggins, A.D. 1973. Interpretation of serological tests for *Mycoplasma gallisepticum.* World Poul. Sci. J. 29:345. It is important to note with respect to this whole section that the specificity of many diagnostic tests vary from population to population depending upon the prevalence in the population of other diseases that give false positive reactions to the test. Thus, test specificity is often an unknown quantity.

5. Modified from data supplied by Dr. Wayne Martin, Ontario Veterinary College, University of Guelph, Canada.

6. Nicoletti, P. 1969. Further evaluation of serological test procedures used to diagnose brucellosis. Am. J. Vet. Res. 30:1811.

7. Marchevsky, N. 1974. Errors in prevalence estimates in population studies: a practical method for calculating real prevalence. Zoonosis 16:98.

8. See Farooq, M., Hairston, N.G., and Samaan, S.A. 1966. The effect of area-wide snail control on the endemicity of bilharziasis in Egypt. Bull. W.H.O. 35:369.

9. These ratios have been applied to the analysis of rabies data from western Europe by Dr. K. Bögel, W.H.O., Geneva.

10. Hill, A.B. 1971. *Principles of Medical Statistics.* Oxford University Press, New York.

11. From Deevey, E.S. 1947. Life tables for natural populations of animals. Q. Rev. Biol. 22:283 (after data from Murie, A. 1944. The wolves of Mount McKinley. *In*: Fauna of the National Parks of the U.S. National Park Service. Fauna Series No. 5, U.S. Department of the Interior, Washington, D.C.).

12. A "busy" table is one that presents unnecessarily fine distinctions (large numbers of categories).

13. Information about the Termatrex system as used for processing clinical data was supplied by Dr. John Reif, School of Veterinary Medicine, University of Pennsylvania. Some uses for marginal punched cards are described in Schwabe, C.W., and Davis, L.R. 1954. Marginal punched cards in veterinary research. Am. J. Vet. Res. 15:634.

14. The formula contains B, which is the value of B under the null hypothesis. In this example, the hypothesis is that B = 0, so the null hypothesis is rejected only if the test statistic forces its rejection. In other situations, it may be useful to test the hypothesis that B is some non-zero value.

15. Recall that $SE_{(p)} = \sqrt{\dfrac{p(1-p)}{n}}$.

16. The temptation to compare all possible pairs with a series of ordinary t-tests should be resisted vigorously.

An Answer to a Text Problem: Toxicological Analysis. One lot of cottonseed hulls (which was practically used up) was without toxic amounts of known poisons. A second lot of hulls, which was used beginning December 9 or 10, was heavily contaminated with parathion. This analysis required 2½ days to obtain.

Chapter 6

1. Burridge, M., Utterback, W.W., and Riemann, H.P. 1975. Methods of spread of velogenic viscerotropic Newcastle disease virus in the southern California epidemic of 1971-73. Avian Dis. 191:666.

2. MacMahon, B. and Pugh, T.F. 1970. *Epidemiology, Principles and Methods.* Little, Brown and Co., Boston.

3. Martin, S.W., Schwabe, C.W., and Franti, C.E. 1975. Dairy calf mortality rate: influence of meteorologic factors on calf mortality rate in Tulare County, California. Am. J. Vet. Res. 36:1105; Martin, S.W., Schwabe, C.W., and Franti, C.E. 1975. Dairy calf mortality rate: the association of daily meteorological factors and calf mortality. Can. J. Comp. Med. 39:377.

An Answer to a Text Problem: Feeds Fed to Cattle. Animals in different pens were in different stages of finishing. Feeds were stored in several buildings at the periphery of the complex and were mixed in three different buildings. On the several days prior to and during the outbreak, the following feedstuffs were fed in each pen:

Barley	All pens
Wheat	1-8, 11-14, 31-45, 53-56
Sorghums	1-14, 24-32, 47-55
Beet molasses	9, 12-14, 51-54
Dried beet pulp	21-26, 30-38, 53-56
Cottonseed cake	1-14, 39-47, 53-55
Tankage	9-10, 12-18
Sorghum fodder	18-26, 47-55
Cottonseed hulls	2-9, 12-18, 25, 43-47, 55
Sorghum silage	1-9, 12-20, 46-56
Hay	All pens

Chapter 7

1. Pathologists interested in this area of epidemiology refer to it as geographic pathology.

2. Davis, D.E. 1950. The rat population of New York. 1949. Am. J. Hyg. 52:147.

3. The simple formula given is seldom used in practice. Various modifications are described in Southwood, T.R.E. 1968. *Ecological Methods.* Methuen and Company, Ltd., London.

Beck, A. (1973. *Ecology of Stray Dogs.* York Press, Baltimore) describes a photographic "capture" technique used to estimate free-ranging urban dog populations; another technique based on dog registration data is given by Anvik, J.O., Hague, A.E., and Rahaman, A. 1974. (Can. Vet. J. 15:219).

4. Example from Southwood (1968), *op. cit.*

5. This general subject is discussed at some length in Siegfried, A. 1965. *Routes of Contagion.* Harcourt, Brace and World, Inc., New York.

6. This episode has been well described by Mack, R. 1965. The great cattle plague epidemic of the 1890's. Paper presented before the Section of Comparative Medicine, Royal

Society of Medicine, London, 17 March (mimeographed manuscript available from the author); Branagan, D., and Hammond, J.A. 1965. Rinderpest in Tanganyika: a review. Bull. Epizoot. Dis. Afr. 13:225; and Pankhurst, R. 1966. The great Ethiopian famine of 1888-1892: a new assessment. J. Hist. Med. 21:95.

7. A helpful reference for this general subject is Smith, L.P. 1970. Weather and Animal Diseases. World Meteorological Organization Tech. Note No. 113.

8. Tinline, R.R. 1972. Lee wave hypothesis for the initial pattern of spread during the 1967-8 foot-and-mouth epizootic. *In* Medical Geography. McGlashan, N.D. (Ed.). Methuen and Company, Ltd., London, p. 301.

9. Learmonth, A.T.A. 1972. Atlases in medical geography 1950-70: a review. *In* Medical Geography. McGlashan, N.D. (Ed.) *op. cit.*

10. Forster, F. 1972. Use of a demographic base map for presentation of real data in epidemiology. *In* Medical Geography. McGlashan, N.D. (Ed.) *op. cit.*

11. See Armstrong, R.W. 1972. Computer mapping in medical geography. *In* Medical Geography. McGlashan, N.D. (Ed.). *op.cit.*

12. Sokal, R.R., and Sneath, P.H.A. 1963. *Principles of Numerical Taxonomy.* Freeman, San Francisco.

13. The reader is referred to Remington, R.D., and Schork, M.A. 1970. *Statistics with Applications to the Biological and Health Sciences.* Prentice-Hall, Inc., Englewood Cliffs, for details on fitting the Poisson distribution to data (p.119) and for testing goodness-of-fit (p. 246).

14. See the following:

Knox, G. 1964a. The detection of space-time interactions. Appl. Stat. 13:25.

Knox, G. 1964b. Epidemiology of childhood leukemia in Northumberland and Durham. Br. J. Prev. Soc. Med. 18:17.

Barton, D.E., David, F.N., and Merrington, M. 1965. A criterion for testing contagion in time and space. Ann. Hum. Genet. 29:97.

Mantel, N. 1967. The detection of disease clustering and a generalized regression approach. Cancer Res. 27:209.

Lloyd, S., and Roberts, C.J. 1973. A test for space clustering and its application to congenital limb defects in Cardiff. Br. J. Prev. Soc. Med. 27:188.

Kraus, J.F., et al. 1976. Unusual incidence of human leukemia in a rural northern California county (unpublished manuscript).

15. If three cases, say A, B, and C, are found such that A and B are adjacent, as are B and C, then it is likely that A and C will also be closely arrayed in time and space. Furthermore, in the example, the *sample* consisted of the 96 cases, and there were 4560 *pairs* of cases, so the sample size has not been increased in some miraculous way.

An Answer to a Text Problem: Map of Distribution of Deaths by Pen by Day

Number in upper left corner = Number of pen

Numerator = deaths on December 11 (in parentheses = deaths on December 12)

Denominator = animals in lot at beginning of December 11. (See page 286).

Chapter 8

1. Hippocrates wrote "In the same manner, when one comes into a city to which he is a stranger, he ought to consider its situation, how it lies as to the winds and the rising sun . . . and concerning the water which the inhabitants use, whether it be marshy or soft, or hard, and running from elevated and rocky situations, and then if saltish . . . . For if he knows all [these types of] things well . . . he cannot miss knowing when he comes into a strange city either the diseases peculiar to the place or the particular nature of common

diseases . . . and . . . as the season and year advance, he can tell what epidemic diseases will attack the city . . . and what each individual will be in danger of experiencing . . . . "

2. Readers are referred to the *International Journal of Biometeorology,* to publications of the World Meteorological Organization, and to such detailed references as the following: Licht, S. (Ed.) 1964. *Medical Climatology.* Elizabeth Licht, Publisher, New Haven, Connecticut; Tromp, S.W. (Ed.) 1963. *Medical Biometeorology.* Elsevier, Amsterdam; Shaw, R.H. (Ed.) 1967. *Ground Level Climatology,* Am. Assoc. Adv. Sci., Washington; and Platt, R.B., and Griffith, J.E. 1964. *Environmental Measurement and Interpretation.* Doubleday, New York. Another particularly useful reference is Munn, R.E. 1970. *Biometeorological Methods.* Academic Press, New York.

3. The Roman veterinary writer, Marcus Terentius Varro, wrote in the 1st century B.C. that "sickness is caused by the fact that the animals are suffering from heat or from cold, or else from excessive work, or, on the other hand, lack of exercise . . . . "

4. Naftalin, J.M. and Howie, J.W. 1949. Hepatic changes in young pigs reared in a cold damp environment. J. Pathol. 61:319.

5. Smith, L.P. 1970. Weather and animal diseases. World Meteorological Organization Tech. Note No. 113.

6. See, for all of these, Munn (1970). *op. cit.* (Note 2).

7. Ollerenshaw, C.B. and Smith, L.P. 1967. Meteorological factors and forecasts of helminthic disease. Adv. Parasitol. 7:283.

8. Kingscate, B.F. 1970. Correlation of bedrock type with the geography of leptospirosis. Can. J. Comp. Med. 34:31.

9. Levine, N.D. 1963. Weather, climate and the bionomics of ruminant nematode larvae. Adv. Vet. Sci. 8:215.

10. Many veterinarians would maintain that comfortable and happy animals are healthier and more profitable animals. See, on this subject, Fox, M. 1972. Demonstrating humane values. *In* What Should A Veterinarian Do? Schwabe, C.W. (Ed.). Centaur Press, Davis.

An Answer to a Text Problem: Organic Phosphorus Analysis. Parathion was found in the cottonseed hulls. This analysis required three days to obtain.

Chapter 9

1. See the papers by Webster, L.T. 1933. Inherited and acquired factors in resistance to infection. I. Development of resistant and susceptible lines of mice through selection breeding. J. Exp. Med. 57: 793; 1933. Inherited and acquired factors in resistance to infection. II. A comparison of mice inherently resistant or susceptible to *B. enteritidis* infection. J. Exp. Med. 57:819; and 1937. Inheritance of resistance of mice to enteric bacterial and neurotropic virus infection. J. Exp. Med. 65:261.

2. LeRiche, W.H., and Milner, J. 1971. *Epidemiology as Medical Ecology.* Churchill Livingstone, Edinburgh, p. 185.

3. Scrimshaw, N.S., Taylor, C.E., and Gordon, J.E. 1968. Interactions of nutrition and infection. W.H.O. Monograph No. 57, Geneva.

4. See Murphy, E.A. 1972. The application of genetics to epidemiology. *In* Trends in Epidemiology. Schwart, G.T. (Ed.) Charles C Thomas, Springfield; Stormont, C. 1958. Genetics and disease. Adv. Vet. Sci. 4:137; Freeden, H.T. 1963. Genetic aspects of disease resistance. Can. Vet. J. 4:219.

5. Binns, W., James, L.F., Shupe, T.L., and Thacker, E.T. 1962. Cyclopian-type malformation in lambs. Arch. Environ. Health. 5:106; Binns, W., Schupe, T.L., Keeler, R.F., and James, L.F. 1965. Chronologic evaluation of teratogenicity in sheep fed *Veratrum californicum.* J. Am. Vet. Med. Assoc. 147:839.

1 $\frac{3(2)}{800}$	**12** $\frac{110(324)}{600}$	**21** $\frac{0(0)}{900}$	**30** $\frac{0(2)}{700}$	**39** $\frac{0(0)}{900}$	**48** $\frac{0(0)}{800}$
2 $\frac{0(0)}{700}$	**13** $\frac{0(0)}{0}$	**22** $\frac{0(0)}{0}$	**31** $\frac{0(0)}{800}$	**40** $\frac{0(0)}{900}$	**49** $\frac{0(0)}{700}$
3 $\frac{0(0)}{600}$	**14** $\frac{312(179)}{900}$	**23** $\frac{0(0)}{900}$	**32** $\frac{0(0)}{800}$	**41** $\frac{0(0)}{800}$	**50** $\frac{0(0)}{900}$
4 $\frac{0(0)}{900}$	**15** $\frac{1(0)}{600}$	**24** $\frac{1(0)}{800}$	**33** $\frac{0(0)}{900}$	**42** $\frac{0(0)}{700}$	**51** $\frac{0(0)}{900}$
5 $\frac{0(0)}{900}$	**16** $\frac{0(0)}{800}$	**25** $\frac{522(182)}{800}$	**34** $\frac{0(0)}{0}$	**43** $\frac{0(0)}{700}$	**52** $\frac{0(0)}{1100}$
6 $\frac{0(0)}{800}$	**17** $\frac{0(0)}{900}$	**26** $\frac{6(7)}{400}$	**35** $\frac{2(0)}{900}$	**44** $\frac{0(0)}{800}$	**53** $\frac{1(0)}{700}$
7 $\frac{0(0)}{700}$	**18** $\frac{218(421)}{700}$	**27** $\frac{0(0)}{900}$	**36** $\frac{0(0)}{900}$	**45** $\frac{0(0)}{900}$	**54** $\frac{2(0)}{800}$
8 $\frac{0(0)}{800}$	**19** $\frac{0(0)}{600}$	**28** $\frac{0(0)}{900}$	**37** $\frac{0(0)}{800}$	**46** $\frac{2(0)}{800}$	**55** $\frac{197(108)}{600}$
11 $\frac{0(0)}{900}$	**20** $\frac{0(0)}{900}$	**29** $\frac{0(0)}{800}$	**38** $\frac{0(0)}{700}$	**47** $\frac{264(74)}{700}$	**56** $\frac{21(2)}{900}$

9
$$\frac{160(182)}{400}$$

10
$$\frac{0(0)}{1000}$$

6. Hutt, F.B. 1965. The utilization of genetic resistance to disease in domestic animals. Genetics To-Day. Proc. 11th Cong. Gen. 3:775. Pergamon Press, London.

7. Gray, D.P. 1964. Aleutian disease: a slowly progressing viral disease of mink. Curr. Top. Microbiol. Immunol. 40:9; see also National Institute of Neurological Diseases and Blindness Monograph No. 2, 1964; Leader, R.W. 1964. Lower animals, spontaneous disease and man. Arch. Pathol. 78:390; and Wilson, H.C. 1963. Aleutian disease: a review. Vet. Rec. 75:991; Hemmingsen, B. 1964. Genetically conditioned hypergammaglobulinemia in mink. Nord. Vet. Med. 16:881.

8. It is of interest that some of these institutions were founded as veterinary hospitals during the reign of the Indian Buddhist Emperor Asoka in the 3rd century B.C.

9. This list is modified from that of MacMahon, B., and Pugh, T.F. 1970. *Epidemiology. Principles and Methods.* Little, Brown and Co., Boston, p. 131.

10. This problem is slightly modified from one originating in the National Center for Disease Control, Atlanta, Georgia; a few of the data are fictitious.

An Answer to a Text Problem: Treatment for Parathion Poisoning.
　Atropine
　Prolidoxime

Chapter 10

1. The actual census numbers and deaths given here are fictitious, but they are consistent with the case-fatality rate calculations provided by Fenner, F., and Ratcliffe, F.N. 1965. *Myxomatosis.* Cambridge University Press, New York.

2. These latter data are from Ph.D. studies of Dr. Paulo Brant, University of California, Davis.

An Answer to a Text Problem: Toxicological Analysis of Tissues. Unless a particular class of toxins or chemicals were suggested by you in your request, a minimum of three weeks would be required for a report. If you have a more specific request of the laboratory, look up the particular toxin or chemical in the index.

Chapter 11

1. The answer in the second part is quite small (17), so the wise investigator will use more animals. These calculations are based on the assumption that *exactly* 9.0% of cases will have pigmented eyelids, as will 50.02% of controls. Since the vagaries of random sampling can produce some variation in these percentages, extra animals would normally be included in each group when the sample size calculation leads to such small-sized samples. Furthermore, the possibility of type II error was not included in the sample size calculation.

2. This may also be possible in some types of prospective cohort studies, but the retrospective approach is usually more attractive in the early stages of exploration of a problem (see MacMahon, B. 1972. Concept of multiple factors, *In* Multiple Factors in the Causation of Environmentally Induced Disease. Lee, D.H.K. and Kotin, P. (Eds.). Academic Press, New York).

3. Mantel, N., and Haenszel, W. 1959. Statistical aspects of the analysis of data from retrospective studies of disease. J. Natl. Cancer Inst. 22:719; Cornfield, J., and Haenszel, W. 1960. Some aspects of retrospective studies. J. Chronic Dis. 11:523.

4. In selecting case and control groups for retrospective study, we do *not* require a and c to be small relative to b and d.

5. This discussion of analyses of significance for relative risk values was prepared by Dr. A.D. Wiggins of this department.

6. Calculation of variance of $\log_e R_e$ gives a 95% confidence interval for R_e of 0.91 - 15.64. The null hypothesis cannot be refuted.

7. Calculation of variance $\log_e R_a$ yields a 95% confidence interval of R_a = 0.956 - 16.98; i.e., the null hypothesis that eye pigmentation was *not* demonstrably a determinant of SCC is sustained.

8. See Armitage, P. 1971. *Statistical Methods in Medical Research.* John Wiley & Sons, Inc., New York.

9. Willeberg, P. 1975. A case-control study of some fundamental determinants in the epidemiology of feline urological syndrome. Nord. Vet. Med. 27:1.

10. Nielsen, S.W., Schroder, J.D., and Smith, D.L.T. 1954. The pathology of osteogenic sarcoma in dogs. J. Am. Vet. Med. Assoc. 128:28.

11. Brodey, R.S., Sauer, R.M., and Medway, W. 1963. Canine bone neoplasms. J. Am. Vet. Med. Assoc. 143:541.

12. Cohen, D., Booth, S., and Sussman, O. 1959. An epidemiological study of canine lymphoma and its public health significance. Am. J. Vet. Res. 20:1026 (with addtional mimeographed data from Dr. Cohen).

13. Priester, W.A. 1965. Breed distributions in canine populations. J. Am. Vet. Med. Assoc. 146:971.

14. Tjalma, R.A. 1966. Canine bone sarcoma: estimation of relative risk as a function of body size. J. Natl. Cancer Inst. 36: 1137.

15. Data from Sanyaolu, S.A. 1975. A retrospective study of canine osteosarcoma: analysis of data from 13 United States and Canadian colleges of veterinary medicine (March, 1964, through May, 1973). Research study submitted for the degree of Master of Preventive Veterinary Medicine, University of California, Davis.

An Answer to a Text Problem: Water Source. Water is piped directly from an irrigation canal approximately 1/2 mile from the feedlot complex and is distributed from this source by a piped supply to all but pens 9 and 10. Pens 9 and 10 both receive piped water from a nearby drilled well.

Chapter 12

1. This problem uses the data and approach of Martin, S.W., and Wiggins, A.D. 1973. A model of the economic costs of dairy calf mortality. J. Am. Vet. Med. Assoc. 34:1027. This life table (with slightly different notation than described in this book) is shown in Problem 20 in Chapter 15.

2. Hird, D.W., Henrickson, R.V., and Hendrickx, A.G. 1975. Infant mortality in *Macaca mulatta*: neonatal and post-neonatal mortality at the California Primate Research Center, 1968-1972. J. Med. Primatol. 4:8.

3. On the other hand, the odds ratio could be an interesting tool in itself.

4. Data kindly supplied by Dr. Paul Blachmer, Ontario, California.

5. Data from a trial by Dr. Michael Huffman and C.W. Schwabe.

6. Fasal, E., Jackson, E.W., and Klauber, M.R. 1966. Mortality in California veterinarians. J. Chronic Dis. 19:293.

An Answer to a Text Problem: Vaccination History. Animals in lot 25 were vaccinated for blackleg on December 9. There were no other mass vaccinations in the preceding week.

Chapter 13

1. Armitage, P. 1971. *Statistical Methods in Medical Research.* John Wiley & Sons, Inc., New York.

2. Martin, S.W., Schwabe, C.W., and Franti, C.E. 1975. Dairy calf mortality rate: influence of meteorological factors on calf mortality rate in Tulare County, California. Am. J. Vet. Res. 36:1105.

3. Nie, N., et al. 1975. *SPSS. Statistical Package for the Social Sciences.* 2nd ed. McGraw-Hill Book Co., New York;

see also Dixon, W.J. (Ed.) 1974. *Biomedical Computer Programs*. University of California Press, Berkeley.

4. From a Ph.D. thesis by Dr. Michael Burridge, University of California, Davis.

5. Franti, C.E., Wiggins, A.D., Lopez-Nieto, E., and Crenshaw, G. 1974. Factor analysis: a statistical tool useful in epizootiologic research, with an example from a study of diarrhea in dairy calves. Am. J. Vet. Res. 35:649. Lopez-Nieto, E., Crenshaw, G., Franti, C.E., and Wiggins, A.D. 1972. A San Joaquin and Tulare County study of diarrhea in dairy calves. Calif. Agric. 26(6):7.

6. Cattell, R.B. 1965. Factor analysis: an introduction to essentials. I. The purpose and underlying models. Biometrics 21: 190.

7. Thurstone, L.L. 1974. *Multiple Factor Analysis*. University of Chicago Press, Chicago.

8. There are many existing computer-based statistical programs for constructing linear discriminant functions, including the BMD series from the University of California, Los Angeles (Dixon, W.J. in note 3). In using such programs, epidemiologists should endeavor to ascertain whether their data conform to the mathematical restrictions inherent in the particular program.

9. Data from a study by Kellar, J., Marra, R., and Martin, S.W. Ontario Veterinary College, University of Guelph, Ontario.

An Answer to a Text Problem: Tissue Analyses for Organic Phosphorus Compounds. Degradation products of parathion in liver, kidneys, and stomach contents. This analysis required three days to obtain.

Chapter 14

1. See, in particular, Florra, S.H. 1972. Report of the 1972 Committee on Livestock Identification. Proc. 70th Annual Meeting, U.S. Anim. Health Assoc., p. 27; Johnson, J.B., and Farrell, R.K. 1974. Individual animal identification. J. Anim. Sci. 38:1323, and Majeau, H.L. 1972. Passive animal identification system. Proc. Horse Identification Seminar, Washington State University, Pullman, Washington, Dec. 8-9, 1972, p.13.

2. There have been a number of previous efforts in veterinary medicine, but none had been widely accepted before S.N.V.D.O.

3. Yang, W.Y. 1969. A Statistical Analysis of Death Rates of Farm Animals in Canada. Canada Department of Agriculture, Ottawa.

4. Some of these efforts are reviewed in Committee on Animal Health. 1966. A Historical Survey of Animal Disease Morbidity and Mortality Reporting. National Academy of Sciences, National Research Council, Publication 1346, Washington, D.C., and in Hourrigan, J.C. 1960. Animal Morbidity and Mortality Reporting Programs as Carried on in the Department of Agriculture, *In* Comparative Medicine in Transition. Stafseth, H.J. (Ed.). University of Michigan, Ann Arbor.

5. This section is based in part upon material organized by Dr. Stephen Acres, formerly of this department and now at the Western College of Veterinary Medicine, University of Saskatchewan.

6. Diesch, S.L., Martin, R.B., Johnson, D.W., and Christensen, L.T. 1975. Proc. 78th Annual Meeting, U.S. Anim. Health Assoc., p.3.

7. The user of medical records for epidemiological purposes is referred for details of this system to Weed, L.L. 1971. *Medical Records, Medical Education, and Patient Care*. Western Reserve University, Press-Yearbook Medical Publishers, Inc., Chicago.

8. Dorn, C.R., Taylor, D.O.N., Frye, F.L., and Hibbard, H.H. 1968. Survey of animal neoplasms in Alameda and Contra Costa Counties, California. I. Methodology and description of cases. J. Natl. Cancer Inst. 40:295.

9. Data supplied by Dr. Michael Vaida of the Registry and this department.

10. Dorn, C.R., Taylor, D.O.N., Schneider, R., Hibbard, H.H., and Klauber, M.R. 1968. Survey of animal neoplasms in Alameda and Contra Costa Counties, California. II. Cancer morbidity in dogs and cats from Alameda County. J. Natl. Cancer Inst. 40:307; Schneider, R. 1970. Comparison of age, sex and incidence rates in human and canine breast cancer. Cancer 26:419; Schneider, R. 1972. Feline malignant lymphoma: environmental factors and the occurrence of this viral cancer in cats. Intl. J. Cancer 10:345; Schneider, R. 1972. Human cancer in households containing cats with malignant lymphomas. Int. J. Cancer 10:338; Taylor, D.O.N., Dorn, C.R., and Luis, O.H. 1969. Morphologic and biologic characteristics of the canine cutaneous histiocytoma. Cancer Res. 29:83; Dorn, C.R., Taylor, D.O.N., and Hibbard, H.H. 1967. Epizootiologic characteristics of canine and feline leukemia and lymphoma. Am. J. Vet. Res. 28:993; Schneider, R. and Vaida, M. 1975. Survey of canine and feline populations: Alameda and Contra Costa Counties, CA, 1970. J. Am. Vet. Med. Assoc. 166:481.

11. Description of this program was provided by Dr. Roger Ruppanner of this department.

12. Beals, T.L. 1969. Use of Market Cattle Testing Program samples to measure prevalence of *Anaplasma*-infected beef cattle in northern California. Research Report for the Master of Preventive Veterinary Medicine degree, University of California, Davis; Utterback, W.W., Stewart, L.M., Beals, T.L., and Franti, C.E. 1972. Anaplasmosis survey in northern California: prevalence of complement fixing antibodies in cattle by herd location. Am. J. Vet. Res. 33:257.

13. Ruppanner, R. 1972. Measurement of disease in animal populations based on interviews. J. Am. Vet. Med. Assoc. 161:1033.

14. Hutton, N.E. (Chm.) 1974. *A Nationwide System for Animal Health Surveillance*. National Academy of Sciences, Washington, D.C. See also Ingram, D.G., Mitchell, W.R., and Martin, S.W. (Eds.) 1975. *Animal Disease Monitoring*. Charles C Thomas, Springfield.

15. Discussed in Hess, A.D., and Hayes, R.O. 1967. Seasonal dynamics of western encephalitis virus. Am. J. Med. Sci., (March): 333.

16. See Trevino, G.S. 1975. Foreign animal disease control programs in the United States. J. Am. Vet. Med. Assoc. 167:459.

An Answer to a Text Problem: Unusual Events. No unusual happenings for the immediate area or vicinity were recorded.

Chapter 15

1. Schwabe, C.W., and Ruppanner, R. 1972. Animal diseases as contributors to human hunger; problems of control. World Rev. Nutr. Diet. 15:185.

2. Hutton, N.E. (Chm.) 1974. *A Nationwide System for Animal Health Surveillance*. National Academy of Sciences, Washington, D.C. (also discussed by Morris[5]).

3. Weisbrod, B.A., Andreane, R.L., Baldwin, R.E., Epstein, E.H., and Kelly, A.C. 1973. *Diseases and Economic Development. The Impact of Parasitic Disease on St. Lucia.* University of Wisconsin Press, Madison.

4. McCauley, E.H. 1975. The contribution of veterinary service to the dairy enterprise income of Minnesota farmers: production function analysis. J. Am. Vet. Med. Assoc. 165:1094.

5. These subjects are discussed also in Morris, R.S. 1969. The economic evaluation of a dairy preventive medicine programme. Victorian Vet. Proc. 1968-69: 59; Wragg, S.R. 1970. The economics of intensive livestock production. Vet. Rec. 86:33; McCauley, E.H. 1971. The management ap-

proach in the livestock producer/ veterinarian relationship. Vet. Med./Small Anim. Clin. 66:454, 455, 458, 460.

6. Morris *op. cit.* in 5.

7. Some are summarized in Schwabe, C.W., and Ruppanner, R. 1972. *op. cit.* in 1. See also Note 20.

8. Morris, R.S. 1969. Mastitis control within a preventive medicine programme. Victorian Vet. Proc. 1968-69:56.

9. Ross, J.G. 1970. The economics of *Fasciola hepatica* infection in cattle. Br. Vet. J. 126:13.

10. Esslemont, R.J. 1974. Economic and husbandry aspects of the manifestation and detection of oestrus in cows. A.D.A.S. Q. Rev. 12:175. Ministry of Agriculture, Fisheries and Food, London, England.

11. Certain aspects of this problem of research priorities have been discussed meaningfully in Morris, R.S. 1969. The economics of research. A viewpoint on priorities. Victorian Vet. Proc. 1969-70:28.

12. Mishan, E.T. 1971. *Economics for Social Decision. Elements of Cost-Benefit Analysis*. Praeger Publishers, New York.

13. Mishan, E.T. 1971. *Cost-Benefit Analysis. An Introduction*. Praeger Publishers, New York.

14. This section is modified from illustrations provided by Dr. Richard Howitt, Department of Agricultural Economics, University of California, Davis, 1974.

15. Jahnke, H.E. 1974. The economics of controlling tsetse flies and cattle trypanosomiasis in Africa, examined for the case of Uganda. Ifo-Institute für Wirtschaftforschung, Weltforum Verlag, München. The approach used in this study was published by Little, I.M.D., and Mürless, J.A. 1969. Manual of industrial project analysis in developing countries. Vol. II. Social cost-benefit analysis, Organization for Economic Cooperation and Development, Paris.

16. Power, A.P., and Harris, S.A. 1970. A cost-benefit evaluation of alternative control policies for foot-and-mouth disease in Great Britain. J. Agric. Econ. 24:573.

17. This problem draws on an example found in Martin, S.W., and Wiggins, A.D. 1973. A model of economic costs of dairy calf mortality. Am. J. Vet. Res. 34:1027.

18. Loew, F.M. 1974. A theoretical effect of fever on feed efficiency in livestock. Can. Vet. J. 15:298.

19. Stoll, N.R. 1947. This wormy world. J. Parasitol. 33:1.

20. The following publications contain additional information related to animal health economics. They do not represent an attempt to make a complete bibliography:

Anderson, B.P. 1970. One year of total herd health programming. Vet. Econ. 11:27.

Amiel, D.K., and Moodie, E.W. 1973. Dairy herd wastage in southeastern Queensland. Aust. Vet. J. 49:69.

Bailey, P.J., and Bishop, A.H. 1972. Effect of age at weaning and post-weaning stocking rate on the growth of autumn-born calves. Aust. J. Exp. Agric. and Anim. Hus. 12:579.

Barfoot, L.W., Cote, J.F., Stone, J.B., and Wright, P.A. 1971. An economic appraisal of a preventive medicine program for dairy herd health management. Can. Vet. J. 12:2.

Bens, R.J. 1971. The economics of preventive medicine and swine production. Can. Vet. J. 12:186.

Brook, A.B. 1970. The role of the practicing veterinary surgeon in modern pig husbandry. Vet. Rec. 87:310.

Christian, M.K., Baker, J.R., and Gardner, T.W. 1973. Observations on disease during the first two years of operation of a large pig-fattening unit. Vet. Rec. 93:153.

Ciordia, H., Baird, P.M., Neville, W.E., and McCampbell, H.C. 1972. Internal parasitism of beef cattle on winter pastures: effects of initial level of parasitism on beef production. Am. J. Vet. Res. 33:1407.

Clarkson, M.R. 1973. Long-range planning for animal disease control programs. University of Wisconsin, Madison. Workshop paper.

Cockburn, W.C. 1964. The implications of large-scale programmes for the control of infectious disease. W.H.O., Geneva.

Cote, J.F. 1963. Herd health practice. Can. Vet. J. 4:181.

Curtis, R.A. 1967. An epizootiological study of respiratory infections in cattle. M.Sc. Thesis. University of Guelph, Ontario.

Dirks, V.A. et al. 1971. Association of veterinary medical services with reporting of bovine leukemia in selected Minnesota dairy herds. Am. J. Vet. Res. 32:551.

Ekesbo, J. 1973. Animal health, behavior and disease prevention in different environments in modern Swedish animal husbandry. Vet. Rec. 93:36.

Gibson, T.E. 1973. Recent advances in the epidemiology and control of parasitic gastroenteritis in sheep. Vet. Rec. 92:469.

Gordon, R.F. 1971. The economic effect of ill health. Vet. Rec. 89:496.

Griliches, Z. 1964. Research, expenditures, education and the aggregate agriculture production equation. Am. Econ. Rev. 6:961.

Grunsell, C.S., Penny, R.H.C., Wragg, S.R., and Allcock, J. 1969. The practicability and economics of veterinary preventive medicine. Vet. Rec. 84:26.

Herschler, R.C., Miracle, C., Crowl, B., Dunlap, T., and Judy, J.W. 1964. The economic impact of a fertility control and herd management program on a dairy farm. J. Am. Vet. Med. Assoc. 145:672.

Leech, F.B.A. 1971. A critique of the methods and results of the British national surveys of disease in farm animals. I. Discussion of the surveys. Br. Vet. J. 127:511.

Leech, F.B.A. 1971. A critique of the methods and results of the British national surveys of disease in farm animals. II. Some general remarks on population surveys of farm animal disease. Br. Vet. J. 127:587.

Maclean, C.W. 1969. Intensive beef production and the veterinarian. Vet. Rec. 85:208.

Morris, R.S. 1969. Assessing the economic value of veterinary services to primary industry. Aust. Vet. J. 45:295.

Morris, R.S., and Blood, D.C. 1969. The economic basis of planned veterinary services to individual farms. Aust. Vet. J. 45:337.

Morris, R.S. 1971. Economic aspects of disease control programs for dairy cattle. Aust. Vet. J. 47:358.

Morris, R.S. 1972. Some theoretical considerations in the management of agricultural ecosystems. Seminar presented at Dept. Agric., University of Reading.

Morrow, D.A. 1966. Analysis of herd performance and economic results of preventive dairy herd health programs. Part I. Vet. Med. 61:474. Part II. Vet. Med. 61:577.

Morrow, D.A. and Smith, R.S. 1968. Financial data summary of 58 veterinary practices, 1967-68. Dept. Agric. Econ. A.E. Res. 268, Cornell University, New York.

Morrow, D.A. and Smith, R.S. 1968. Comparative financial analysis of 29 veterinary practices, 1966-1967. Dept. Agric. Econ. A.E. Res. 262, Cornell University, New York.

Mullenax, C.H., Plaxico, J.S., and Spain, J.M. 1969. Analysis of alternative beef production system in Los Llanos Orientales de Colombia. Interna Document Centro Internacional de Agriculture Tropical, Colombia.

Nesbitt, G.H. et al. 1970. Evolution of certain factors related to subclinical parasitism in cattle in Argentina. Am. J. Vet. Res. 31:981.

Pay, N.G. 1965. The effect of disease on a large pig-fattening enterprise. Vet. Rec. 77:642.

Reid, G.K.R. 1968. Economic aspects of the sheep industry

in the pastoral zone. Q. Rev. Agric. Econ. 21(1). Bur. Agric. Econ., Canberra A.C.T.

Report of consultations on socioeconomic aspects of zoonoses. 1972. W.H.O., V.P.H./73.2, United Kingdom.

Roberts, S.J., and DeCamp, C.E. 1965. Study of a planned preventive health program for dairy herds. Vet. Med. 60:771.

Rogers, L.F. 1972. Economics of replacement rates in commercial beef herds. J. Anim. Sci. 34(6):921.

Smith, H.J., and Calder, F.W. 1972. The development, clinical signs and economic losses of gastrointestinal parasitism in feeder cattle on irrigated and nonirrigated dikeland and upland pasture. Can. J. Comp. Med. 36:380.

VanHouweling, C.D. 1957. The economic importance of mastitis. Proc. 61st Annual Meeting U.S. Livestock Sanitary Assoc., St. Louis, p. 171.

Weaver, A.D. 1971. Solar penetration in cattle: its complications and economic loss in one herd. Vet. Rec. 89:288.

Wragg, S.R. 1971. Changes in the level of money expenditure and real investment by farmers in veterinary services and medicines between 1954/55 and 1968/70. Vet. Rec. 89:458.

An Answer to a Text Problem: Necropsy Findings. Animals began to die on December 11. On necropsy, the only observable changes were pulmonary edema and, in some animals, a marked enteritis. Cause of death was considered to be respiratory failure.

Chapter 16

1. Ackoff, R.L. 1962. *Scientific Method: Optimizing Applied Research Decisions.* John Wiley & Sons, Inc., New York.

2. The following references provide useful additional summaries of the general notions of model building: Bailey, N.T.J. 1957. *The Mathematical Theory of Epidemics.* Charles Griffin and Co., Ltd., London; Bartlett, M.S. 1955. *Stochastic Processes.* Cambridge University Press, Cambridge; Greenwood, M. 1935. *Epidemics and Crowd Diseases.* Williams and Norgate, London; Bailey, N.T.J., Sendov, B. and Tsanev, R. (Eds.). 1974. *Mathematical Models in Biology and Medicine.* North-Holland Publishing Co., Amsterdam.

3. Note that C is simply a symbol designating mathematically the homogeneous mixing that is assumed to occur.

4. For additional details, see Bailey, N.T.J. (1957). *op. cit.*

5. Armitage, P. 1953. A note on the epidemiology of malaria. Trop. Dis. Bull. 50:890; MacDonald, G. 1953. The analysis of malaria epidemics. Trop. Dis. Bull. 50:871-889; Morris, R.E. 1972. The use of computer modeling techniques in studying the epidemiology and control of animal disease. Proc. Int. Summer School on Computers and Research in Animal Nutrition and Veterinary Medicine (Arne Madson and Preben Willeberg, Eds). Frederiksberg Bogtrykkeri, Copenhagen; Ross, R. 1915. Some *a priori* pathometric equations. Br. Med. J. 1:546; Ross, R. 1916. An application of the theory of probabilities to the study of *a priori* pathometry, I. Proc. R. Soc., A. 92:204; Ross, R. 1917. An application of the theory of probabilities to the study of *a priori* pathometry, II. Proc. R. Soc., A. 93:212; Ross, R. and Hudson, H.P. 1917. An application of the theory of probabilities to the study of *a priori* pathometry, III. Proc. R. Soc., A. 93:225; Hugh-Jones, M.E. 1976. A simulation model of the spread of foot-and-mouth disease through the primary movement of milk. J. Hyg. 77:1.

6. Abbey, H. 1952. An examination of the Reed-Frost theory of epidemics. Hum. Biol. 3:201; Soper, H.E. 1929. The interpretation of periodicity in disease prevalence. J. R. Stat. Soc. 92:34.

7. This model was developed by Martin, S.W., and Wiggins, A.D. 1973. A model of the economic costs of dairy calf mortality. Am. J. Vet. Res. 34:1027.

8. This model was designed by A.D. Wiggins, C.W. Schwabe, and C. Hjerpe.

9. Kelker, D. 1973. A random walk epidemic simulation. J. Am. Stat. Assoc. 68:821.

10. The data for use in this model were supplied by Dr. R. J. Farnsworth, College of Veterinary Medicine, St. Paul, Minnesota.

11. Model developed by W.W. Miller, H.P. Riemann, M. Richards, R.K. Anderson, and E. Fuller (to be published).

An Answer to a Text Problem: Chemotherapy. There were no other mass treatments with drugs in the preceding week. No spraying or dipping with insecticides had been carried out for several weeks.

Chapter 17

1. Further discussion of the subject and a lengthier bibliography may be found in Schwabe, C.W., and Ruppanner, R. 1972. Animal diseases as contributors to human hunger. Problems of control. World Rev. Nutr. Diet. 15:185.

2. This subject is addressed in much greater detail in W.H.O./F.A.O. 1975. *Veterinary Contributions to Public Health Practice.* W.H.O. Tech. Report Series 573, Geneva; Hubbert, W.T., McCulloch, W.F., and Schnurrenberger, P.R. (Eds.) 1975. *Diseases Transmitted from Animals to Man*, 6th ed. Charles C Thomas, Springfield; Schwabe, C.W. 1969. *Veterinary Medicine and Human Health*, 2nd ed. The Williams & Wilkins Co., Baltimore; and Riemann, H., and Bryan, F. (Eds.) *Food-borne Infections and Intoxications*, 2nd ed. Academic Press, New York.

3. W.H.O./F.A.O. 1975. (See Note 2).

4. For lengthier discussion of this area of application, see Schwabe, C.W. 1972. *What Should A Veterinarian Do?* Centaur Press, Davis.

5. Similar national roles have been fulfilled, as examples, by South Africa's Onderstepoort Institute for Veterinary Research and Iran's Razi Institute, both unequalled for long periods of time by human medical research institutes in those countries.

6. Some veterinarians in public and private practice have also been content to neglect facing such complicated problems squarely by blaming them on that amorphous demon "management factors."

7. Nathan Sinai, a leading American veterinarian, organized and directed in Stockton, California, one of the world's first rural health departments. Later, as professor in the School of Public Health of the University of Michigan, he pioneered in development of the fields of medical and public health economics.

An Answer to a Text Problem: Signs and Symptoms. On December 10 many cattle in a number of pens began to show the following signs: salivation, lachrymation, "colic," and muscle spasms. Some animals developed diarrhea. Animals began to die on December 11. No records were kept of numbers of cattle that showed signs but recovered.

INDEX